FRONTIERS IN HEADACHE RESEARCH

Volume I

Migraine and Other Headaches

The Vascular Mechanisms

Frontiers in Headache Research Series

Volume 1: Migraine and Other Headaches: The Vascular Mechanisms
J. Olesen, editor; 384 pp.; 1991.

FRONTIERS IN HEADACHE RESEARCH

Volume I

Migraine and Other Headaches

The Vascular Mechanisms

Editor

Jes Olesen

Professor of Neurology
University of Copenhagen, and
Department of Neurology
University Hospital of Copenhagen
Gentofte Hospital
Copenhagen, Denmark

RAVEN PRESS

Raven Press, Ltd., 1185 Avenue of the Americas, New York, New York 10036

© 1991 by Raven Press, Ltd. All rights reserved. This book is protected by copyright. No part of it may be reproduced, stored in a retrieval system, or transmitted, in any form or by any means, electronic, mechanical, photocopying, or recording, or otherwise, without the prior written permission of the publisher.

Made in the United States of America

Library of Congress Cataloging-in-Publication Data

Migraine and other headaches : the vascular mechanisms / editor, Jes Olesen.
    p.   cm.—(Frontiers in headache research ; vol. 1)
  Includes bibliographical references.
  Includes index.
  ISBN 0-88167-795-7
  1. Migraine. 2. Cluster headache. 3. Cerebral circulation.
I. Olesen, Jes. II. Series.
  [DNLM: 1. Headache. 2. Migraine. WL 344 M6356]
RC392.M572 1991
DNLM/DLC
for Library of Congress   91-13860
                                                                                                 CIP

    The material contained in this volume was submitted as previously unpublished material, except in the instances in which credit has been given to the source from which some of the illustrative material was derived.
    Great care has been taken to maintain the accuracy of the information contained in the volume. However, neither Raven Press nor the editors can be held responsible for errors or for any consequences arising from the use of the information contained herein.
    Materials appearing in this book prepared by individuals as part of their official duties as U.S. Government employees are not covered by the above-mentioned copyright.

9 8 7 6 5 4 3 2 1

This book is dedicated to Professor Niels A. Lassen. He has been a continuous source of inspiration for young scientists and an exceptional teacher. He has greatly stimulated the research of cerebral blood flow in Denmark and around the world. He invented the first method for regional measurements of cerebral blood flow in humans and later provided a large part of the theoretical background to further develop such methods. He remains a driving force in the construction of ever-improving equipment. Without these contributions, we would know much less about the cerebral circulation in migraine and other headaches.

Acknowledgment

This publication has been made possible by an educational grant from Glaxo Holdings p.l.c.

Contents

1. Introduction 1
   Jes Olesen

I   **Methods** 3

2. Cerebral Blood Flow Measured by Xenon 133 Using the Intraarterial Injection Method or Inhalation Combined with SPECT in Migraine Research 5
   Niels A. Lassen and Lars Friberg

3. Inhalation or Intravenous Injection of Xenon 133 and External Stationary Detectors 15
   Jarl Risberg

4. Utility of the Retained Tracer Complex Technetium 99m-HMPAO for Measurements of Regional Cerebral Blood Flow 23
   Allan R. Andersen

5. Stable Xenon CT-CBF Methodology for Studying Vascular Headaches 29
   John Stirling Meyer, Jun Kawamura, and Yasuo Terayama

6. Comparison of rCBF by SPECT and Stationary Detectors Using Xenon 133 35
   Torben Schroeder and Sissel Vorstrup

7. Radiation Doses with Xenon-133, Xenon-127, and TC-99m HMPAO 43
   Søren Holm

8. Methods: Discussion Summary 47
   Niels A. Lassen

II   **Interictal Studies in Migraine with Aura** 51

9. Interictal rCBF Studies with ^{133}Xe or ^{99m}Tc-HMPAO and SPECT in Patients Suffering from Migraine with Aura ... 53
   Lars Friberg, Ida Nicolic, Jes Olesen, Helle Iversen, Bjørn Sperling, Niels A. Lassen, and Peer Tfelt-Hansen

CONTENTS

10. Brain Imaging with ^{99m}Tc-HMPAO and SPECT in Migraine with Aura: An Interictal Study 61
    Hans-Peter Schlake, Ingolf G. Böttger, Karl-Heinz Grotemeyer, Ingo W. Husstedt, and Otmar Schober

11. ^{99m}Tc-d,1-HMPAO SPECT in Migraine with Aura in the Headache-Free Interval 65
    E. Suess, P. Wessely, G. Koch, and I. Podreka

12. The Effects of Aging on Cerebral Blood Flow in Patients with Migraine Equivalents 71
    Wendy M. Robertson, Nabih M. Ramadan, Steven R. Levine, Lonni R. Schultz, and K. M. A. Welch

13. Interictal Studies in Migraine with Aura: Discussion Summary... 75
    Olaf B. Paulson

III The Onset of Migraine Attacks with Aura 77

14. Migraine with Aura: Onset of the Attack: Intracarotid Xenon 133 Method 79
    Tom Skyhøj Olsen

15. Reversible Hemispheric Ischemia in a Patient with Migraine... 89
    Ken Nagata, Kazunari Fukushima, Eriko Yokoyama, Yuichi Satoh, Yasuhito Watahiki, Yutaka Hirata, Fumio Shishido, and Iwao Kanno

16. Onset of Migraine Attacks with Aura: Discussion Summary... 95
    Olaf B. Paulson

IV Spontaneous Attacks of Migraine with Aura................ 97

17. ^{99m}Tc-HMPAO Studies in Migraine with Aura............... 99
    Paul T. G. Davies and Tim J. Steiner

18. Stable Xenon CT-CBF Measurements in Migraine Patients with Aura... 105
    John Stirling Meyer, Jun Kawamura, and Yasuo Terayama

CONTENTS

19. Xenon 133 Cerebral Blood Flow Measurements in Migraine with Aura... 115
   John Stirling Meyer, Jun Kawamura, and Yasuo Terayama

20. Xenon 133 SPECT Studies in Migraine with Aura......... 121
   Jes Olesen and Lars Friberg

21. Migraine with Aura: Discussion Summary.................. 131
   T. J. Steiner

V Mechanisms of Migraine with Aura......................... 135

22. Mechanisms of Migraine with Aura: Primary Ischemia... 137
   Tom Skyhøj Olsen

23. Links Between Cortical Spreading Depression and Migraine: Clinical and Experimental Aspects 143
   Martin Lauritzen

24. Receptors on Sensory Fibers Provide a Locus for Antimigraine Drug Action...................................... 153
   Michael A. Moskowitz

25. Extracellular Changes of Aspartate and Glutamate During Generation and During Propagation of Cortical Spreading Depressions in Rats 161
   Dieter Scheller, Ulrike Heister, Karin Dengler, and Frank Tegtmeier

26. Noninvasive DC Recordings from the Skull and the Skin During Cortical Spreading Depression: A Model of Detection of Migraine... 167
   Alfred Lehmenkühler, Frank Richter, Dieter Scheller, and Erwin-Josef Speckmann

27. Changes in Cerebral Blood Flow Associated with Cortical Spreading Depression in the Cat 171
   Richard Piper, Geoffrey Lambert, John Duckworth, and James Lance

28. Effects of Spreading Depression on Physiological Activation of the Cerebral Cortex in the Cat 177
   Richard Piper

29. Hypercapnic but Not Neurogenic Cortical Vasodilatation is Blocked by Spreading Depression in Rat 181
   Peter J. Goadsby, Jacques Seylaz, and Sima Mraovitch

30. Magnetoencephalographic Signals During and Between Migraine Attacks: Possible Relationship to Spreading Cortical Depression 187
Gregory L. Barkley, Norman Tepley, John E. Moran, Sandra Nagel-Leiby, and K. M. A. Welch

31. Mechanisms of Migraine with Aura: Discussion Summary... 195
John Stirling Meyer and Michael A. Moskowitz

VI Interictal Studies of Migraine Without Aura 197

32. Regional Cerebral Blood Flow Patterns in Migraine Without Aura: An Interictal SPECT Study 199
Lars Friberg, Bjørn Sperling, Jes Olesen, Helle Iversen, Ida Nicolic, Peer Tfelt-Hansen, and Niels A. Lassen

33. ^{99m}Tc-d,1-HMPAO SPECT in Migraine Without Aura 203
P. Wessely, E. Suess, G. Koch, and I. Podreka

34. Brain Imaging with ^{99m}Tc-HMPAO and SPECT in Migraine Without Aura: An Interictal Study................ 209
Hans-Peter Schlake, Ingolf G. Böttger, Karl-Heinz Grotemeyer, Ingo W. Husstedt, and Otmar Schober

35. Age-Related Changes in Cerebral Blood Flow in Patients with Migraine... 213
Wendy M. Robertson, K. M. A. Welch, Steven R. Levine, and Lonni R. Schultz

36. Interictal Studies of Migraine Without Aura: Discussion Summary... 217
Jes Olesen

VII Attacks of Migraine Without Aura 219

37. ^{99m}Tc-HMPAO Studies in Migraine Without Aura 221
T. J. Steiner and Paul T. G. Davies

38. CT-CBF and ^{133}Xe CBF Studies in Migraine Without Aura.. 227
John Stirling Meyer, Jun Kawamura, and Yasuo Terayama

39. Xenon-133 SPECT Studies in Migraine Without Aura 237
Jes Olesen and Lars Friberg

40.	^{99m}Tc-HMPAO SPECT in Migraine Attacks Without Aura and Effect of Sumatriptan on Regional Cerebral Blood Flow .... *Michael D. Ferrari, Joost Haan, J. A. Koos Blokland, Pieter Minnee, Koos H. Zwinderman, and Pramod R. Saxena*	245
41.	Attacks of Migraine Without Aura: Discussion Summary *Jes Olesen and John Stirling Meyer*	249
VIII	**Transcranial Doppler Studies in Migraine**	**251**
42.	Principles of Transcranial Doppler Measurements .... *Rune Aaslid*	253
43.	Transcranial Doppler Studies During Migraine and Other Headaches .... *Andreas Thie*	263
44.	Transcranial Doppler Measurement of Blood Flow Velocity Changes in the Middle Cerebral Artery During Experimentally Induced Headache .... *Thomas-Martin Wallasch and Hartmut Göbel*	275
45.	Cerebrovascular Reactivity During Valsalva Test in Migraine.. *Thomas-Martin Wallasch and Martin Reinecke*	279
46.	Orthostatic Cerebrovascular Reactivity in Migraine .... *Martin Reinecke, Thomas-Martin Wallasch, M. Schütz, and H. D. Langohr*	283
47.	Blood Flow Velocity Changes and Vascular Reactivity During Migraine Attacks Without Aura: A Transcranial Doppler Study.. *C. P. Zwetsloot, J. F. V. Caekebeke, J. C. Jansen, J. Odink, and M. D. Ferrari*	289
48.	Transcranial Doppler Studies: Discussion Summary ...... *Rolf Nyberg-Hansen*	293
IX	**Cluster Headache**	**295**
49.	^{99m}Tc-HMPAO Study During Cluster Headache Period and in Acute Attacks.. *Rachel Hering, E. G. M. Couturier, Paul T. G. Davies, and T. J. Steiner*	297

50. Brain Imaging with ^{99m}Tc-HMPAO and SPECT in
Episodic Cluster Headache: An Interictal Study............ 301
*Hans-Peter Schlake, Ingolf G. Böttger,
Karl-Heinz Grotemeyer, Ingo W. Husstedt, and
Otmar Schober*

51. CT-CBF and ^{133}Xe Inhalation Cerebral Blood Flow
Studies in Cluster Headache................................... 305
*John Stirling Meyer, Jun Kawamura, and
Yasuo Terayama*

52. Cerebral Blood Flow Response to Oxygen in
Cluster Headache.. 311
Jan Erik Hardebo and Erik Ryding

53. Cluster Headache: Discussion Summary.................... 315
Jes Olesen

X   Other Headaches and Effects of Antimigraine Drugs...... 317

54. Regional Cerebral Blood Flow in Chronic
Tension-Type Headache 319
Allan R. Andersen, Michael Langemark, and Jes Olesen

55. Decrease of Pourcelot Index in the Middle Cerebral
Artery During Post–Lumbar Puncture Headache.......... 323
Hartmut Göbel and Thomas-Martin Wallasch

56. Nitroglycerin-Induced Headache and
Intracranial Hemodynamics 327
Helle K. Iversen, Søren Holm, and Lars Friberg

57. Sumatriptan Increases the Cranial Blood Flow Velocity
During Migraine Attacks: A Transcranial Doppler Study   331
*Jo F. V. Caekebeke, C. P. Zwetsloot, J. C. Jansen,
Pramod R. Saxena, and Michel D. Ferrari*

58. Effect of Sumatriptan on Pial Vessel Diameter
In Vivo.. 335
*Patrick P. A. Humphrey, H. E. Connor, C. M. Stubbs,
and W. Feniuk*

59. The Effect of Ergotamine on Human Cerebral Blood
Flow and Cerebral Arteries..................................... 339
*Peer Tfelt-Hansen, Bjørn Sperling, and
Allan R. Andersen*

60.	Other Headaches and Effects of Migraine Drugs: Discussion Summary... *Jes Olesen*	345
61.	Conclusions and Prospects for the Future................ *Jes Olesen*	347
Subject Index		351

Contributors

Rune Aaslid *Department of Neurosurgery, University of Berne, Inselspital, CH-3010 Berne, Switzerland*

Allan R. Andersen *Department of Neurology, Rigshospitalet, Blegdamsvej 9, DK-2100 Copenhagen Ø, Denmark*

Gregory L. Barkley *Neuromagnetism Laboratory, Department of Neurology, Henry Ford Hospital, 2799 West Grand Boulevard, Detroit, MI 48202*

J. A. Koos Blokland *Department of Radiology, University Hospital, P.O. Box 9600, 2300 RC Leiden, The Netherlands*

Ingolf G. Böttger *Department of Nuclear Medicine, Westfälische Wilhelms-Universität, Albert-Schweitzer-Str. 33, D-4400 Münster, Germany*

Jo F. V. Caekebeke *Department of Clinical Neurophysiology, University Hospital, Rijnsburgerweg 10, 2333 AA Leiden, The Netherlands*

H. E. Connor *Department of Neuropharmacology, Glaxo Group Research Ltd., Park Road, Ware, Hertfordshire SG12 0DP, England*

E. G. M. Couturier *Academic Unit of Neuroscience, Charing Cross and Westminster Medical School, The Reinolds Building, St. Dunstans Road, London W6 8RP, England*

Paul T. G. Davies *Academic Unit of Neuroscience, Charing Cross Hospital, Fulham Palace Road, London W6 8RP, England*

Karin Dengler *Janssen Research Foundation, Raiffeisenstr. 8, D-4040 Neuss 21, Germany*

John Duckworth *Institute of Neurological Sciences, University of New South Wales, Prince Henry Hospital, Anzac PDE, Little Bay, Sydney, Australia 2036*

W. Feniuk *Department of Neuropharmacology, Glaxo Group Research Ltd., Park Road, Ware, Hertfordshire SG12 0DP, England*

Michel D. Ferrari *Department of Neurology, University Hospital Leiden, P.O. Box 9600, 2300 RC Leiden, The Netherlands*

Lars Friberg *Department of Clinical Physiology and Nuclear Medicine, Bispebjerg Hospital, Bispebjerg Bakke 23, DK-2400 Copenhagen NV, Denmark*

Kazunari Fukushima *Department of Neurology, Research Institute for Brain and Blood Vessels, 6-10 Senshu-Kubota-Machi, Akita 010, Japan*

Peter J. Goadsby *The National Hospital for Neurology and Neurosurgery, Maida Vale, London WC1N 3BG, England*

Hartmut Göbel *Department of Neurology, University of Kiel, Niemannsweg 147, D-2300 Kiel 1, Germany*

Karl-Heinz Grotemeyer *Department of Neurology, Westfälische Wilhelms-Universität, Albert Schweitzer Str. 33, D-4400 Münster, Germany*

Joost Haan *Department of Neurology, University Hospital, P.O. Box 9600, 2300 RC Leiden, The Netherlands*

Jan Erik Hardebo *Department of Neurology, Medical Cell Research, University Hospital of Lund, S-221 85 Lund, Sweden*

Ulrike Heister *Janssen Research Foundation, Raiffeisenstr. 8, D-4040 Neuss 21, Germany*

Rachel Hering *Academic Unit of Neuroscience, Charing Cross and Westminster Medical School, The Reynolds Building, St. Dunstan's Road, London W6 8RP, England*

Yutaka Hirata *Department of Neurology, Research Institute for Brain and Blood Vessels, 6-10 Senshu-Kubota-Machi, Akita 010, Japan*

Søren Holm *Department of Clinical Physiology and Nuclear Medicine, Bispebjerg Hospital, Bispebjerg Bakke 23, DK-2400 Copenhagen NV, and Department of Neurology, Rigshospitalet, DK-2100 Copenhagen, Denmark*

Patrick P. A. Humphrey *Pharmacology Division, Glaxo Group Research, Ltd., Park Road, Ware, Hertfordshire, SG12 0DP, England*

Ingo-Wilhelm Husstedt *Department of Neurology, Westfälische Wilhelms-Universität, Albert Schweitzer Str. 33, D-4400 Münster, Germany*

Helle K. Iversen *Department of Neurology, Gentofte Hospital, University of Copenhagen, Niels Andersens Vej 65, DK-2900 Copenhagen Hellerup, Denmark*

J. C. Jansen *Department of Neurology, University Hospital, Rijnsburgerweg 10, 2333 AA Leiden, The Netherlands*

Iwao Kanno *Department of Radiology and Nuclear Medicine, Research Institute for Brain and Blood Vessels, 6-10 Senshu-Kubota-Machi, Akita 010, Japan*

CONTRIBUTORS

Jun Kawamura *Cerebral Blood Flow Laboratory, Veterans Affairs Medical Center, and Department of Neurology, Baylor College of Medicine, 2002 Holcombe Building, Houston, Texas 77030*

Gabriele Koch *Neurologische Universitätsklinik Universität Wien, Währinger Gürtel 18-20, A-1090 Vienna, Austria*

Geoffrey Lambert *Institute of Neurological Sciences, University of New South Wales, Prince Henry Hospital, Anzac PDE, Little Bay, Sydney 2036, Australia*

James Lance *Institute of Neurological Sciences, University of New South Wales, Prince Henry Hospital, Anzac PDE, Little Bay, Sydney 2036, Australia*

Michael Langemark *Department of Neurology, Gentofte Hospital, University of Copenhagen, Niels Andersens Vej 65, DK-2900 Copenhagen, Denmark*

H. D. Langohr *Klinik fur Neurologie und Neurophysiologie, D-6400 Fulda, Germany*

Niels A. Lassen *Department of Clinical Physiology and Nuclear Medicine, Bispebjerg Hospital, Bispebjerg Bakke 23, DK-2400 Copenhagen NV, Denmark*

Martin Lauritzen *Department of General Physiology and Biophysics, The Panum Institute, University of Copenhagen, Blegdamsvej 3C, DK-2200 Copenhagen N, Denmark*

Alfred Lehmenkühler *Institut für Physiologie, Westfälische-Wilhelms-Universität, Robert-Koch-Str. 27a, D-4400 Münster, Germany*

Steven R. Levine *Center for Stroke Research, Department of Neurology, Henry Ford Hospital, 2799 West Grand Boulevard, Detroit, Michigan 48202*

John Stirling Meyer *Cerebral Blood Flow Laboratory, Veterans Affairs Medical Center, and Department of Neurology, Baylor College of Medicine, 2002 Holcombe Building, Houston, Texas 77030*

Pieter Minnee *Department of Neurology, University Hospital, P.O. Box 9600, 2300 RC Leiden, The Netherlands*

John E. Moran *Physics Department, Oakland University, Rochester, Michigan, and Neuromagnetism Laboratory, Department of Neurology, Henry Ford Hospital, 2799 West Grand Boulevard, Detroit, Michigan 48202*

Michael A. Moskowitz *Department of Neurosurgery and Neurology, Massachusetts General Hospital, Harvard Medical School, 32 Fruit Street, Boston, Massachusetts 02114*

Sima Mraovitch *Laboratoire de Physiologie et Physiopathologie Cerebrovasculaire, INSERM U. 182, CNRS U.A. 641, Universite VII, Paris, France*

Ken Nagata *Department of Neurology, Research Institute for Brain and Blood Vessels, 6-10 Senshu-Kubota-Machi, Akita 010, Japan*

Sandra Nagel-Leiby *Neuromagnetism Laboratory, Department of Neurology, Henry Ford Hospital, 2799 West Grand Boulevard, Detroit, Michigan 48202*

Ida Nicolic *Institute of Pathophysiology, Medical School, University of Novi Sad, Hajduk Veljkova 7-9, 21000 Novi Sad, Yugoslavia*

Rolf Nyberg-Hansen *Department of Neurology, The National Hospital, University of Oslo, 0027 Oslo 1, Norway*

J. Odink *Department of Clinical Biochemistry, TNO-CIVO Institutes, Poabus 250, 3700 AJ Zeist, The Netherlands*

Jes Olesen *Department of Neurology, Gentofte Hospital, University of Copenhagen, Niels Andersens Vej 65, DK-2900 Copenhagen, Denmark*

Tom Skyhøj Olsen *Department of Clinical Physiology and Nuclear Medicine, Bispebjerg Hospital, Bispebjerg Bakke 23, DK-2400 Copenhagen NV, Denmark*

Olaf B. Paulson *Department of Neurology, Rigshospitalet, University of Copenhagen, Blegdamsvej 9, DK-2100 Copenhagen Ø, Denmark*

Richard Piper *Institute of Neurological Sciences, University of New South Wales, Prince Henry Hospital, Anzac PDE, Little Bay, Sydney, Australia 2036*

Ivo Podreka *Neurologische Universitätsklinik, Universität Wien, Währinger Gürtel 18-20, A-1090 Vienna, Austria*

Nabih M. Ramadan *Center for Stroke Research, Department of Neurology, Henry Ford Hospital, 2799 West Grand Boulevard, Detroit, Michigan 48202*

Martin Reinecke *Praxisgemeinschaft Nordwest Zentrum, Postfach 550180, D-6000 Frankfurt/Main 55, Germany*

Frank Richter *Institut fur Physiologie, Friedrich-Schiller-Universitat, 0-6900 Jena, Germany*

Jarl Risberg *CBF Laboratory, Department of Psychiatry, University Hospital, S-221 85 Lund, Sweden*

Wendy Robertson *Center for Stroke Research, Department of Neurology, Henry Ford Hospital, 2799 West Grand Boulevard, Detroit, Michigan 48202*

Erik Ryding *Department of Clinical Neurophysiology, University Hospital of Lund, S-221 85 Lund, Sweden*

Yuichi Satoh *Department of Neurology, Research Institute for Brain and Blood Vessels, 6-10 Senshu-Kubota-Machi, Akita 010, Japan*

Pramod R. Saxena *Department of Pharmacology, Erasmus University, Rotterdam, The Netherlands*

Dieter Scheller *Institut für Experimentelle Medizin, Janssen Research Foundation, Raiffeisenstr. 8, W-4040 Neuss (Rosellen), Germany*

Hans-Peter Schlake *Department of Neurology, Westfälische Wilhelms-Universität, Albert Schweitzer Str. 33, D-4400 Münster, Germany*

Otmar Schober *Department of Nuclear Medicine, Westfälische Wilhelms-Universität, Albert Schweitzer Str. 33, D-4400 Münster, Germany*

Torben Schroeder *Department of Vascular Surgery, Rigshospitalet, University of Copenhagen, Blegdamsvej 9, DK-2100 Copenhagen Ø, Denmark*

Lonni R. Schultz *Center for Stroke Research, Department of Biostatistics, Henry Ford Hospital, 2799 West Grand Boulevard, Detroit, Michigan 48202*

Michael Schütz *Psychiatrische Klinik, Universität Marburg, Rudolf Bultmann Str. 8, 3550 Marburg, Germany*

Jacques Seylaz *Laboratoire de Physiologie et Physiopathologie Cerebrovasculaire, INSERM U. 182, CNRS U.A. 641, Universite VII, Paris, France*

Fumio Shishido *Department of Radiology and Nuclear Medicine, Research Institute for Brain and Blood Vessels, 6-10 Senshu-Kubota-Machi, Akita 010, Japan*

Erieh-Josef Speckmann *Institut für Physiologie, University of Münster, Robert-Koch-Str. 27a, W-4400 Münster, Germany*

Bjørn Sperling Department of Clinical Physiology and Nuclear Medicine, Bispebjerg Hospital, Bispebjerg Bakke 23, DK-2400 Copenhagen NV, Denmark

T. J. Steiner Academic Unit of Neuroscience, Charing Cross and Westminster Medical School, St. Dunstan's Road, London W6 8RP, England

C. M. Stubbs Department of Neuropharmacology, Glaxo Group Research Ltd., Park Road, Ware, Hertfordshire SG 12 0DP, England

Erhard Suess Neurologische Universitätsklinik, Universität Wien, Währinger Gürtel 18-20, A-1090 Vienna, Austria

Frank Tegtmeier Janssen Research Foundation, Raiffeisenstr. 8, D-4040 Neuss 21, Germany

Norman Tepley Physics Department, Oakland University, Rochester, Michigan, and Neuromagnetism Laboratory, Department of Neurology, Henry Ford Hospital, 2799 West Grand Boulevard, Detroit, MI 48202

Yasuo Terayama Cerebral Blood Flow Laboratory, Veterans Affairs Medical Center, and Department of Neurology, Baylor College of Medicine, 2002 Holcombe Building, Houston, Texas 77030

Peer Tfelt-Hansen Department of Neurology, Bispebjerg Hospital, Bispebjerg Bakke 23, DK-2400 Copenhagen NV, Denmark

Andreas Thie Department of Neurology, University of Hamburg, Martinistr. 52, D-2000 Hamburg 20, Germany

Sissel Vorstrup Department of Neurology, Rigshospitalet, University of Copenhagen, Blegdamsvej 9, DK-2100 Copenhagen Ø, Denmark

Thomas-Martin Wallasch Department of Neurology, Christian-Albrechts University, Niemannsweg 147, D-2300 Kiel, Germany

Yasuhito Watahiki Department of Neurology, Research Institute for Brain and Blood Vessels, 6-10 Senshu-Kubota-Machi, Akita 010, Japan

K. M. A. Welch Center for Stroke Research, Department of Neurology, Henry Ford Hospital, 2799 West Grand Boulevard, Detroit, Michigan 48202

Peter Wessely Neurologische Universitätsklinik, Universität Wien, Währinger Gürtel 18-20, A-1090 Vienna, Austria

Eriko Yokoyama Department of Neurology, Research Institute for Brain and Blood Vessels, 6-10 Senshu-Kubota-Machi, Akita 010, Japan

C. P. Zwetsloot   *Department of Clinical Neurophysiology, University Hospital, Rijnsburgerweg 10, 2333 AA Leiden, The Netherlands*

Koos H. Zwinderman   *Department of Medical Statistics, University Hospital, P.O. Box 9600, 2300 RC Leiden, The Netherlands*

Preface to the Series

Among the adult population, 16% are migraine sufferers and 71% have had tension-type headache. The burden on society in terms of work days lost, health care costs, and the amount of suffering by the victims is enormous. Headache disorders have not been taken seriously, however. Patients try to hide that they suffer from migraine or other headaches because they are afraid of being accused of faking or because the disorders are often regarded as more or less psychiatric. Lack of knowledge and inconsistencies in published research work have turned many medical scientists away from the study of these disorders. Over the last decade headache research has, however, been burgeoning. Unfortunately, this has not yet had significant impact on general medicine or on the neurological disciplines. It is the aim of this forthcoming series of books entitled *Frontiers in Headache Research* to demonstrate the major advances made in our understanding of headache.

Each book in this series focuses on a major field of headache research. The scope is multidisciplinary, involving both the medical and the basic sciences. Each topic is introduced by one or more overview chapters by leading experts. Thereafter, the newest developments are presented in short articles. Finally, each topic closes with a summary of the discussions by the chairpersons. These summaries provide a state-of-the-art presentation, sometimes indicating consensus, sometimes highlighting differing views. They will prove useful for readers who want a quick and unbiased update.

Jes Olesen

Preface

More than anything else, studies of the cephalic vascular system have contributed toward an understanding of the mechanisms of migraine and other headaches. This development began more than 20 years ago but has accelerated, especially within the last decade. This book gives a comprehensive account of what we know today, but also exposes large areas of ignorance and controversies which, as in all the young areas of science, are quite numerous. Conclusions can be drawn, however, and distinctive patterns are appearing.

The discussion summaries after each section, written by leading experts, will guide the nonexpert through what may occasionally appear to be a jungle of opposing views. At the end of the book is my summary of where we stand today—an abstract to the whole book—and that is, perhaps, where reading should start.

I am sure it will come as a welcome surprise to many that so much is known about vascular headache mechanisms and that research into these mechanisms is gaining increasing support. Furthermore, the understanding of vascular migraine mechanisms now goes hand in hand with the development of new drugs that are both more effective and much more specific than currently available treatments.

Jes Olesen

Migraine and Other Headaches:
The Vascular Mechanisms,
edited by Jes Olesen.
Raven Press, Ltd., New York © 1991.

1
Introduction

Jes Olesen

Department of Neurology, University of Copenhagen, Gentofte Hospital, DK-2900 Copenhagen, Denmark

Migraine has been one of the most difficult yet most rewarding areas of regional cerebral blood flow (rCBF) research. The difficulties are clinical as well as methodological. Clinically, proper description of patients was difficult when, previously, no universal agreement existed about required clinical characteristics to make the diagnosis or the necessity of subdividing patients according to whether or not they had an aura. This aspect eased up after the advent of the operational diagnostic criteria of the International Headache Society (1), which should be strictly adhered to in future studies. Having described and classified patients properly, the next problem is their heterogeneity. Not only are patients with aura and without aura quite different, but those with aura range from having a pure visual aura lasting 20 min and no further symptoms to having very severe, long-lasting hemiplegic attacks. In migraine without aura, attacks vary in severity and mild attacks may be difficult to distinguish from tension-type headache.

In each patient, the type and severity of attacks may differ over time, and many patients have attacks with aura as well as attacks without aura. The laterality of the aura and of the headache usually changes between attacks. It is therefore absolutely necessary to describe the symptomatology of the actually studied attack and to ascertain that this attack fulfills the criteria of the International Headache Society. But even studying a single attack is difficult because it evolves over time. Exact timing is essential, but patients do not present at the same time after onset of the attack and thus may be difficult to compare.

It is not easy to persuade patients to come into the hospital during an attack. They feel miserable, are nauseated and vomit, and prefer to stay at home. Furthermore, even if they are willing to come, the minimum time delay is usually in the order of one hour before they can reach the CBF laboratory. The necessary equipment must be ready, staffed, and cleared of other patients when the migraineur arrives. Physical facilities and medical expertise to treat the patient must be available, often at odd hours. Having coped with all these difficulties and requirements, measurements are then made of a phenomenon that develops over time and spreads out topographically within the brain. Exact timing of measurements in relation to both the onset and termination of aura symptoms and headache is essential. Ideally, the patient should be followed with repeated measurements to disclose these dynamic changes. Many confusing reports in the literature come about because patients studied at different times with different clinical characteristics are lumped together. When it comes to publishing, the heterogeneity makes tabulation difficult so that the presentation of multiple case histories is often necessary (2,3,4).

The technical problems of studying migraine are considerable. As will be apparent later, the blood flow abnormalities are mostly focal, in some are confined to midline structures (the primary visual cortex), and they are mostly cortical. The degree of rCBF changes is debatable but obviously not as large as with ischemic cerebrovascular disease and, therefore, more difficult to measure. The abnormalities are not stationary but change in each region over time, only with certain intervals of constancy. The time of onset and duration of these periods of constancy of rCBF abnormalities vary from patient to patient. Thus, the ideal method in migraine is atraumatic, easy to handle at short notice and odd hours, allows repeated measurements three or four times in the individual patient, has a high spatial resolution, is insensitive to Compton scatter, should be able to separate cerebral and extracerebral blood flow, requires a short measurement time, and allows the patient to rest comfortably without being restrained in order to be able to cope with vomiting. Exact repositioning should be possible in order to compare studies at different times of the attack to studies outside of attack. Obviously no method is available that fulfills all these requirements. Each has its merits and its drawbacks, which will be discussed in the first chapter of this book. Methodological aspects should always be taken into account when evaluating published studies.

How rewarding research in this area has been, despite all difficulties, hopefully will be apparent from reading this book.

REFERENCES

1. Headache Classification Committee of the International Headache Society. Classification and diagnostic criteria for headache disorders, cranial neuralgias and facial pain. *Cephalalgia* 1988; 8[Suppl 7]:1–96.
2. Andersen AR, Friberg L, Olsen TS, and Olesen J. SPECT demonstration of delayed hyperemia following hypoperfusion in classic migraine. *Arch Neurol* 1988; 45:154–159.
3. Lauritzen M, Skyhøj Olsen T, Lassen NA, and Paulson OB. The changes of regional cerebral blood flow during the course of classical migraine attacks. *Ann Neurol* 1983; 13:633–641.
4. Olesen J, Larsen B, and Lauritzen M. Focal hyperemia followed by spreading oligemia and impaired activation of rCBF in classic migraine. *Ann Neurol* 1981; 9:344–352.

PART I
Methods

2

Cerebral Blood Flow Measured by Xenon 133 Using the Intraarterial Injection Method or Inhalation Combined with SPECT in Migraine Research

Niels A. Lassen and Lars Friberg

Department of Chemical Physiology/Nuclear Medicine, Bispebjerg Hospital, DK-2400 Copenhagen NV, Denmark

The most widely used ^{133}Xe method for measuring cerebral blood flow (CBF) is based on inhalation or intravenous (iv) injection of the tracer combined with external detection over the brain using one or more stationary scintillating detectors. This technique was proposed by Hadley L. Conn, Jr., in 1955 based on studies using radioxenon in dogs (1). Conn reported his results at a meeting in the United States and was allegedly criticized rather severely by Seymour S. Kety, who argued that the counts recorded over the head did not solely arise from the brain but also from extracerebral structures. Conn, accepting the critique, so we may surmise, never published a full report. Thus, only a brief abstract remains to document his early study (1), that followed the same approach as Hardin B. Jones's pioneer studies in man involving the inhalation of gamma-emitting isotopes of other noble gases (2).

Mallett and Veal, independent of Conn's study, proposed in 1963 the same ^{133}Xe inhalation method and applied it to the measurement of CBF in humans, where extracerebral contamination of the head curve is much less of a problem than in the dog (3). Nevertheless, as an approach to the measurement of regional CBF, the conventional ^{133}Xe inhalation technique is rather crude, because tissue layers in the depth are superimposed. Thus, even counts from the contralateral hemisphere are recorded ipsilaterally albeit in attenuated form due to absorption, as discussed by Risberg elsewhere in this volume. This brief account of the early history of the conventional ^{133}Xe inhalation method is provided because it puts into perspective and clarifies essential features of the two other ^{133}Xe methods for measuring CBF in humans.

^{133}Xe AS A TRACER OF CBF

According to the basic principles developed in particular by Kety, inert and freely diffusable molecules can be used as tracers for tissue blood flow, because their uptake and release from the tissue depends only on flow and solubility (4).

The concept of solubility may need a brief explanation. The important parameter is the *relative solubility* or more precisely the ratio of the solubility in the brain to that of the blood. This solubility ratio, λ, defines or describes the capacity of the tissue relative to that of the blood to dissolve the tracer:

$$\lambda = \frac{\text{concentration in 1 g of brain at equilibrium}}{\text{concentration in 1 ml of blood at equilibrium}} \text{ ml/g}$$

The solubility of ^{133}Xe in a complex physical system as 1 g of brain or blood depends on chemical composition, that is, content of water, proteins, and lipids. Knowing the composition one can calculate λ. The essential feature or "secret" of using inert gases as tracers of CBF is, as Kety recognized, the fair degree of constancy of the gross physiochemical composition of brain tissue and blood with regard to content of water, protein, and lipids.

A specific point to emphasize in this context is that the solubility in the brain is practically independent of variations in the blood volume per gram of brain. This volume is so small, 2–3%, that even if it should double (as with severe vasodilatation), then it would still account for only a negligible part of the tissue. Moreover, the solubility in blood and in brain tissue (without blood) is almost the same. Hence the effect of variations in blood volume on λ is further minimized. Therefore, because the freely diffusable inert tracers dissolve in the entire tissue mass—in the tissue proper and in the blood volume of the tissue—these tracers are fundamentally superior to tracers that remain inside the vessels because they are unable to cross the blood-brain barrier. For such tracers, as, for example, radiolabeled human serum albumin, only the local plasma volume serves as the dilution space. As this volume can vary considerably with flow, it follows that λ can no longer be considered as a constant.

Many different inert, freely diffusable tracers can be used for measuring CBF. Kety and Schmidt in 1945 introduced nitrous oxide, N_2O, for measuring average CBF based on arterial and cerebral venous blood samples (5), while Lassen and Munck in 1955 applied Krypton 85 to the same approach (6). In animal studies ^{14}C-labeled tracers as ethanol, butanol, or iodo-antipyrine are widely used because they afford excellent spatial resolution using the autoradiographic technique. In man, external counting of gamma or positron emitting tracers are used for assessing regional CBF. Among the inert gamma-emitting gases, only ^{133}Xe is more widely used. ^{127}Xe and ^{127m}Xe offer advantages, but these cyclotron-produced tracers are much more costly.

[133]Xe has a half-life of 5.5 days, so that it need only be supplied once a week to be available whenever needed. It is not an ideal tracer for external detection, because its gamma radiation is so soft and has so low an energy (81 KeV) that absorption and scatter in the brain and in the skull occur to a considerable extent. Because of the effective elimination via the lungs, ^{133}Xe results in only a small radiation exposure, typically less than 1/10 of that of slowly eliminated tracers as Technetium 99m in the form of pertechnetate used for bone scans or hexa-methyl-propylene-amine-oxime (HMPAO), used for showing the distribution of CBF (see the chapter by Andersen in this volume).

THE INTRAARTERIAL ^{133}Xe INJECTION CBF METHOD

This method is based on the rapid injection of a bolus of saline containing the tracer via the internal carotid or vertebral artery, a principle first described by Lassen and Ingvar in 1961 (7–10). As the ^{133}Xe reaches the brain, it diffuses across the capillary walls and distributes (dissolves) in the tissue. It is subsequently washed out (cleared) from the tissue by unlabeled arterial blood arriving after the bolus. Because of the effective elimination via the lungs, the tracer recirculates to only a negligible degree.

According to the principles mentioned in the previous section, the clearance rate k is proportional to the blood flow f and inversely proportional to solubility coefficient λ; that is, $k = f/\lambda$. As λ can be considered as a constant—in the cerebral cortex it is about 0.83 ml/g and in the white matter about 1.50 ml/g—one can calculate f as the product $k \cdot \lambda$. This is the basis for calculating cortical CBF from the initial, steepest slope of a semilogarithmic plot of the clearance curve as recorded by one or more scintillation detectors placed over the side of the head (10). The measurement can be repeated several times with an interval of about 10 min, because it is easy to correct for the small amount of radioactivity remaining from a previous injection at 10 min. Routinely we perform a series of four to six measurements in a study. In this way one can measure precisely the CBF response at rest and after various stimuli in many regions. We currently use a battery of 254 detectors each looking at approximately 1 cm^2 of brain surface (11).

Injecting ^{133}Xe via the internal carotid artery eliminates labeling of skin or bone. Thus, the extracerebral contamination that affects the conventional ^{133}Xe inhalation method and the airway artifact is avoided. In addition, superposition of tissue layers and Compton scatter is less of a problem because only one hemisphere is being labeled, eliminating interhemispheric crosstalk. Thus, for several important reasons, the intraarterial method is much more precise than the conventional ^{133}Xe inhalation procedure.

The intraarterial method is used much less today because of the trauma involved in the intraarterial catheterization and injections. Therefore, as cerebral angiography as a clinical tool is used much less frequently because of the advent of CT and MR imaging, the possibility of obtaining CBF maps by injecting ^{133}Xe before or after angiography is limited. In migraine research, where angiography is now used only in exceptional, severe, and clinically atypical migraine attacks, the intracarotid ^{133}Xe method is virtually obsolete.

Nevertheless, the technique is of basic interest in migraine research mainly because in more than one-half of all migraineurs the procedure of catheterizing and injecting the internal carotid artery will provoke a migraine attack (Figs. 1 and 2). The provoked symptoms start with aural symptoms 15 to 30 min after the first injection of the angiographic contrast medium or the ^{133}Xe-containing saline. The aural symptoms last about 1 hr and are in most cases followed by throbbing headache located at the side of the injection or having a bilateral localization. This strange phenomena, which emphasizes the vascular pathogenesis of migraine with aura, has allowed detailed studies of what appears to mimic precisely a spontaneous migraine attack and is discussed by Olsen and Lauritzen elsewhere in this volume.

THE TOMOGRAPHIC ^{133}Xe CBF METHOD

This approach was described by Lassen and coworkers in 1978 (12) and in a series of subsequent methodological studies (13–16). The method is entirely atraumatic, being based on the same inhalation or iv route of tracer application as the conventional ^{133}Xe technique. However, two of the main errors of that technique are eliminated due to the tomographic principle, namely, extracerebral contamination and superposition of tissue layers including intrahemispheric cross-talk.

Essential for this technique was the development of a specialized tomographic device that was highly sensitive and rotated quickly enough to allow dynamic tomographic recordings. The instrument, the TOMOMATIC (Medimatic, Inc.), is the only commercially available brain-dedicated single photon emission computed tomography (SPECT) system specifically designed for ^{133}Xe tomography as well as for the tomography of other low to medium energy radioisotopes as Technetium 99m or Iodine 123.

The TOMOMATIC instrument has a sensitivity about 15 times that of a conventional rotating gamma camera. This gain in sensitivity is obtained by the system having four camera heads that rotate close to the head and by using converging collimators in the Z direction (axially). This convergence means, therefore, that a contiguous set of slices is not obtained in a single study. Typically three slices are seen, each with a thickness of 1.7 cm and with a distance between the midslice planes of 4.0 cm, so that an "unseen" slice of 2.3 cm in thickness separates the three slices.

The high intrinsic sensitivity is important because a high counting rate during the 1 min of scanning is a necessity for accurate tomographic image

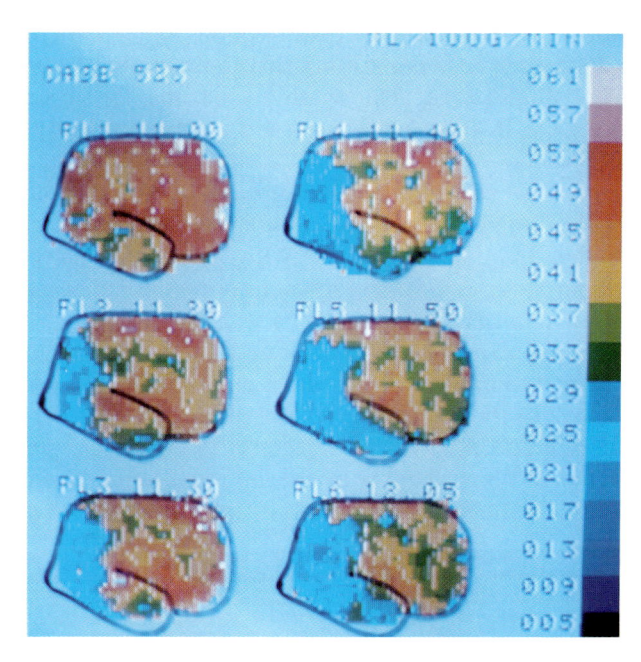

FIG. 1. ^{133}Xe intracarotid injection method. In this patient suffering from migraine, the investigative procedure (the intracarotid injection of saline) provoked a migraine attack.

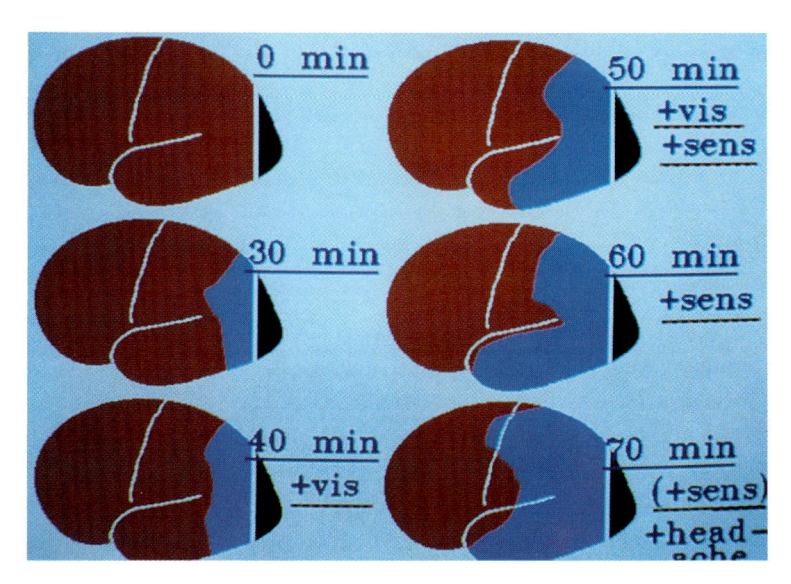

FIG. 2. Diagrammatic representation of the results obtained in the study depicted in Fig. 1. The image is turned mirror-wise so that the anterior end now points to the left. The development of visual (vis) and sensory (sens) aural symptoms as well as of headache is indicated.

reconstruction. The inhalation of ^{133}Xe lasts 1.0 to 1.5 min. We prefer the longer inhalation time in order to improve the counting statistics per unit dose of ^{133}Xe administered. During this time and for three subsequent 1-min intervals the instrument records the arrival and early wash-out of radioactivity.

The mathematical principles involved in calculating CBF tomographically from the observed radioisotope images differ only slightly from those of the conventional nontomographic method. With ^{133}Xe tomography the shape of the arterial input curve is assessed by monitoring the radioactivity over the lung or in end-expiratory (alveolar) air.

CBF tomography using ^{133}Xe is well suited for migraine research (Fig. 3). The absorbed radiation dose is very low, approximately 0.6 mSv/scan, or equivalent to two to three diagnostic x-ray photographs of the lung. It lasts only 4 to 4½ min and involves no injections or blood sampling. It is well tolerated by the patients. This is of special importance during a migraine attack, where the patient's general level of tolerance to all external stimuli tends to be very low.

The following shortcomings may be noted:

1. Even though superimposition of tissue layers is eliminated, the fairly gross resolution of 1.2–1.7 cm in the plane and 1.7 cm axially should be stressed.
2. Due to absorption in the tissue of the weak gamma emission, the deeper structures are not well visualized. In migraine the blood flow changes are largely confined to the cortex.
3. The problem of scattered radiation in the brain implies that one cannot accurately measure focal low flow values. This is an important point because it means that it is not easy to ascertain if ischemic flow levels are actually reached, that is, levels of cortical flow below approximately 23 ml/100 g/min. As the scatter effect always causes an overestimation of flow, it is our conclusion that the low measured values, reaching down below 30 ml/100 g/min in many cases, strongly suggest ischemia. The postattack hyperemia now becoming apparent in many severe cases points to the same conclusion (17).
4. ^{133}Xe taken up by the extracerebral tissues plays a minor role. The only serious contamination stems from the upper airways: the nasal cavity and the sinuses. This distorts flow calculation in the low frontal lobe in the midline, but in migraine the flow changes are mainly in the cortex of the convexity, regions where extracerebral contamination is negligible.
5. As with the other ^{133}Xe methods, a constant CBF is assumed during the study.

The validity of this assumption may be checked by the simultaneous recording of the velocity of the blood in the major intracranial arteries using the

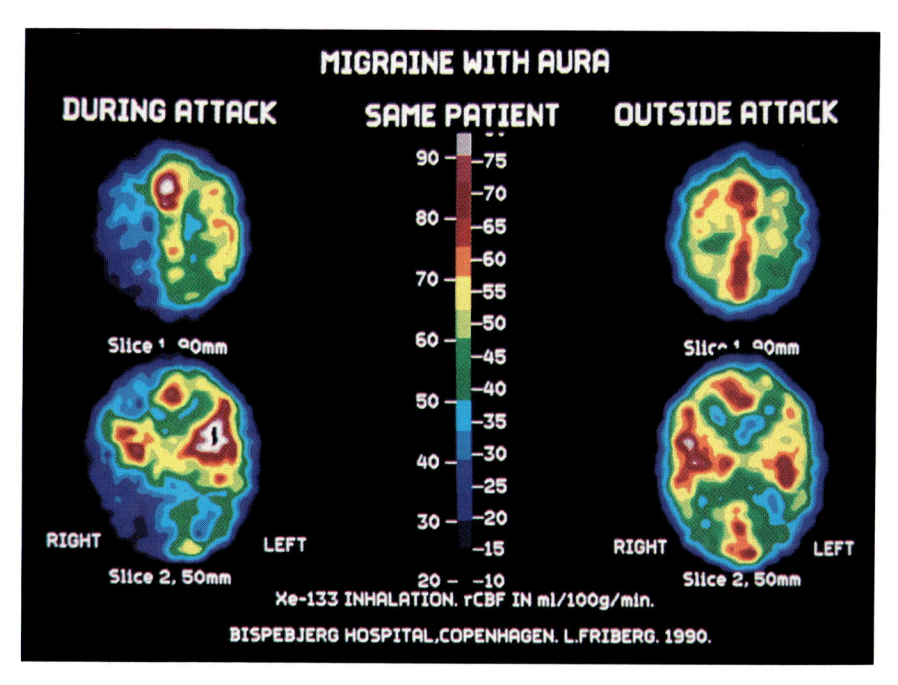

FIG. 3. ¹³³Xe tomography CBF during aural phase of an attack of migraine and of the same patient outside an attack.

transcranial doppler, a combined approach that has much to offer (see Friberg).

DISCUSSION: COMPARISON TO OTHER CBF METHODS

Of the two methods mentioned, only ¹³³Xe tomography can be considered of practical value in relation to migraine research. But, ¹³³Xe tomography demands costly and specialized equipment available, perhaps, in only 50 clinical centers worldwide. What then? Should one rather use the less costly nontomographic ¹³³Xe inhalation approach that in principle is so similar? It is our impression that this can indeed be a sensible recommendation because it appears that on a scientific level the conventional ¹³³Xe technique still has much to offer migraine research: The method can, with a suitable number of detectors (32 on either side of the head), give gross localization and is well suited for repeated measurements. Nevertheless, in particular, the tomographic technique is intrinsically superior because of the possibility of enhanced ¹³³Xe uptake in the extracerebral tissues including the temporal muscles.

Other tomographic CBF methods are available. Clearly, positron tomography is currently the "ultimate" technique. But because of the formidable problems of logistic nature, it is nearly impossible to study an acute, evanescent state as a migraine attack by positron emission tomography (PET). For all the obvious interest, not least in the context of deciding if ischemia (severe "misery" perfusion) exists in the migrainous aura, it is disappointing but understandable that only reports of a very few patients have been published (18). Clearly, therefore, PET is not usable or useful in migraine research. The same applies apparently to CBF tomography by the "cold" xenon-enhanced computed tomography (CT) scanning technique. This technique is rather cumbersome and no reports on results obtained in migraine are available.

Thus, at the present time only the other SPECT techniques based on brain retained tracers, in particular ^{99m}Tc-HMPAO, are applicable (Fig. 4). This approach, discussed by Andersen elsewhere in this volume, is used in a number of studies on migraine and lies outside the scope to discuss, beyond stating that indeed HMPAO tomography is practical and, although giving only relative values (flow distribution), is a useful tool in clinical brain research.

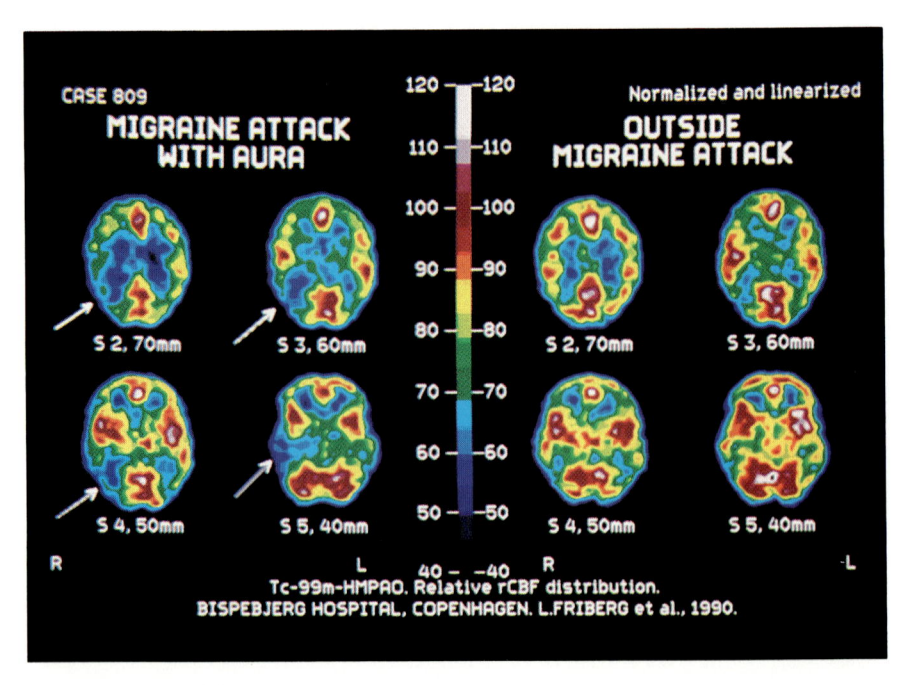

FIG. 4. ^{99m}Tc-HMPAO tomograms of CBF distribution during a severe attack of migraine with aura and of the same patient outside an attack.

REFERENCES

1. Conn, Jr, HL. Measurement of organ blood flow without blood sampling. *J Clin Invest* 1955; 34:916–917.
2. Jones HB. Respiratory system, nitrogen elimination. In: Glasser O, ed. *Medical Physics*. Chicago: Year Book Medical Publishers, 1950; 2:855–871.
3. Mallett BL and Veal N. Investigation of cerebral blood flow in hypertension, using radioactive-Xenon inhalation and extracranial recording. *Lancet* 1963; 1:1081–1082.
4. Kety SS. The theory and applications of the exchange of inert gas at the lunds and tissues. *Pharmacol Rev* 1951; 3:1–41.
5. Kety SS and Schmidt CF. The determination of cerebral blood flow in man by the use of nitrous oxide in low concentration. *Am J Physiol* 1945; 143:53–66.
6. Lassen NA and Munck O. The cerebral blood flow in man determined by the use of radioactive Krypton. *Acta Physiol Scand* 1955; 33:30–49.
7. Lassen NA and Ingvar DH. The blood flow of the cerebral cortex determined by radioactive Krypton-85. *Experientia* 1961; 17:42–45.
8. Høedt-Rasmussen K, Sveinsdottir E, and Lassen NA. Regional cerebral blood flow in man determined by intra-arterial injection of radioactive inert gas. *Circ Res* 1966; 18:237–247.
9. Høedt-Rasmussen K, Skinhøj E, Paulson O, et al. Regional cerebral blood flow in acute apoplexy: The "Luxury Perfusion Syndrome" of brain tissue. *Arch Neurol* 1967; 17:271–281.
10. Olesen J, Paulson OB, and Lassen NA. Regional cerebral blood flow in man determined by the initial slope of the clearance of intra-arterially injected ^{133}Xe. *Stroke* 1971; 2:519–540.
11. Sveinsdottir E, Larsen B, Rommer P, and Lassen NA. A multidetector scintillation camera with 254 channels. *J Nucl Med* 1977; 18:168–174.
12. Lassen NA, Sveinsdottir E, Kanno I, Stokely EM, and Rommer P. A fast moving, single photon emission tomograph for regional cerebral blood flow studies in man. *J Comput Assist Tomogr* 1978; 2:661–662.
13. Kanno I and Lassen NA. Two methods for calculation of regional cerebral blood flow from emission computed tomography of inert gas concentration. *J Comput Assist Tomogr* 1979; 3:71–76.
14. Stokely EM, Sveinsdottir E, Lassen NA, and Rommer P. A single photon dynamic computer-assisted tomograph (DCAT) for imaging brain function in multiple cross-sections. *J Comput Assist Tomogr* 1980; 4:230–240.
15. Celsis P, Goldman T, Henriksen L, and Lassen NA. A method for calculating regional cerebral blood flow from emission computed tomography of inert gas concentrations. *J Comput Assist Tomogr* 1981; 5:641–645.
16. Shirahata N, Henriksen L, Vorstrup S, Holm S, Lauritzen M, Paulson OB, and Lassen NA. Regional cerebral blood flow assessed by ^{133}Xe inhalation and emission tomography: Normal values. *J Comput Assist Tomogr* 1985; 9:861–866.
17. Andersen AR, Friberg L, Olsen TS, and Oleson F. Delayed hyperemia following hypoperfusion in classic migraine. Single photon emission computed tomographic demonstration. *Arch Neurol* 1988; 45:154–159.
18. Herold S, Gibbs JM, Jones AKP, Brooks DJ, Frackowiak RSJ, and Legg NJ. Oxygen metabolism in migraine. *J Cereb Blood Flow Metab* 1985; 5[Suppl. 1]:S445–S446.

3

Inhalation or Intravenous Injection of Xenon 133 and External Stationary Detectors

Jarl Risberg

CBF Laboratory, Department of Psychiatry, University Hospital, S-221 85 Lund, Sweden

The measurement of the regional cerebral blood flow (rCBF) by inhalation of ^{133}Xe and recording of the gamma radiation by means of multiple external stationary scintillation detectors were suggested and tried during the 1960s by Mallet and Veall (1). However, the technique was severely criticized (2). It was considered to give erroneous flow values due to contamination of the recordings by radiation originating from extracranial tissues and recirculation of the isotope. Similar problems were also considered to affect the somewhat later suggested method based on intravenous (iv) injection of ^{133}Xe (3). The methodological problems were eventually solved, however, mainly through the thorough work of Obrist and collaborators (4,5). From about 1975 the two nontraumatic rCBF techniques were generally considered to be reliable and valid and became widely used in research and in the clinic. Their ability to provide quantitative and repeatable measures of rCBF makes them still useful methods in the study of cerebral hemodynamics. Their noninvasiveness and the relatively low radiation exposure (comparable to a chest x-ray) make them still possible to use in most countries in research involving normal volunteers.

BASIC METHODOLOGY

The Classic Obrist Method

The standard methodology implies that the tracer is administered either by inhalation during 1 min or by a short-lasting iv injection. The clearance of the isotope is then followed by multiple (up to 254) scintillation detectors during 10 min of normal air breathing. The arterial concentration of the tracer is estimated by monitoring the radiation from a continuous sample of the air in the air passages. The end-tidal values of this air curve are used to estimate the arterial input function, which is of crucial importance for an accurate determination of the flow level. The method of analysis, as suggested by Obrist (5), implies the fitting of the curve to a two-compartment model. The fast clearing part of the curve is assumed to represent gray matter blood flow and the second compartment is considered to represent cerebral white matter with contamination of extracranial tissues. A correction for the recirculation of the isotope is made throughout the recording period by means of deconvolution. The original Obrist method also involves the exclusion of the first 90–120 sec from the analysis (delayed start fit time) in order to limit the influence of radiation from the air passages. (This artifact will be dealt with in more detail later.)

Noncompartmental Flow Indices

The two-compartment analysis is theoretically the most proper way to calculate flow. The method has a severe disadvantage, however, for measurements made in patients with subnormal flow levels and/or brain pathology because the mathematical solution becomes unstable when the gray matter flow level is below about 50 ml/100 g/min (6). There is simply not enough information for a stable and valid separation of the two compartments if the gray and white matter flow values are close. Another reason for instability is the presence of abnormal tissues. Such tissues might have flow levels in between the "fast" and the "slow" and might be included at random in either compartment. This problem, called "slippage," might cause large and erroneous variations of the flow levels measured with the two-compartment analysis.

Slippage is avoided by the use of flow indices, which depend less on a paper compartmental separation. Several such indices have been suggested. One of the most commonly used noncompartmental flow measures for the inhalation technique is the Initial Slope Index (ISI), as originally suggested by the present author (6). It is calculated from the slope of the first 2–3 min of the recirculation corrected curve and is immune to slippage because it is based on the two compartments combined. It is dominated by gray matter flow, somewhat influenced by white matter flow, and only slightly contaminated by extracranial blood flow. Similar flow indices are also used for the iv technique.

FEATURES AND LIMITATIONS

Spatial Resolution

The region of measurement depends on four factors: (a) the geometric field of view of the detector, (b) the absorption of the photons emitted by the isotope, (c) the pattern of distribution of isotope in the tissue, and (d) the recording of scattered photons.

The geometric field of view of a scintillation detector is determined by the size and shape of the collimator. The distribution of count rates from a point source moving through water (similar to brain tissue regarding absorption of photons) in front of the detector will show the highest counts along the center line and close to the crystal and gradually declining values at distant and/or peripheral positions.

The absorption of photons in the brain tissue is thus the main factor limiting the influence from more distant brain structures. Superficial cortical layers close to the detector will have the largest influence on the recordings with gradually decreasing contributions from deep structures. Most of the photons emitted by the xenon isotope (81 KeV) from medial and more distant structures will be absorbed, limiting the contribution from the contralateral hemisphere to about 20% of the counts recorded (7).

The pattern of distribution of isotope in the tissue recorded is also important when defining the region of measurement. A certain subvolume of tissue will influence the curve recorded in proportion to its content of isotope. The tracer concentration is determined by the blood flow of the subvolume and its tissue/blood partition coefficient (λ). An instantaneous arrival of isotope (intracarotid injection) will give a distribution of tracer that is proportional to its flow, whereas an extended input of tracer will end with saturation, in which case the concentration is proportional to λ. The inhalation and iv methods described here involve a rather short-lasting bolus input, and the distribution of tracer is thus mainly flow-related. This means that a subvolume of tissue with high perfusion has a considerably greater influence on the recorded curve than a subvolume of slowly perfused tissue of similar size. The methods are thus more sensitive to hyperemia than to ischemia. The most dramatic example is the low sensitivity to cerebral infarcts. Surrounding, better-perfused tissues will totally dominate the recording, with erroneously high flow values for the region of the infarct as a result (the "look through" effect).

The recording of scattered photons (Compton scatter) will also influence the spatial resolution. Compton scatter is the phenomenon of a photon colliding with an atom in the brain, losing some of its energy, and continuing its flight with a change of direction. This means that some of the counts recorded by the detector originate from Xe atoms outside the geometric field of measurement. The Compton scatter often can be efficiently discriminated electronically because of its lower energy. It is an unfortunate feature of ^{133}Xe that the energy lost in the collision is very small and the scattered photons are thus very close in energy to the "good" photons. The proportion of scattered photons recorded has been estimated to be about 25% (7).

Despite these resolution-limiting factors, there is ample evidence that the techniques still are able to record rather narrowly localized cortical events. This is especially true when recording systems like the Cortexplorer with 254 scintillation detectors are used (8). The spatial resolution for such a system is about 1 cm for the cortical mantle.

Temporal Resolution

The measurement of blood flow with the present techniques implies that the level of perfusion is stable during the period of recording. The basic principle of the method thus excludes the recording of transient or very short-lasting flow changes. Only the average flow during the period of registration can be recorded. The shortest period of recording required to obtain a reliable flow value is 4–5 min using any of the initial slope indices. A new recording cannot be made, however, until the concentration of the tracer has approached baseline values. Using present standard routines, the shortest time interval between recordings is about 20 min (9). The second and following measurements are then preceded by a recording of remaining activity lasting for 5 min.

Inherent Measurement Errors

The coefficient of variation of the hemispheric mean flow values in repeated studies of resting normal subjects has been reported to be 10–12% for gray matter flow (bicompartmental analysis) and about 8% for ISI (10,11). It is not possible to determine exactly how much of this variation is caused by real physiologic changes of rCBF and how much is the error of measurement. The hemispheric averages are determined with great precision, especially with multiprobe systems. Global and regional right–left asymmetries have low error because they are unaffected by errors in the estimation of the input function. An asymmetry of 5% or more for the hemispheric means has been found to be significantly different from the normal, whereas an asymmetry of at least 10% is needed for significance regarding a regional asymmetry (10,11).

The Air Passage Artifact

The air passage artifact is caused by the presence of isotope in the nasopharyngeal passages, which influences the recordings primarily by scattered photons. Measurements made in regions close to the air passages (e.g., frontotemporal areas) will be heavily influenced during the period of inhalation (or immediately after iv injection). If an uncorrected curve is analyzed the result will be a marked overestimation of flow. This artifact is somewhat more pronounced for the inhalation method than for the iv technique because of the higher concentration of isotope in the inhaling phase of the respiratory cycle for the former method. The earliest attempt to minimize the influence of this artifact was to omit the first 90–120 sec of the curve in the calculation of flow (5). Several correction methods have since then been suggested and implemented. Some of them (8,9,12) check for variations in the shape of the head curves, which are synchronous with tracer variations in the air passages. These synchronous changes are used to calculate a weighting factor for the artifact for each region and the artifact is then removed by subtraction (its shape is known—it is similar to that of the air curve). This correction method is safe (never overcorrects) and accurate, provided the early part of the head curve is sampled with high time resolution (ideally 0.2 sec). This is needed for exact information about the rapid fluctuations of the head curve, which are synchronous with changes of tracer concentration in the air passages. Unfortunately, this rapid sampling for the head curves is only possible with the more modern type of rCBF equipment (Cortexplorer). Another approach is the introduction of the artifact size as an unknown in the equation for the curve (13,14). With this correction the total curve from start of inhalation/injection can be utilized in the calculation of flow.

Contamination from Extracerebral Tissues

The extracerebral influence on the recordings has been a topic of much discussion throughout the development of the nontraumatic ^{133}Xe methods (1,2,4). A fairly small influence of the tracer in extracerebral tissues has, however, been convincingly demonstrated by Obrist and coworkers (4,5). They showed that the blood flow of skin, muscles, and bone is low and does not contaminate the gray matter flow (if this is not extremely low). Some contamination of white matter blood flow is present, however, which makes interpretation of the slow flow compartment as white matter flow questionable. The interpretation of the slow flow parameter becomes especially complicated if the intracerebral and extracerebral flow levels change in different directions (as might be the case in patients with headache). Since the major research and clinical interest so far has been focused on cortical blood flow, the limitation regarding white matter flow has been of minor practical importance.

Technical Errors

Isotope leak from the mask or mouthpiece is the most common technical artifact. The leaking gas will be efficiently recorded by the detectors, and a severe leak might ruin the study. The most dangerous leak is the small one, however. It is difficult to detect by visual inspection, but might still distort the recording and cause erroneously high or low flow values. There is some risk that the operator is fooled by this artifact. Most modern rCBF systems do, however, have built-in warning systems for leaks. A leak often can then be eliminated before it has caused any damage.

ACKNOWLEDGMENT

Supported by the Swedish Medical Research Council (4969).

REFERENCES

1. Mallett BL and Veall N. The measurement of regional cerebral clearance rates in man using xenon-133 inhalation and extracranial recordings. *J Clin Sci* 1965; 29:179–191.
2. Jensen KB, Høedt-Rasmussen K, Sveinsdottir E, Stewart BM, and Lassen NA. Cerebral blood flow evaluated by inhalation of 133-Xe and extracranial recording: A methodological study. *J Clin Sci* 1966; 30:485–494.
3. Austin G, Horn H, Rouhe S, and Hayworth W. Description and early results of an intravenous radioisotope technique for measuring regional cerebral blood flow in man. *Eur Neurol* 1972; 8:43–51.
4. Obrist WD, Thompson HK, King CH, and Wang HS. Determination of regional cerebral blood flow by inhalation of 133-xenon. *Circ Res* 1967; 20:124–135.
5. Obrist WD, Thompson HK, Wang HS, and Wilkinson WE. Regional cerebral blood flow estimated by 133-xenon inhalation. *Stroke* 1975; 6:245–256.
6. Risberg J, Ali Z, Wilson EM, Wills EL, and Halsey JH. Regional cerebral blood flow by 133-xenon inhalation. Preliminary evaluation of an initial slope index in patients with unstable flow compartments. *Stroke* 1975; 6:142–148.
7. Bolmsjö M. Hemisphere cross-talk and signal overlapping in bilateral rCBF-measurements using Xe-133. In: Bolmsjö M. *The physical and psychological aspects of xenon isotopes in nuclear medical applications,* 1981. Thesis, Lund.
8. Risberg J. Development of high-resolution two-dimensional measurement of regional cerebral blood flow. In: Wade J, et al., eds. *Impact of functional imaging in neurology and psychiatry.* London: John Libbey & Co., 1987; 35–43.
9. Risberg J. Regional cerebral blood flow measurements by 133-Xe-inhalation: Methodology and applications in neuropsychology and psychiatry. *Brain Lang* 1980; 9:9–34.
10. Blauenstein UW, Halsey JH, Wilson EM, Wills EL, and Risberg J. 133 Xenon inhalation method, analysis of reproducibility: Some of its physiological implications. *Stroke* 1977; 8:92–102.
11. Prohovnik I, Håkansson K, and Risberg J. Observations on the functional significance of regional cerebral blood flow in resting normal subjects. *Neuropsychologia* 1980; 18:203–217.

12. Nilsson B, Ryding E, and Ingvar DH. Quantitative airway artefact compensation at regional cerebral blood flow measurements with radioactive gases. *J Cerebr Blood Flow Metab* 1982; 2:73–78.
13. Hazelrig JB, Katholi CR, Blauenstein UW, Halsey JH, Wilson EM, and Wills EL. Total curve analysis of regional cerebral blood flow with 133-Xe inhalation: Description of method and values obtained with normal volunteers. *IEEE Trans Biomed Eng* 1981; 28:609–616.
14. Prohovnik I, Knudsen E, and Risberg J. Accuracy of models and algorithms for determination of fast compartment flow by non-invasive 133-Xe clearance. In: Magistretti P, ed. *Functional radionuclide imaging of the brain*. New York: Raven Press, 1983; 80–95.

Migraine and Other Headaches:
The Vascular Mechanisms,
edited by Jes Olesen.
Raven Press, Ltd., New York © 1991.

4

Utility of the Retained Tracer Complex Technetium 99m-HMPAO for Measurements of Regional Cerebral Blood Flow

Allan R. Andersen

Department of Neurology, Rigshospitalet, DK-2100 Copenhagen, Denmark

Three-dimensional measurements of regional cerebral blood flow (rCBF) in humans using single photon emission computer tomography (SPECT) became possible several years ago. The first brain-dedicated SPECT system was designed to detect the brain activity after inhalation or injection of the diffusible tracer ^{133}Xe. Afterward a number of techniques using SPECT, positron emission tomography (PET), or computed tomography (CT) were developed in an effort to obtain methods with more accurate measurements of CBF or with a higher spatial resolution. The recent development of new SPECT tracers that are retained in the brain and trapped in proportion to regional blood flow has allowed high resolution static imaging with SPECT without some of the drawbacks inherent to the previous ^{133}Xe techniques. These new tracers do not require a dynamic brain-dedicated SPECT system, but can also be used with a conventional rotating gamma camera; thus, routine SPECT studies of rCBF have now become more widespread. The ^{123}I labeled amines constituted the breakthrough for the use of retained tracers of rCBF by SPECT. ^{99m}Tc-D,L-hexa-methyl-propylene-amine-oxime (HMPAO) has better radiation characteristics for SPECT imaging, acceptable radiation exposure, lower cost as compared to the ^{123}I complexes, and daily availability all together favoring HMPAO's use for routine clinical studies.

Using ^{99m}Tc-HMPAO with a single-head conventional rotating gamma camera, a resolution of about 15 mm (FWHM) axially and in the plane can be obtained, whereas brain-dedicated scanners yield a resolution of about 9–10 mm (FWHM).

METHOD

The lipophilic tracer complex (^{99m}Tc-HMPAO) is unstable and converts rapidly from the lipophilic form, which passes the blood-brain barrier (BBB), to a hydrophilic form that is unable to pass the BBB and is trapped in the brain. A review of the tracer kinetics has been published elsewhere (1) but a brief summary is presented next.

The conversion from the lipophilic to the hydrophilic form takes place during the transport of the tracer from the intravenous (iv) injection site to the brain. The fraction of activity in the lipophilic form and thus available for extraction across the BBB is less in the cerebral microvessels as compared to the cubital vein. The input function to the brain is therefore hard to obtain, as the conversion continues in the vials even after arterial blood sampling, unless the blood is collected in octanol (1). The instability of the tracer complex is thus both the key to the retention of the complex and to the difficulties in estimating the input function necessary for quantitated rCBF measures.

^{99m}Tc-HMPAO is distributed initially like rCBF but an early backdiffusion (brain to blood) is seen, in essence lasting only 2–3 min. The backdiffusion is flow-dependent, leading to a preferential loss of activity from the high flow regions of the brain. The distribution images might be rather influenced by backdiffusion. This can be corrected for by the algorithm of Lassen et al. (2). This correction is valid within normal flow ranges but the highest flow rates that may be achieved during brain activation or epileptic seizures are somewhat underestimated. The algorithm corrects the distribution images to relative CBF images using an internal region for reference. The algorithm was developed to omit the cumbersome arterial sampling and it works well (1). After correction, rCBF as measured by HMPAO is usually given in activity measures or in relative flow. The retention in the brain is stable when the early back diffusion has ceased, and only a small loss of tracer (0.4% per hr) is observed in most human cases during the next 24 hr. It can be concluded that many aspects of the kinetics of ^{99m}Tc-HMPAO are known, and the complex can be used for rCBF measurements using SPECT. Examples demonstrating the utility are given below with emphasis on the benefit obtained from the stability of the distribution image obtained combined with the short fixation time. Combining these characteristics, it is evident that "frozen" images of short-lasting blood flow changes can be measured hours after the event. This is of special interest in patients with seizures or migraine with aura.

CLINICAL APPLICATION

Normal Aging

The development of ^{99m}Tc-HMPAO increased the potential of SPECT for studying the effects of normal aging and atrophy on regional cerebral blood flow. In a recent study from our laboratory (3), 53 carefully screened healthy volunteers with ages ranging from 20–90 years were presented. The contributions of age, sex, and atrophy to variations in global CBF were studied. Cortical atrophy was the only significant determinant for global CBF, accounting for 27% of its variance. There was no significant correlation of global CBF with ventricular size, Evans' ratio, sex, or age. There was a preferential decline of CBF in the frontal cortex with advancing age, and the side-to-side asymmetry ratio of several regions of interest, most of all the frontotemporal cortex, increased with age. Subcortical CBF decreased with advancing cortical atrophy, and the relative area of the subcortical low flow region in midbrain levels increased with age. All subjects had normal CT scans without any focal or periventricular abnormalities (3). In patients with suspected degenerative dementia disorders, a SPECT scan is often the only study that is be abnormal. Thus, failure to recognize the pronounced but variable changes in rCBF with age in healthy humans may lead to overinterpretation of SPECT scans with a consequent overdiagnosis of dementia disorders.

Studies of stroke and dementia profit from the static retention qualities of ^{99m}Tc-HMPAO. Concerning stroke and other cerebrovascular diseases, the "expected" results for a flow tracer have been reported. Stroke cases show abnormal flow regions of hypoactivity and hyperactivity (luxury perfusion) and remote changes in the contralateral cerebellar hemisphere or ipsilateral thalamic or capsula interna (diashisis). None of these or other stroke patients at present have been reported to present with a low or high flow region in a scan obtained early after iv injection of ^{99m}Tc-HMPAO because redistribution was reverted into a flow region of the opposite extreme a few hours later.

Studies aiming at the classification of demented patients using ^{99m}Tc-HMPAO SPECT are of major interest. Preliminary reports have been published. A number of SPECT studies have aimed at characterizing a typical perfusion pattern in Alzheimer's disease (AD). The most consistent finding seemed to be a significant bilateral reduction of rCBF in posterior temporoparietal regions, in most studies with a meaningful correlation to the results of some of the psychometric tests. However, in only few of the studies are the results supported by parametric data and comparison to age-matched control subjects. These controlled studies consistently found a bilateral reduction of rCBF in posterior temporoparietal regions to be the most striking feature in AD, although asymmetric cases were also mentioned.

Vascular dementia (VD) is a complex of different disorders, whose diagnosis should be based primarily on structural imaging techniques, especially magnetic resonance imaging (MRI). There are only a few studies with ^{99m}Tc-HMPAO in VD. They included only patients with multiple infarcts to demonstrate the ability of the technique to differentiate AD from patients with VD, in whom posterior flow reductions were not seen (4). Waldemar et al. (4) studied 17 patients with vascular dementia, only a very few of whom had multiple cortical infarcts as the only structural abnormality. More than half of the patients had structural changes similar to those reported in subacute arteriosclerotic encephalopathy. In published cases patients with frontal lobe dementia of non-Alzheimer type have shown reduced tracer uptake in the anterior cerebral hemispheres.

High resolution CBF studies of the central parts of the human brain have been performed. CBF changes have been demonstrated in the basal ganglia of patients with Parkinson's disease whereas patients with Huntington's chorea have been shown to have a characteristic low flow of the head of the caudate nucleus.

ACUTE, ATTACK-WISE CHANGES OF rCBF

The labeling period of the brain, essentially lasting only 2 min, and the long retention have made routine studies of rCBF possible during epileptic attacks and interictally. The patient can be injected at the department during the seizure. Treatment can be initiated and the patient can be studied 1–2 hr later. This appears to be important for the focal diagnosis in temporal lobe epilepsy and of initial changes in aura migraine, especially in cases with no structural lesions when studied by MRI or CT and no side localization by electroencephalography (EEG).

Twenty-eight epileptic patients have been studied by our group. They exhibit therapy-resistant simple or complex partial seizures with or without secondary generalization. The patients have been studied by SPECT as a part of a presurgical evaluation program, interictal SPECT studies, CT, MRI scannings, and 16-channel scalp EEG recordings. Intracranial electrodes were not used. When the interictal neuroimaging studies were performed the patient data were analyzed and discussed. If the data were incongruent, an ictal video-EEG monitored SPECT study was performed. The attacks are provoked by reducing the antiepileptic medication for a few days before the stipulated day of ictal SPECT. We injected 0.7–0.9 GBq of ^{99m}Tc-HMPAO within seconds after the onset of the attack, and the patients were brought to the SPECT unit after intensive antiepileptic therapy had been resumed.

In 24 of the 28 patients studied, we observed an obvious low flow region in one temporal lobe using ^{99m}Tc-HMPAO. The low flow regions were well demarcated from normal tissue and in many cases involved higher (parietal and frontal) ipsilateral regions of the brain. In 13 patients a smaller region of low flow was observed in the contralateral (mirror) temporal lobe.

SPECT was superior to CT and MRI for visualizing the focal epileptogenic region suggested by the EEG. In five of the MRI-negative and CT-negative cases a consistent diagnosis was made by combining the results of the EEG and SPECT. So far, side localization has been impossible in only one patient. In all ictal studies the activity increased up to 45% of the control values of the contralateral hemisphere comprising rather larger regions. All had large hyperperfused regions of interest at the site where the interictal studies showed a low flow region interictally. The results correspond closely to those presented by using PET (5) because a significant focal rCBF change is demonstrated in about 75% of the patients using ^{99m}Tc-HMPAO, ^{133}Xe, or iodinated amines.

SHORTCOMINGS OF RETAINED TRACERS

A few shortcomings are evident when a retained tracer such as ^{99m}Tc-HMPAO is compared to a freely diffusible inert gas such as ^{133}Xe. Repeated studies in the same patient can be performed with an interval as short as 20 min using ^{133}Xe because this tracer is rapidly washed out. It is also an inherent consequence of the excellent retention of ^{99m}Tc-HMPAO that a second study within hours after a first injection is jeopardized by the high background from the first study. This, combined with the decrease of extraction (E) and lower fractional retention (R) of tracer with increased CBF, may explain why the attempts to show focal rCBF changes during normal brain activation until now have been rather unsuccessful. A second drawback with respect to clinical utility of ^{99m}Tc-HMPAO as compared to ^{133}Xe SPECT is the lack of studies documenting an increased uptake of ^{99m}Tc-HMPAO after CO_2 stimulation, a procedure known to increase CBF. This is probably also due to the decreasing E and R rates at high flow values and the increased cardiac output induced by CO_2. SPECT imaging using ^{99m}Tc-HMPAO, however, does not have the inherent errors of the ^{133}Xe SPECT: the airway artefact and the poor resolution of deep brain structures. Therefore, the two methods supplement each other: ^{133}Xe inhalation for easy, repeatable, and quantitative measurements of rCBF and ^{99m}Tc-HMPAO for high resolution static imaging in relative flow units.

APPLICATION FOR MIGRAINE STUDIES

It may be concluded that the following perspectives are obvious for rCBF measurements using SPECT and HMPAO in migraine. HMPAO is a well-described tracer of rCBF using conventional SPECT. Studies of patients during attacks can be performed because the tracer complex is built in within 2–3 min after the iv injection. The tracer injection may thus be performed at the emergency unit, but the data acquisition may be postponed until the nausea, headache, and vomiting has stopped hours later. Low flow regions and (later) high flow regions should be seen during the course of a migraine with aura attacks as it has earlier been demonstrated using ^{133}Xe. With a split-dose technique injecting one-third of the total activity first and two-thirds an hour later, HMPAO may be used for the analysis of parts of the sequential flow events during the migraine attack. ^{133}Xe, however, is obviously superior with respect to these repeated studies. More than two studies on the same day are probably not recommendable using HMPAO. Because of the better radiation characteristics of ^{99m}Tc for SPECT as compared to ^{133}Xe, better in-plane and axial resolution is obtainable using HMPAO. Quantitated rCBF values are hard to obtain with HMPAO, as the arterial input curve is difficult to obtain. Semiquantitative estimates are easy to obtain using the algorithm of Lassen et al (2). This algorithm corrects the distribution images of HMPAO to a closer correlation with true rCBF (1) and makes the images easier to interpret. If SPECT images of rCBF with HMPAO in migraine with aura do not correspond to earlier results using ^{133}Xe, the following pitfalls should be considered: poor shape of the SPECT device, low purity of the HMPAO (by too late injection after mixing of tracer with eluate or bad eluate from ^{99m}Tc source), poor timing of injection with respect to onset of symptoms (1), or poor classification of the attack of the patient.

ACKNOWLEDGMENTS

This study was supported by the Danish Medical Research Council, the Lundbeck Foundation, and the Danish Hospital Foundation for Medical Research, region of Copenhagen, The Faroe Islands, and Greenland.

REFERENCES

1. Andersen AR. Tc99m-d,l-hexamethylpropyleneamineoxime (Tc99m-HMPAO): Basic kinetic studies of a tracer of cerebral blood flow. *Cerebrovasc Brain Metab Rev* 1989; 1:288–318.
2. Lassen NA, Andersen AR, Friberg L, and Paulson OB. The retention of Tc99m-d,l-HMPAO in the human brain after intracarotid bolus injection. A kinetic analysis. *J Cereb Blood Flow Metab* 1988; 8:S13–S22.
3. Waldemar G, Hasselbalch SG, Andersen AR, Delecluse F, Johnsen A, and Paulson OB. Tc99m-HMPAO and SPECT of the brain in normal aging. *J Cerebr Blood Flow Metab* (in press).
4. Waldemar G, Larsson HB, Lassen NA, and Paulson OB. Tomographic measurements of regional cerebral blood flow by SPECT in vascular dementia. In: *Cerebral ischemia and dementia*. Springer-Verlag, Berlin-Heidelberg (in press).
5. Engel J. The role of neuroimaging in the surgical treatment of epilepsy. *Acta Neurol Scand* 1988; [Suppl 117]:84–89.

5

Stable Xenon CT-CBF Methodology for Studying Vascular Headaches

John Stirling Meyer, Jun Kawamura, and Yasuo Terayama

Cerebral Blood Flow Laboratory, Veterans Affairs Medical Center, and Department of Neurology, Baylor College of Medicine, Houston, Texas 77030

Investigations of cephalic blood flow have provided interesting information concerning the pathophysiology and pathogenesis of "vascular headaches." In the past decade, several tomographic methods have become available for three-dimensional imaging of local cerebral blood flow (LCBF). This chapter describes the xenon-enhanced computed tomographic method for imaging LCBF during inhalation of low concentrations of xenon gas as the indicator and using high resolution, rapid x-ray transmission computed tomographic (CT) scanners for imaging purposes.

METHODS

Theoretical Background

Xenon gas is a lipid-soluble x-ray contrast indicator that absorbs transmitted x-rays, so that both their location and concentration may be detected and quantified with high resolution CT scanners. Xenon rapidly crosses the blood-brain barrier and diffuses freely through brain tissues. After inhalation of xenon gas, time-dependent changes of its concentrations in different brain tissues cause directly proportional changes in CT or Hounsfield numbers. Local changes of tissue concentrations of xenon gas over time are used to measure local cerebral blood flow according to the basic monoexponential equation described by Kety (1). According to Kety's model, time-dependent increases of diffusible indicator of the brain may be represented by the formula:

$$Ci(T) = \lambda i k i \int_0^T Ca(t)\, e^{-ki(T-t)} dt \qquad (1)$$

where T is the time given after starting inhalation of xenon, $C_i(T)$ are the regional enhancements for different regions of interest in brain tissue measured as changes in CT numbers determined at time T, λ_i is the blood-brain partition coefficient for xenon, and k_i is the flow rate constant. Since arterial input function $C_a(t)$ is approximated by the equation:

$$C_a(t) = C_{amax}(1 - e^{-rt}) \qquad (2)$$

where $C_a(t)$ is the arterial xenon concentration at time t, C_{amax} is the arterial xenon concentration at infinity, and r is the rate constant for arterial saturation with xenon. Since arterial or end-tidal input functions $C_a(t)$ are approximated by equation (2), equation (1) can be solved analytically by the following formula:

$$C_i(T) = k_i \lambda_i C_{amax}[k_i^{-1}(1 - e^{-k_iT}) - (k_i - r)^{-1}(e^{-rT} - e^{-k_i})] \qquad (3)$$

where k_i is estimated by unweighted, nonlinear, least-squares fitting utilizing a computer program. Lλ values are calculated from tissue and blood ΔH values are estimated at saturation during inhalation of Xe by utilization of Kelcz et al.'s formula (2). LCBF is then calculated by:

$$LCBF = \lambda_i k_i$$

Procedure for Xe CT-CBF Measurement

Xe CT-CBF measurements are performed using a Siemens SOMATOM DR Version H CT scanner (Siemens Medical Systems, Inc., Iselin, New Jersey). Settings for the instrument during scanning were 540 mAs, 96 KV, 8 mm thickness, and 5 sec scanning times. Desired concentrations of xenon and oxygen to be inhaled are selected (27% xenon in oxygen is recommended) by means of a specially designed xenon gas delivery system (Enhancer 3000, Diversified Diagnostic Products, Inc., Houston, Texas), which uses a closed rebreathing system. Two baseline noncontrasted CT scans are performed at 1-min intervals before switching to the xenon mixture. Seven serial scans are then made at 1-min intervals while the brain is being saturated with 27% stable xenon gas.

End-tidal xenon concentrations are monitored by means of a thermoconductivity analyzer mounted within the Enhancer console. End-tidal xenon concentrations have been shown to be in equilibrium with those of the arterial blood by the use of a conversion constant (2). End-tidal partial pressure values for xenon are thereby converted to equivalent changes in CT numbers for arterial blood.

Calculation of LCBF values on cross-sectional images of the brain are then performed by a series of programs using a desk-top computer (3,4).

Reproducibility

To quantify short-time drift during LCBF measurements, scannings of water, iodine mixtures, and a CT skull phantom were repeated 11 times at 1-min intervals. CT numbers during serial scanning of water and the CT skull phantom were 4.3 ± 0.2 and 128.8 ± 0.2, respectively. There was no systematic increase in the CT values throughout scanning.

SUBJECTS

The population studied consisted of 32 neurologically normal volunteers aged between 20 and 88 years with and without vascular headaches. Selection of normal volunteers required the following criteria: (a) normal neurological examination and normal Cognitive Capacity Screening Examination, (b) absence by history of any neurological or psychological disorder other than vascular headache, and (c) exclusion by CT or magnetic resonance imaging (MRI) of any intracranial abnormalities other than age-related cerebral atrophy.

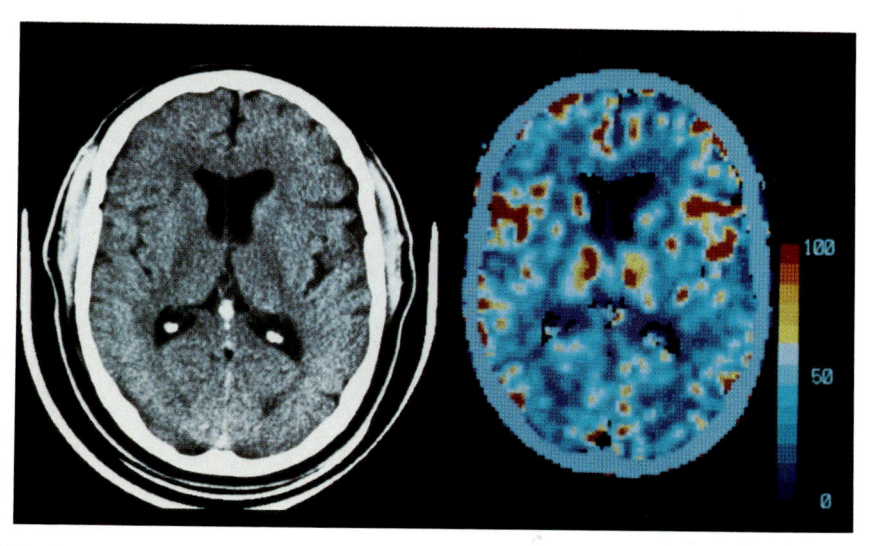

FIG. 1. Noncontrast CT image of the brain and corresponding LCBF map recorded from a 59-year-old normal male volunteer.

TABLE 1. *LCBF and Lλ values among volunteers*

Regions	LCBF (ml/100 g/min)	Lλ
Frontal cortex	51.6 ± 10.8	1.03 ± 0.13
Temporal cortex	49.8 ± 12.0	1.07 ± 0.09
Occipital cortex	47.0 ± 14.4	1.04 ± 0.10
Caudate nucleus	54.1 ± 14.6	1.01 ± 0.11
Putamen	53.2 ± 14.9	1.07 ± 0.14
Thalamus	59.5 ± 16.5	1.13 ± 0.13
Frontal white	15.9 ± 3.6	1.56 ± 0.10
Occipital white	18.9 ± 4.0	1.48 ± 0.11
Internal capsule	25.6 ± 5.9	1.54 ± 0.11

RESULTS

Fig. 1 displays a nonenhanced CT image and corresponding LCBF and Lλ maps measured in a 59-year-old normal male volunteer (#P73).

Table 1 shows LCBF and Lλ values for 32 normal volunteers aged from 20–88 years. Mean LCBF values for gray matter are significantly higher than those for white matter, and mean Lλ values for gray matter are significantly lower than those for white matter.

Results of the relationships between advancing age and LCBF values are illustrated in Fig. 2. It is apparent that LCBF values for cortical and subcortical gray matter significantly decline with advancing age.

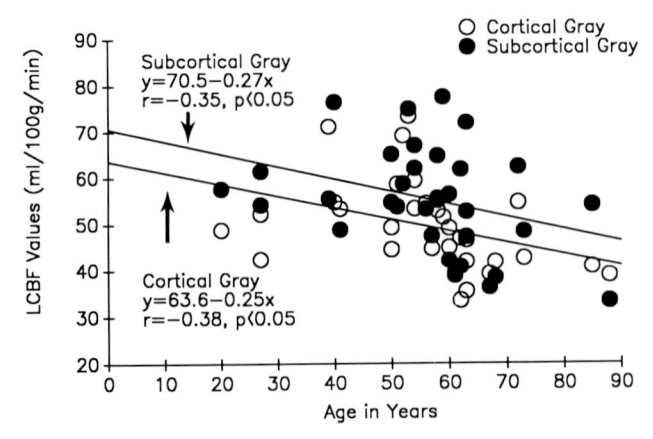

FIG. 2. Age-related declines in mean LCBF values for cortical and subcortical gray matter measured among 32 neurologically normal volunteers aged between 20 and 88 years old. Both lines of regression are statistically significant.

DISCUSSION

There are distinct advantages of the Xe CT-CBF method over conventional ^{133}Xe clearance techniques. They are: (a) it offers high resolution cross-sectional images of local cerebral blood flow in three dimensions including all cortical and subcortical brain structures, which may be precisely correlated with brain anatomy, (b) values for the local partition coefficients, necessary for LCBF calculations, are actually measured rather than assumed, and (c) problems due to Compton scatter, contamination by extracranial blood flow, and residual isotope noise are eliminated.

Xenon gas exerts subanesthetic effects, particularly if the concentrations used exceed 35% (5). Inhalation of lower concentrations of xenon gas (27%) were used in the present study, which minimizes any potential subanesthetic effects. Improved collimation of modern CT scanners reduces scattered radiation to the scalp, cornea, and lens of the eye. The radiation dose to the center of the brain is estimated to be 19 rads per LCBF measurement. Exposure is limited to narrow slices of the head and brain, which are relatively radioresistant structures. The effect of xenon on cerebral circulation has been evaluated by a number of investigators. In our laboratory, ^{133}Xe measurements of gray and white matter are in good agreement with CT-CBF measures in the same individuals. Microsphere studies in animal models have indicated either no alteration in CBF or less than 17% homogeneous increases of CBF in all brain regions (6,7).

There have been many reports concerning changes in CBF among patients with vascular headache, but results have been inconsistent. The discrepancy appears to be caused by several factors, which include selection of patients, the duration and timing of CBF measurements in relation to the stage of the attack, whether headaches are spontaneously induced, and methods used for CBF measurements. It is preferable to use a methodology that can measure LCBF values for subcortical brain structures as well as the cerebral cortex since some hypotheses concerning the pathogenesis of vascular headache are based on changing neuronal activity involving different brain regions. We have applied the Xe CT-CBF method for LCBF measurements and have reported cortical and subcortical hyperperfusion during spontaneously occurring migraine and cluster headache (8,9). Our results support Wolff's vascular theory rather than the theory of spreading cortical depression as offered by Olesen et al. (10).

In summary, Xe CT-CBF methodology appears to be useful for pathophysiological studies of vascular headaches. This method provides three-dimensional information concerning LCBF in patients suffering from vascular headache with high resolution, excellent anatomical correlation, and using Lλ values that are measured rather than assumed.

REFERENCES

1. Kety SS. The theory and applications of the exchange of inert gas at the lungs and tissues. *Pharmacol Rev* 1955; 3:1–41.
2. Kelcz F, Hilal SK, Hartwell P, and Joseph PM. Computed tomographic measurement of the xenon brain-blood partition coefficient and implications for regional cerebral blood flow: A preliminary report. *Radiology* 1978; 127:385–392.
3. Meyer JS, Shinohara T, Imai A, et al. Imaging local cerebral blood flow by Xenon-enhanced computed tomography—Technical optimization procedures. *Neuroradiology* 1988; 30:283–292.
4. Imai A, Meyer JS, Kobari M, Ichijo M, Shinohara T, and Oravez WT. LCBF values decline while Lλ values increase during normal human aging measured by stable xenon-enhanced computed tomography. *Neuroradiology* 1988; 30:463–472.
5. Winkler S and Turski P. Potential hazards of Xenon inhalation. *Am J Neuroradiol* 1985; 6:974–975.
6. Gur D, Yonas H, Jackson DL, et al. Measurement of cerebral blood flow during xenon inhalation as measured by the microspheres method. *Stroke* 1985; 16:871–874.
7. Panos PP, Fatouros R, Kishmore PRS, et al. Comparison of improved stable xenon/CT method for cerebral blood flow measurements with radiolabeled microspheres technique. *Radiology* 1985; 158:334.
8. Kobari M, Meyer JS, Ichijo M, Imai A, and Oravez WT. Hyperperfusion of cerebral cortex, thalamus and basal ganglia during spontaneously occurring migraine headache. *Headache* 1989; 29:282–289.
9. Kobari M, Meyer JS, Ichijo M, and Kawamura J. Cortical and subcortical hyperperfusion during migraine and cluster headache measured by Xe CT-CBF. *Neuroradiology* 1990; 32:4–11.
10. Olesen J, Larsen B, and Lauritzen M. Focal hyperemia followed by spreading oligemia and impaired activation of rCBF in classic migraine. *Ann Neurol* 1981; 9:344–352.

6

Comparison of rCBF by SPECT and Stationary Detectors Using Xenon 133

*Torben Schroeder and †Sissel Vorstrup

Departments of Vascular Surgery and †Neurology,
Rigshospitalet, DK-2100 Copenhagen, Denmark

Noninvasive ^{133}Xe measurements of CBF using ^{133}Xe technique and stationary detectors are widely used for examination of patients with cerebrovascular disease. The development of a compact mobile unit using the intravenous (iv) injection of ^{133}Xe has extended the applicability of the method and made repeated bedside measurements possible. However, with respect to focal flow reductions, the information obtainable by stationary detectors is limited, since blood flow recorded from ischemic areas are heavily influenced by radiation emanating from the surroundings owing to the "look-through" phenomenon and owing to Compton scatter (1). The three-dimensional approach as applied in single photon emission tomography circumvents to a great extent the problems caused by superimposition of tissue layers (2). To test the performance of the mobile 10-detector equipment in patients with cerebrovascular disease, cerebral blood flow (CBF) was measured at rest and after vasodilation with acetazolamide and compared with those values obtained by dynamic emission tomography.

METHODS

Patients

After informed consent, 16 patients with cerebrovascular disease were investigated. The median age of the 10 women and 6 men was 56 years, ranging from 31–76 years. Twelve patients had suffered ischemic strokes and four transient ischemic attacks. Four-vessel angiography showed bilateral severe

---

This chapter is an extract of a paper previously published in *J Cereb Blood Flow Metab* 1986;6:739–746.

(>75% diameter reduction) stenosis of the internal carotid artery in eight patients, unilateral severe stenosis in five, and the remaining three patients showed no or only minor changes at the carotid bifurcations. Computer-assisted tomography showed a hypodense area, taken as an infarction in 11 patients.

Measurements of CBF

At the time of examination, the patients were neurologically stable and the stroke patients were studied at least 10 weeks after the acute onset. Baseline CBF was measured with both methods in all patients and in eight patients the study was repeated 20 min after iv administration of 1 g of the potent vasodilator acetazolamide (3).

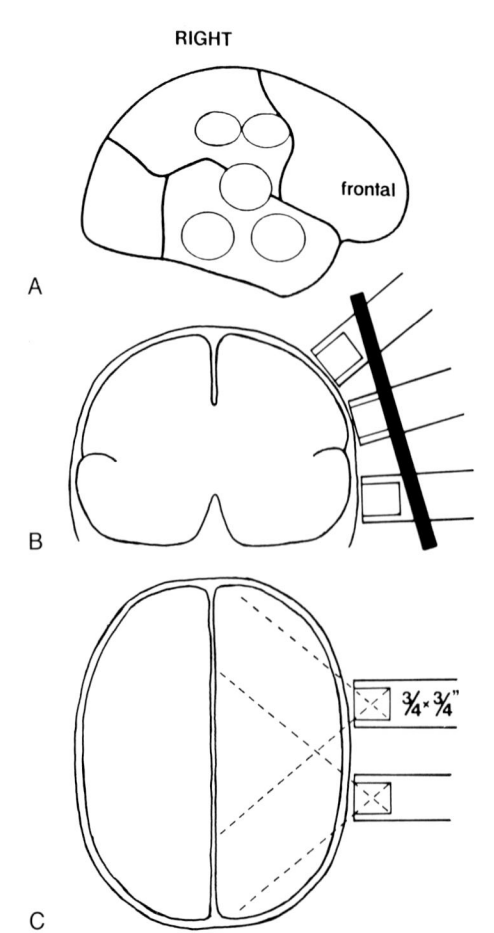

FIG. 1. Collimation and positioning of the stationary detectors: lateral (**A**), coronal (**B**), and transverse (**C**) views. Five-detector holder is shown in B. (From Schroeder et al., ref. 6, with permission.)

Stationary detector CBF studies were performed with a mobile 10-detector system using the iv ^{133}Xe technique (Novo Cerebrograph 10a), as previously described (4). Five detectors covered each middle cerebral territory, as shown in Fig. 1. After iv injection of a bolus of 10–20 mCi ^{133}Xe in saline clearance was recorded throughout 11 min. From a tight-fitted face mask, air samples were drawn continuously for estimation of the arterial input curve. Data were analyzed according to a two-compartment algorithm to which a linear correction term for air passage artifact was added. CBF was expressed as the fast compartment flow, F_g, and as the initial slope index, ISI, the latter calculated from the monoexponential slope between 30 and 90 sec the deconvoluted clearance curve. In this study we have considered only the hemispheric CBF, expressed as F_g, and ISI calculated as the average value of all five detectors without any attempt to evaluate the results of the individual detector.

Tomographic CBF measurements were performed with a dynamic single photon emission tomograph (Tomomatic 64) using ^{133}Xe inhalation (5). During ^{133}Xe inhalation lasting 1.5 min and the following 3 min tomographic pictures of the isotope distribution were obtained. These pictures, along with the arterial input profile estimated by a single lung detector, permitted calculation of CBF by a deconvolution procedure. In this study we used only the middle of three slices, placed approximately 5 cm above the orbitomeatal plane. For reason of comparison, the hemispheric CBF measured with the tomograph was determined, as shown in Fig. 2. In both methods the side-

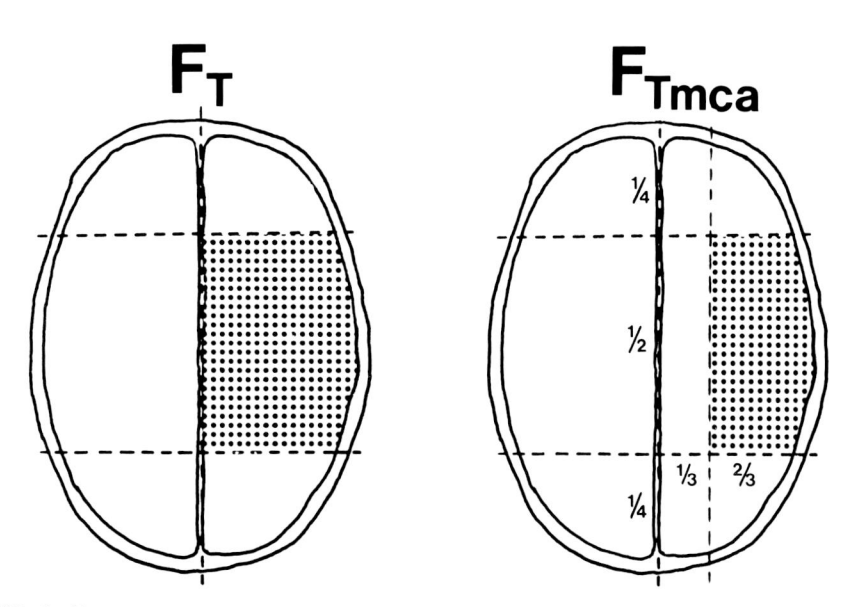

FIG. 2. Tomographic regions of interest for calculation of hemispheric CBF, F_T (*left*) and middle cerebral artery territory CBF, F_{Tmac} (*right*). (From Schroeder et al., ref. 6, with permission.)

TABLE 1. CBF mean values (SD) obtained in 16 baseline and 8 acetazolamide studies

	Baseline CBF (ml/100 g^{-1}/min^{-1})	Acetazolamide (ml/100 g^{-1}/min^{-1})	Flow increase (%)
Emission tomography			
F_T	56 ± 10	71 ± 13	18 ± 9
F_{Tmca}	56 ± 11	69 ± 17	19 ± 13
Stationary detectors			
F_g	52 ± 17	76 ± 27	28 ± 25
ISI	39 ± 11	54 ± 16	27 ± 18

to-side CBF asymmetry was determined as the interhemispheric flow difference as a percentage of mean CBF.

The arterial blood pressure and the end-expiratory CO_2 concentration were registered with each measurement. Corrections for CO_2 changes were not performed. The dependence of results obtained in the two methods was expressed in terms of the correlation coefficient, r, and the relationship estimated in linear regression analysis.

RESULTS

The CBF results measured at baseline conditions and after acetazolamide are shown in Table 1. The tomographic F_T is correlated with the stationary detector F_g in Fig. 3, left and with ISI in Fig. 3, right. The correlation coefficient between the tomograph CBF and the stationary CBF indexes F_g and ISI was 0.80 and 0.82, respectively ($p < 0.0001$). Regression analysis showed that both stationary detector CBF indexes underestimated low-flow values relative to F_T. At high flow, F_g yielded values equal to or higher than F_T, whereas ISI remained lower than F_T but increased in parallel to the F_T values. Correlation of the middle cerebral territory tomographic CBF, F_{Tmca} (Fig. 2), with F_g and with ISI gave practically identical results.

Correlating the stationary detector ISI asymmetry with the tomographically determined F_T and F_{Tmca} asymmetry revealed a correlation coefficient of 0.95 (Fig. 4). The slopes of the regression lines were 1.2 and 1.6, respectively, and the lines practically passed through the origin. In other words, the stationary detector ISI yielded 83% of the asymmetry obtained with F_T and 63% of the F_{Tmca} asymmetry. Similar results were obtained with stationary detector F_g, the correlation being slightly inferior ($r = 0.90$).

DISCUSSION

Comparing the flow levels obtained with the two methods showed that at low flow levels the stationary detectors for both F_g and ISI yielded system-

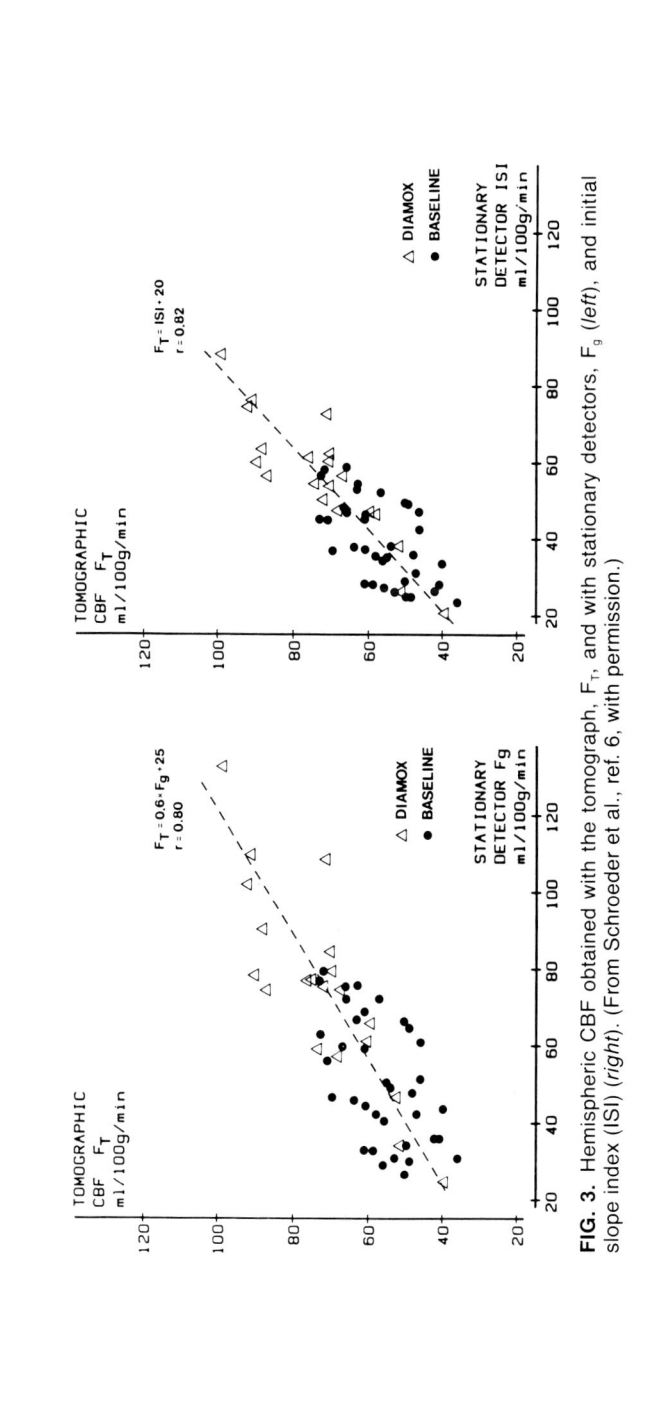

FIG. 3. Hemispheric CBF obtained with the tomograph, F_T, and with stationary detectors, F_g (*left*), and initial slope index (ISI) (*right*). (From Schroeder et al., ref. 6, with permission.)

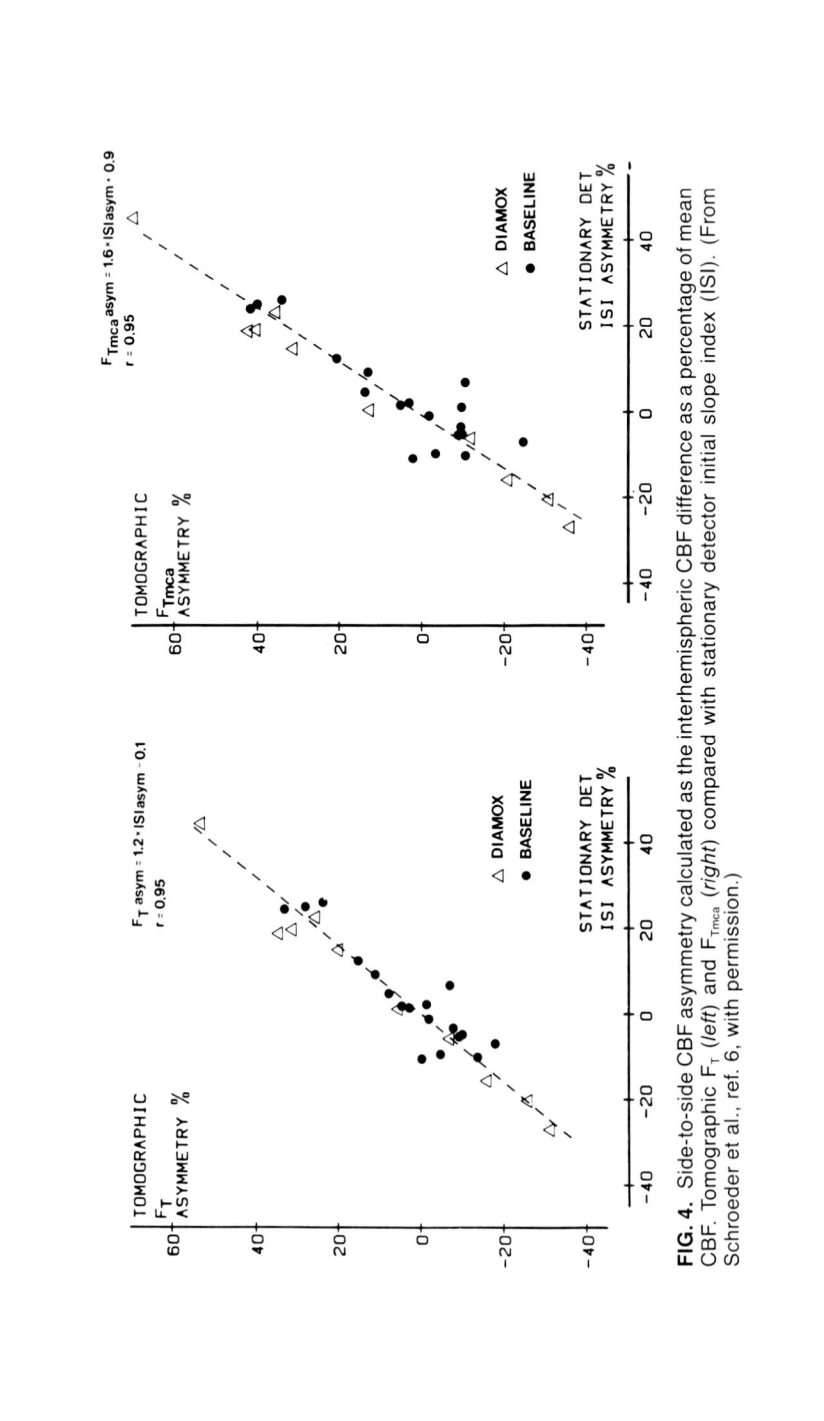

FIG. 4. Side-to-side CBF asymmetry calculated as the interhemispheric CBF difference as a percentage of mean CBF. Tomographic F_T (*left*) and F_{Tmca} (*right*) compared with stationary detector initial slope index (ISI). (From Schroeder et al., ref. 6, with permission.)

atically lower values than did the tomograph. At higher flow levels F_g tended toward higher CBF values than did F_T, whereas ISI increased in parallel to F_T (Fig. 3). By the noninvasive ^{133}Xe CBF techniques, radiation from the air passages distorts the clearance curves, resulting in overestimation of flow. This overestimation will be most pronounced when true flow levels are low. A systemic difference in flow level also may occur in the presence of lung disease, not uncommon in elderly smokers with cerebrovascular disease. Furthermore, gas trapping in parts of the lungs seems to be quite common in healthy elderly people. In these instances the radioactivity of the end-expiratory air underestimates the relative height of the arterial input function to the brain, consequently underestimating CBF. In contrast, with external lung monitoring as used with the tomograph, the input curve is overestimated in these situations.

By comparing flow in a given region or in one hemisphere with the symmetrical region of the opposite hemisphere, the methodological variations are markedly reduced. Accordingly, the side-to-side asymmetries obtained with the two methods were excellently correlated (Fig. 4). On the other hand, approximately 25% of the signal received by a stationary detector placed over one hemisphere will originate from the contralateral hemisphere. Thus, the interhemispheric asymmetry will be smoothed and, according to Bolmsjö (1), detected as only 50% of its true value. In this study, using the same detectors and collimators, the stationary detectors yielded 80–90% of the interhemispheric asymmetry detected by the tomograph (F_T). Comparing the stationary detector device with the emission tomograph, it should be noted that dealing with such relatively large areas as considered in this study does not do full justice to the capacities of the tomograph for detecting focal flow asymmetry. Accordingly, when CBF was calculated from the middle cerebral territory (F_{Tmca}), the asymmetry was systematically more marked. Still, the stationary detector ISI yielded 63% and F_g 74% of this asymmetry.

REFERENCES

1. Bolmsjö M. Hemisphere cross talk and signal overlapping in bilateral regional cerebral blood flow measurements using 133-xenon. *Eur J Nucl Med* 1984; 9:1–5.
2. Lassen NA. Regional cerebral blood flow measurements in stroke: the necessity of a tomographic approach. *J Cereb Blood Flow Metab* 1981; 1:141–142.
3. Vorstrup S, Henriksen L, and Paulson OB. Effects of acetazolamide on cerebral blood flow and cerebral metabolic rate for oxygen. *J Clin Invest* 1984;74:1634–1639.
4. Schroeder T, Holstein PE, Lassen NA, and Engell HC. Measurements of cerebral blood flow by intravenous xenon-133 technique with a mobile system. Reproducibility using the Obrist model compared to total curve analysis. *Neurol Res* 1986;8:237–242.
5. Lassen NA, Henriksen L, and Paulson O. Regional cerebral blood flow in stroke by 133-xenon inhalation and emission tomography. *Stroke* 1981; 12:284–288.
6. Schroeder T, Vorstrup S, Lassen NA, and Engell HC. Noninvasive xenon-133 measurements of cerebral blood flow using stationary detectors compared with dynamic emission tomography. *J Cereb Blood Flow Metab* 1986; 6:739–746.

*Migraine and Other Headaches:
The Vascular Mechanisms*,
edited by Jes Olesen.
Raven Press, Ltd., New York © 1991.

7

Radiation Doses with Xenon-133, Xenon-127, and TC-99m HMPAO

Søren Holm

Department of Clinical Physiology and Nuclear Medicine, Bispebjerg Hospital, DK-2400 Copenhagen, and Department of Neurology, Rigshospitalet, DK-2100 Copenhagen, Denmark

Measurement of regional cerebral blood flow (rCBF) by dynamic single photon emission computed tomography (SPECT) and xenon inhalation was introduced by the Copenhagen group in 1979. More than 5,000 patient studies have now been performed with this method in the CBF Laboratories at Rigshospitalet and Bispebjerg Hospital. Imaging by means of Tc-labeled flow tracers started with the nonretained PnAO in 1983 and the first preliminary high resolution images with the retained hexamethyl-propylene-amine-oxime (HMPAO) were presented in 1985 (1). This chapter deals with basic aspects of the image quality obtained by the various methods.

SPECT images are limited in quality mainly by the number of counts that can be obtained at acceptable radiation absorbed doses and for the retained tracers with reasonable imaging time. Therefore, the dosimetry of tracers for SPECT is a matter of practical concern. In the following the use of ^{133}Xe and ^{127}Xe is discussed for dynamic SPECT, and compared to the use of ^{99m}Tc-labeled compounds for measurement of rCBF by (dynamic or) static methods.

METHODS

A detailed performance and optimization analysis has been made of the instrument (Tomomatic 64) for ^{133}Xe, ^{127}Xe, and ^{99m}Tc (2). The flow algorithm based on Kanno and Lassen (3) was analyzed here in detail with special emphasis on error propagation (noise amplification) and response to changes in gray matter flow. The noise amplification is a consequence of the correction for xenon washout. A similar effect, however, is inherent in the HMPAO-linearization method by Lassen et al. (4). In addition to machine performance and flow algorithm, the dosimetry of the tracers has been reexamined using data from the literature (e.g., ref. 5) adjusted to the actual measuring situations. The different protocols compared are:

1. xenon inhalation, 1.5 min, 750 MBq/l in 4 l bag. Final flow image based on recording in 2.5 min. ("early picture"), scaled by the observed dynamics (4 min)
2. intravenous (iv) injection of 750 MBq Tc-PnAO with image frames of 10 sec
3. iv injection of 750 MBq Tc-HMPAO, 30 min imaging.

In either case, the maximum local dose and the weighted whole body (effective) dose equivalent H_E has been calculated according to the definitions and recommendations of the International Committee of Radiation Protection (6), based on a linear risk model, extrapolating from known effects at much higher levels.

DOSIMETRY

In addition to figures for ^{133}Xe and ^{127}Xe, one must consider the fact that the available ^{127}Xe may contain some ^{129m}Xe, ^{131}Xe, and ^{133}Xe, all of which give higher doses than ^{127}Xe per unit of activity. The contaminants can hereby significantly reduce the inherent advantages of ^{127}Xe; they are of no concern for image quality because all energies are lower than for ^{127}Xe and the incidence of gamma photons is relatively low. The dosimetry values for the two isotopes are shown in Table 1 (per GBq administered).

Thus, the typical ^{133}Xe inhalation study administration of three GBq results in only H_E = 0.6 mSv, or less than 10% of that of a typical ^{99m}Tc-HMPAO study (see below). The absorbed dose to the airway mucosa is in the order of 50 mGy, but the radiosensitivity of this tissue is quite low. For ^{127}Xe the H_E value is reduced to two-thirds for the same nominal activity and the mucosa dose by almost an order of magnitude. If contaminated by 40% ^{129m}Xe, both these advantages disappear.

The dosimetry for the new ^{99m}Tc-labeled brain agents PnAO and HMPAO

TABLE 1.

Nuclide	Absorbed dose to airway mucosa mGy/GBq	Effective dose equivalent H_E mSv/GBq
^{127}Xe	2.1	0.14
^{127}Xe[a]	11	0.20
^{133}Xe	17	0.21

[a]Contaminated by 40% ^{129m}Xe.

TABLE 2.

Nuclide	Form	Amount GBq	Imaging time	Collimator	Number of counts	H_E^a mSv	Counts/ mSv
^{133}Xe	gas	3	2.5 min	LR	7 10^5	0.63	1.1 10^6
^{127}Xe	gas	3	2.5 min	LR	3 10^6	0.42	7.0 10^6
^{99m}Tc	PnAO	0.75	10 sec	LR	1.2 10^5	9.8	1.2 10^4
^{99m}Tc	HMPAO	0.75	30 min	HR	2.2 10^6	9.8	2.2 10^{6b}

[a] Weighted whole body dose equivalent.
[b] Corrected for the different collimator sensitivity (HR).

has been calculated by the manufacturer (Amersham Intl., Amersham, England). The maximal local absorbed dose was found in the bladder wall (90 µGy/MBq injected) assuming no voiding during decay. With voiding intervals of 2 hr this is reduced to 14 µGy/MBq. The effective dose equivalent calculated from these data (by the author) yielded 13 µSv/MBq (10 mSv for a typical study), which is in the same order of magnitude as most other applications of ^{99m}Tc in nuclear medicine. For PnAO, similar dose estimates emerge.

RESULTS

The results for dynamic versus static imaging can now be compared with respect to counts per unit of dose equivalent. Results are summarized in Table 2.

DISCUSSION

The use of ^{127}Xe for brain studies by the inhalation method, instead of ^{133}Xe, has been anticipated to give major advantages in image quality for dynamic SPECT. These expectations were based on the similar use of xenon isotopes for lung scans, and are accounted for by the more than a sixfold increase in counts/mSv. The phantom studies of this work, however, showed that some of the qualitative improvements to be realized within the Tomomatic system require redesigned collimators and additional shielding. This will reduce the measured sensitivity; if the contaminants of ^{127}Xe are also taken into account, the improvement factor of 6 may be reduced to 4 (which, of course, still is important).

In Holm et al. (1) it was shown that ^{99m}Tc-labeled PnAO can be used to perform very fast dynamic, CBF-related imaging over 10-sec periods. Quantification, however, is hardly possible, and compared to the modified substance, HMPAO, the PnAO is obsolete. It is included here merely to highlight the importance of achieving a high "dose equivalent utilization," since the number of counts sampled per unit of dose is extremely low, almost two orders of magnitude below that of the brain-retained HMPAO! HMPAO, intended and used for static imaging, does not range much higher than the xenon isotopes in this respect. If used for 15-min imaging, it is equivalent to ^{133}Xe; if imaging is extended to 1–1.5 hr, it is comparable to ^{127}Xe (Table 2). Therefore, if one could practically and safely administer the higher amounts of xenon and, in addition, handle the higher count rates, then there is no difference in the ultimate resolution that can be obtained. Even for HMPAO (with 6 hr half-life of Tc), still only 10% of the time-activity product can be used for practical imaging; this offsets the gain of a higher photon yield and brain uptake.

Obviously, other factors often are more important for the choice of imaging modality than the (in any case) minimal radiation risk of the subject studied. Although the measured concentrations of xenon isotopes in the air of the examination room on average is far below the limits of "derived air concentration" used in radiation protection, the risk of sudden releases of tenfold GBq of longer-lived ^{127}Xe would have to be carefully evaluated; it seems unlikely, therefore, that very high resolution dynamic studies will be routinely performed. The limitations of availability and, in particular, price point to the same conclusion.

The virtues of the ^{99m}Tc-labeled agents are the availability and the price of ^{99m}Tc and the simple and safe iv administration as well as the possibility of using general-purpose rotating gamma cameras, because the necessary time activity product can be obtained by extending the imaging time. Drawbacks are that quantification is at least difficult and that the dose equivalent for the standard protocol actually is close to (and in some environments exceeds) the limit accepted by health authorities for examination of normal volunteers. A reduction in dose still permits imaging (of lower resolution) but longitudinal studies in one subject cannot be performed with high resolution imaging. Therefore, the two methods are expected to supplement each other: xenon inhalation for easy repeatable and quantitative measurements and Tc agents (HMPAO) for high resolution static imaging.

REFERENCES

1. Holm S, Andersen A, Vorstrup S, et al. Cerebral blood flow measured within 10 seconds using dynamic SPECT and lipophilic technetium-99m compounds, PnAO and HMPAO. *J Cereb Blood Flow Metab* 1985; 5[Suppl 1]:565–566.
2. Holm S. *Dynamic SPECT of the Human Brain for measurement of rCBF*. PhD Thesis, Physics Laboratory, University of Copenhagen, 1988.
3. Kanno I and Lassen NA. Two methods for calculating regional cerebral blood flow. *J Comput Assist Tomogr* 1979; 3:71–76.
4. Lassen NA, Andersen AR, Friberg L, and Paulson OB. The retention of Tc-99m-D,L-HMPAO in the human brain after intra-carotid bolus injection: A kinetic analysis. *J Cerebr Blood Flow Metab* 1988; 8:S13–S22.
5. Atkins HL, Robertson JS, Croft BY, et al. Estimates of radiation absorbed doses from radioxenons in lung imaging. (MIRD report no. 9). *J Nucl Med* 1980; 21:459–465.
6. ICRP Publication 26, *Annals of the ICRP* 1977; 1:3. Oxford, Pergamon Press Ltd.

8

Methods: Discussion Summary

Niels A. Lassen

The intraarterial method using radioactive xenon gives a more reliable measure of the clearance from a given area than the xenon inhalation method, but the obvious limitation inherent in the necessity for an arterial puncture must be stressed. This limitation means that now, when angiography by carotid puncture or catheterization via the femoral artery is getting so much rarer, the intracarotid injection method is obsolete for migraine research.

Of very special interest in the context of migraine is, however, the fact that in about 50% of all migraineurs the injection itself produces a migraine-like attack. The provoked attack mimics the spontaneous attacks of the same patient. Therefore, it was agreed that we may indeed consider them as a provocation of the spontaneous attack. It was seen both in the Copenhagen group and by Dr. Deisenhammer from Austria. These provoked attacks are not confined to injections made via a needle in the neck as used by the Copenhagen group. They also are seen with injections made via a catheter from the femoral artery passed up to the internal carotid or vertebral artery, as was the case in the studies in Austria. There are experiments to show that the nature of the fluid injected does not matter. You can inject blood, saline, or an x-ray contrast medium.

It is of crucial importance to know if visual symptoms are also common in the provoked attacks. This would be surprising, since it is not obvious how an intracarotid injection (that was used in almost all cases) could reach the primary visual area, which is supposed to be the area affected when visual aural symptoms are manifest. Only in 5–10% of cases where the posterior cerebral artery arises from the carotid system would the striate cortex have its arterioles affected directly by the injection. It was agreed that the provoked auralike symptoms were indeed *not* so commonly visual. Paresthesias of variable and changing location, slight paresis, aphasia, and confusion were typical findings. Moreover, it was mentioned that one should not necessarily ascribe all visual symptoms to alterations in the primary visual cortex: it cannot be excluded that some of them are due to processes in the visual association areas such as area 19, an area supplied by the middle cerebral artery (and an area characteristically involved in the spontaneous attack of migraine with aura).

The mechanism of injection-provoked migraine might involve brief distension of the artery by the rapid injection of 2–3 ml resulting in accentuation of the vasomotion via so-called myogenic mechanisms. Åslid mentioned vasomotion-like responses observed with transcranial doppler on the middle cerebral artery (MCA) after brief carotid occlusion during hyperventilation. And, as Friberg has demonstrated, there is evidence of enhanced vasomotion (vasomotor instability) in migraineurs possibly due to increased oscillatory myogenic responses. Vasomotion is only marked in smaller arterioles. If oscillation of flow velocity in the MCA is seen (Åslid's comments), this must mean synchronous vasomotion of the arterioles, the synchronization being elicited by the brief induced hypotension resulting from the manual compression of the carotid. In all likelihood, the cause of increased cerebrovascular resistance in local brain areas in the early phase of migraine is due to arteriolar contraction, not constriction of the major arteries. This conclusion is tentative but in consonance with the unilateral decrease in blood flow velocity on the affected side measured with transcranial Doppler on the MCA. An arterial narrowing would be seen as an increased velocity.

The discussion then turned to the methodology of regional cerebral blood flow (rCBF) measurements using inhalation or intravenous (iv) injection of ^{133}Xe. With this method the isotope does not arrive in the brain as a compact bolus but as an extended input function, which must be accurately measured. Measuring this input is not easy and constitutes a major source of error. Ideally, one should record directly the arterial blood curve. The end-expired xenon concentration is perhaps the best atraumatic way to estimate the shape of this curve indirectly. One may also record over the chest wall so as to follow the alevolar ^{133}Xe concentration (with some contamination from the tissues of the chest wall). The ^{133}Xe inhalation or iv method is totally atraumatic and is usually carried out over 12 min. It therefore takes a longer time than the intraarterial method, which lasts only 30 sec when using the initial slope approach.

For use in migraine research, the discussion of the side-to-side differences is of special interest. If low flow is unilateral, to what extent will we see this by the inhalation or iv method? Risberg discussed the so-called cross-over phenomenon, that is, that ^{133}Xe in one hemisphere will be seen by a detector positioned externally over the opposite hemisphere, with radiation crossing the midline. It is attenuated by absorption but nevertheless is in the order of 25%, meaning that 25% of counts recorded by a given detector arise from the opposite hemisphere. Risberg stressed that the contralateral contribution is fairly diffuse, as it comes from an extended tissue area. It is in fact a diffuse background activity. Risberg concluded that any actual side-to-side difference would be measured with about half efficiency. With a side-to-side difference of 20%, only 10% will be measured. It was also stressed that because of the very high accuracy obtained by having many detectors and a good count rate, even a 10% asymmetry was easily detectable.

From tomographic studies using ^{133}Xe we know that there is less than a

5% asymmetry of hemispheric flow in normal humans. A comparison of the two ^{133}Xe methods, the nontomographic and the tomographic one, has actually been made by Schroeder and collaborators, and asymmetries are seen, better than many may have thought, with the nontomographic ^{133}Xe inhalation method. When we discuss in the following section the asymmetries and nonasymmetries of rCBF during a migraine attack, we shall indeed look for asymmetries observed by the conventional nontomographic ^{133}Xe inhalation method and take them seriously, even if they are down to about 5%!

What is the best method for studying cerebral blood flow in migraine? This is not easy to say. The atraumatic nature of the ^{133}Xe inhalation methods using both stationary detectors and rotating tomographic devices is attractive. It can be implemented quickly, even more quickly than a technetium hexamethyl-propylene-amine-oxime (HMPAO) study. On the other hand, technetium HMPAO has the advantage that it is firmly retained in the brain for many hours. As the patient comes in, one can give the HMPAO injection and start the treatment. After recovery, one to several hours later, one can image rCBF using the rotating camera or a brain specialized single photon emission computed tomography (SPECT) device without causing undue strain to the patient. Yet, what you see is the distribution of CBF that was present when the patient entered the clinic, that is, when the injection of HMPAO was made. Measuring blood flow is of special interest in the context of transcranial doppler velocity measurements. Changes in recorded velocity can be caused by changes in blood flow, to arterial diameter, or to a combination of both. The interpretation of doppler changes is much more concrete if the blood flow in the area of supply of the insonated artery is known. For such measurements HMPAO is not recommended because it provides only relative flow in different areas of the brain and not changes in total flow.

The "cold" xenon method based on x-ray tomography was presented by Meyer. It has its special advantage in high spatial resolution. This resolution comes to the level of the computed tomography (CT) scan itself. Unfortunately, this is modified by the poor signal-to-noise ratio. Hence, integration over several pixels must be performed in order to reduce the variability. The method is also very sensitive to movement artifacts. With this method one can sample discrete tissues including deep structures such as the thalamus or basic ganglia. But the images shown, and they are hardly the worse cases, are disappointing. The well known difference between blood flow in the cortical rim and basal ganglia as compared to the white matter does not show up as it does with positron emission tomography (PET) or SPECT images of blood flow. Despite the elegance of the method and its 10 years of development, the "cold" xenon method has not reached the accuracy of the isotope tomographic SPECT or PET methods, whose advantages are an excellent signal-to-noise ratio and relative insensitivity to movement artifacts.

PART II
Interictal Studies in Migraine with Aura

Migrane and Other Headaches:
The Vascular Mechanisms,
edited by Jes Olesen.
Raven Press, Ltd., New York © 1991.

9

Interictal rCBF Studies with ^{133}Xe or ^{99m}Tc-HMPAO and SPECT in Patients Suffering from Migraine with Aura

*Lars Friberg, *Ida Nicolic, †Jes Olesen, †Helle Iversen,
*Bjørn Sperling, *Niels A. Lassen, and
‡Peer Tfelt-Hansen

*Department of Clinical Physiology and Nuclear Medicine and ‡Neurology, Bispebjerg Hospital, DK-2400 Copenhagen NV, †Department of Neurology, Gentofte Hospital, University of Copenhagen, DK-2900 Hellerup, Denmark

The basic pathophysiological mechanisms of migraine are still concealed and it is difficult to explain why migraine attacks develop readily in some individuals, once or twice in a lifetime in others, and never affect most of the population. Perhaps there is a continuous scale from marked disposition for migraine to almost no ability to develop an attack.

Migraine attacks with aura are associated with transient, marked focal changes in the cerebral perfusion pattern (1–4). One hypothesis could therefore be that interictally, cerebrovascular regulation is more labile in migraineurs than in nonmigraineurs, facilitating episodes with severe abnormal cerebrovascular response as found during migraine with aura. If so, does the interictal regional cerebral blood flow (rCBF) pattern of migraineurs differ from that of nonmigraineurs?

The rCBF study described here was undertaken to elucidate whether abnormalities of vascular or neuronal origin could be present interictally in patients suffering from migraine with aura. This preliminary report will focus on asymmetrical rCBF distribution among larger symmetrical regions in the two cerebral hemispheres.

PATIENTS AND CONTROLS

According to a prospective, consecutive protocol we examined rCBF in 75 patients that fulfilled the IHS criteria for having solely or predominantly migraine attacks with aura (5). They were all examined at a time when they were completely free from symptoms, including headache types other than migraine. After examination 15 subjects were excluded because either they reported having had a migraine attack less than 5 days before examination or because of a technically unsatifactory examination, including rCBF measurements on a slice level different from OM + 50 mm. Sixty patients are reviewed in this chapter. Fifty patients were studied with the ^{133}Xe inhalation technique (28 women, 22 men, mean age 50 years, range 15–71 years). Ten patients were examined with the intravenous (iv) ^{99m}Tc-hexamethyl-propylene-amine-oxime HMPAO technique (seven women, three men, mean age 36 years, range 22–51 years). Thirty healthy nonmigraineurs served as controls; 10 were examined with the ^{133}Xe inhalation technique (four women, six men, mean age 24, range 20–29 years) and 20 with the iv ^{99m}TC-HMPAO technique (9 women, 11 men, mean age 24, range 20–29 years).

METHODS

The rCBF examination was carried out with a fast rotating, brain dedicated, single photon emission computerized tomograph (SPECT) (Tomomatic 232). rCBF was recorded simultaneously in two slices of the brain, separated by an interslice distance of 40 mm. Each slice was 17 mm thick and the resolution of the instrument was 12 mm in the transverse plane for both types of measurements. During the ^{133}Xe inhalation studies the slice positions were either 10 mm and 50 mm or 50 and 90 mm above the orbitomeatal plane (OM plane). One ^{133}Xe inhalation study lasted 4.5 min. During the first 1.5 min a mixture of atmospheric air and ^{133}Xe was rebreathed in a closed system (with CO_2-absorbers and H_2O-absorbers) from a reservoir containing ^{133}Xe with an activity of approximately 720 MBq/l. The total counts obtained were around 1 ml per slice. Quantitated rCBF values (ml/100 g/min) were obtained from the ^{133}Xe inhalation studies.

^{99m}Tc-HMPAO investigations were performed by administering approximately 550 MBq of the flow tracer intravenously and starting data acquisition 10 min after injection. During the ^{99m}Tc-HMPAO studies rCBF distribution was recorded in eight slices (from OM + 10 mm to OM + 80 mm) by performing four 5-min acquisitions and displacing the camera 10 mm between each acquisition period. A semiquantitated rCBF distribution was obtained from the ^{99m}Tc-HMPAO examinations. Before data analysis all pictures were normalized relative to the mean count rate of their respective cerebellar region, and linearized according to the algorithm described by Lassen et al. (6). All examinations were performed while the patients were lying with closed and covered eyes, in a supine and resting state in a quiet room.

DATA ANALYSIS

Data were analyzed for asymmetries between mirrored regions in the hemispheres in two ways.

An independent visual evaluation by four experienced observers. Data were presented as high quality, color-coded, rCBF pictures of all obtained slice levels, but without personal or diagnostical identifications. A random series of pictures from the 60 patients and the 30 healthy controls were analyzed. Each examiner allotted each picture a score from 1 to 4: 1 = normal, 2 = slight asymmetry, but within normal range, 3 = moderate asymmetry, out of normal range, 4 = asymmetry, clearly abnormal. Adding the scores for all four observers the lowest total rating for one picture was 4 and the highest was 16. We defined rCBF examinations with a total rating score from 4 to 8 as *normal*. Examinations obtaining a total rating score from 9 to 16 we defined as *asymmetrical*. In cases evaluated as asymmetrical the hemisphere containing the lowest perfused region was indicated.

Quantitative, calculating, side-to-side asymmetry indices between a set of symmetric, predefined regions of interest (ROIs) for the slice level OM + 50 mm (Fig. 1). This predefined set of ROIs was superimposed on and proportionally fitted to the outlines of each rCBF pattern. The ROIs corresponded approximately to the supply territories of the large intracranial arteries: anterior (ACA), middle (MCA), and posterior (PCA) cerebral arteries. In addition, the MCA region was subdivided into an anterior and posterior portion. A special "migraine ROI" was defined posteriorly in the region that is affected most frequently by significant hypoperfusion during attacks of migraine with aura. For the two control groups (^{133}Xe and ^{99m}Tc-HMPAO) a mean right-left asymmetry index ± SD was calculated for each ROI. Re-

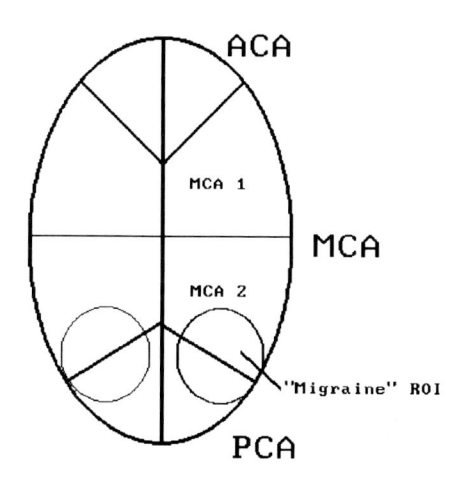

FIG. 1. A schematic drawing of the division of the rCBF slice level 50 mm above the orbito-meatal plane into regions of interest (ROI's). The three main ROI's in each hemisphere represent supply territories of the main intra-cranial arteries: ACA, anterior cerebral artery; MCA, middle cerebral artery; PCA, posterior cerebral artery. The MCA ROI was futhermore analyzed in an anterior (MCA 1) and a posterior (MCA 2) portion. The "migraine" ROI was defined as the area most often affected in our previous studies of migraine with aura (1–4).

gional *asymmetry* in the patients' rCBF distribution was defined as an asymmetry index value below or above 2.5 times the standard deviation from the mean value of the same region in the relevant control group. The referral index values are reported elsewhere (see Friberg et al., this volume).

RESULTS

Visual Evaluation

Among the group of migraine patients with aura, 11 (18%) were scored as having asymmetrical rCBF patterns (total score between 9 and 16). Thus, the remaining 49 (82%) patients were evaluated as normal (total score between 4 and 8). All 30 rCBF patterns from the control group were evaluated as being normal. However, when comparing the individual assessments there was only full consensus of asymmetry among the observers in 4/60 patients with aura (*all* observers scoring 3 or 4). Full interobserver consensus of normality was found in 48/90 patients and controls (*all* observers scoring 1 or 2). Thus, there was absence of agreement among observers in 38/90 (42%) of the evaluated pictures.

Quantitative Evaluation

By quantitated regional analysis and comparison to values of the control material, and considering that asymmetry had to be present in only one ROI, we found asymmetry in 3/10 (30%) of the patients examined with ^{99m}Tc-HMPAO, but in no less than 36/50 (72%) of the patients examined with ^{133}Xe inhalation. The high overall rate of asymmetries in the ^{133}Xe studies was very much influenced by a high incidence of asymmetries between the ACA ROIs, in whom 24/50 (48%) had asymmetry. However, in none of the ^{99m}Tc-HMPAO studied patients did we find significant asymmetries between the ACA ROIs. It is possible that the ^{133}Xe gas in the superior, air-filled sinuses of the cranium can introduce artifacts and asymmetrical scattered radiation to the lowest and most frontal parts of the brain. This could have caused a methodological error of the calculated rCBF values in the chosen ACA ROI of the ^{133}Xe studies, which was not present in the ^{99m}Tc-HMPAO studies. To avoid this possible error we left out the ACA ROIs in the continued analysis. This showed that 27/50 (45%) had asymmetries in one or more ROIs. When more than one hypoperfused ROI was found they were all located in the same hemisphere. The distribution of number of ROIs with asymmetry was: 1 ROI = 12 patients; 2 ROIs = 7, 3 ROIs = 5, 4 ROIs = 2, and 5 ROIs = 1 patient. The large MCA ROI was less frequently affected than MCA1, MCA2, PCA, and "migraine ROI." In 11/27 the asymmetry in smaller ROIs affected mean CBF in the whole hemisphere, causing mean hemisphere asymmetry.

DISCUSSION

Both visual evaluation and quantitated evaluation resulted in a high percentage of patients classified as having focal asymmetries in their interictal rCBF patterns. In this it should be noted that none of the patients had complications of migraine as defined by paragraph 1.6 in the IHS classification (5).

The lowest rate of side-to-side abnormalities was found by visual evaluation (18%). One might consider a visual evaluation preferable, as the human eye is very sensitive to irregularities in visual patterns and because such irregularities do not have to be confined to fixed shapes or predefined intensities. Furthermore, our visual evaluation implied inspection of all examined brain slices in a given patient. The demarcation of hypoperfused regions, the degree of hypoperfusion relative to surrounding tissue, and the degree of asymmetry were much less marked in our migraine patients than in patients with ischemic stroke. The interobserver disagreement in 42% of the cases might reflect the small and borderline nature of the relative flow decreases. It was comforting, however, that all controls were evaluated as normal.

The more rigorous quantitative analysis resulted in a higher rate (45%) of abnormalities. This rate was even higher before we decided to exclude the ACA regions for methodological reasons, as explained above. The rate of asymmetries might be overestimated for several reasons. The ^{133}Xe control material was relatively small and the mean age and age range were lower than that of the patients. Our control group could be considered very homogeneous, giving rise to too narrow confidence limits. Generally, absolute global CBF values are considered to decrease with age, although this might not be the case in migraine patients with aura (7). However, according to our experience and from previous reports of our knowledge, the degree of regional rCBF *asymmetry* does not increase between 24 years (controls) and 36 or 50 years (patients), whereas in the highest age groups there seems to be a tendency for gradually increasing rCBF asymmetries.

There are only a few reports on interictal blood flow in patients suffering from migraine with aura. By quantitated analysis Lauritzen and Olesen (2) could not detect regional asymmetries interictally in 11 patients having migraine with aura when compared to a group of 20 normals. With a less regional, 16-stationary probe method, Levine et al. (8) examined CBF interictally in 15 patients with migraine with aura and/or complicated migraine. They reported a significant anterior-posterior asymmetry within the brain as a whole and in addition an interhemispheric asymmetry when their patient group was compared to a control material of 20 subjects. Lagrèze et al. (9) found abnormal rCBF in 4/8 patients. After visual analysis by one observer Schlake et al. (10) found abnormal regional hypoperfusion in 3/9 patients examined interictally.

It is likely that the cause for the abnormal rCBF asymmetries is local blood flow variations from desynchronized vascular tone regulation. Friberg et al. (4,11,12) have presented evidence that migraineurs with aura studied during an attack often show marked and fairly rapid oscillations in regional CBF, indicating an instability of cerebrovascular tone. Perhaps migraine patients have even interictally patchy and maybe fluctuating increases in cerebrovascular tone. Enhanced vasoconstrictor activity might predispose for the vascular instability and pronounced focal hypoperfusion so typically seen during the aura and early headache phase of a migraine attack with aura (1–4).

The possibility of interictal dysregulation of cerebrovascular tone is supported by CBF studies showing excessive hypernormal responses both during 5% CO_2 and 100% O_2 inhalation among migraine patients when compared to the response of controls (13,14). Likewise, transcranial doppler studies have shown abnormally high velocity responses to CO_2 inhalation (15) and to change in level of physiological activation (16).

REFERENCES

1. Olesen J, Larsen B, and Lauritzen M. Focal hyperemia followed by spreading oligemia and impaired activation of rCBF in classic migraine. *Ann Neurol* 1981; 9:344–352.
2. Lauritzen M and Olesen J. Regional cerebral blood flow during migraine attacks by Xenon-133 inhalation and emission tomography. *Brain* 1984; 107:447–461.
3. Skyhøj Olsen T, Friberg L, and Lassen NA. Ischemia may be the primary cause of the neurological deficits in classic migraine. *Arch Neurol* 1987; 44:156–161.
4. Friberg L. Cerebral blood flow changes in migraine: methods, observations and hypothesis. *Neurology* 1991 (in press).
5. Headache Classification Committee of the International Headache Society. Classification and diagnostic criteria for headache disorders, cranial neuralgias and facial pain. *Cephalalgia* 1988; 8[Suppl 7]:1–96.
6. Lassen NA, Andersen AR, Friberg L, and Paulson OB. The retention of [99mTc]-d, l-HM-PAO in the human brain after intracarotid bolus injection: A kinetic analysis. *J Cerebr Blood Flow Metab* 1988; 8:S13–S22.
7. Robertson WM, Welch KM, Levine SR, and Schultz LR. The effects of aging on cerebral blood flow in migraine. *Neurology* 1989; 39:947–951.
8. Levine SR, Welch KMA, Ewing JR, and Robertson WM. Asymmetrical cerebral blood flow patterns in migraine patients. *Cephalalgia* 1987; 7:245–248.
9. Lagrèze HL, Dettmers C, and Hartmann A. Abnormalities of interictal cerebral perfusion in classic but not common migraine. *Stroke* 1988; 19:1108–1111.
10. Schlake H-P, Böttger IG, Grotemeyer KH, et al. Single photon emission computed tomography with technetium-99m hexamethyl propylamino oxime in the pain-free interval of migraine and cluster headache. *Eur Neurol* 1990; 30:153–156.
11. Friberg L, Skyhøj Olsen T, Roland PE, and Lassen NA. Focal ischemia caused by instability of cerebrovascular tone during attacks of hemiplegia migraine: a regional cerebral blood flow study. *Brain* 1987; 110:917–934.

12. Friberg L and Skyhøj Olsen T. Rapid extreme oscillations of focal cerebral blood flow during the aura phase of migraine. In Clifford Rose F, ed. *New advances in headache research*. London: Smith-Gordon and Company Ltd. Publisher, 1989: 163–167.
13. Sakai F and Meyer JS. Abnormal cerebrovascular reactivity in patients with migraine and cluster headache. *Headache* 1979; 19:257–266.
14. Meyer JS, Zetusky W, Jonsdottir M, and Mortel K. Cephalic hyperemia during migraine headaches. A prospective study. *Headache* 1986; 26:388–397.
15. Thomas TD, Harpold GJ, and Troost BT. Cerebrovascular reactivity in migraineurs as measured by transcranial doppler. *Cephalalgia* 1990; 10:95–99.
16. Thie A, Fuhlendorf A, Spitzer K, and Kunze K. Transcranial doppler evaluation of common and classic migraine. Part 1. Ultrasonic features during the headache-free period. *Headache* 1990;30:201–208.

10

Brain Imaging with ^{99m}Tc-HMPAO and SPECT in Migraine with Aura: An Interictal Study

*Hans-Peter Schlake, †Ingolf G. Böttger, *Karl-Heinz Grotemeyer, †Ingo W. Husstedt, and †Otmar Schober

*Departments of *Neurology and †Nuclear Medicine, Westfälische Wilhelms-Universität, D-4400 Münster, Germany*

In a previous study with iodoamphetamine (^{123}I-IMP) and single photon emission computed tomography (SPECT) we demonstrated alterations of cerebral perfusion and/or metabolism in patients suffering from migraine with aura during the interictal state (1). In "hemiplegic migraine" the observed regions of decreased tracer uptake corresponded mostly to the topography of transient neurologic symptoms during migraine attack. Cerebral blood flow asymmetries in migraine patients during the pain-free interval have also been demonstrated by means of ^{133}Xe inhalation technique (2,3).

We extended our regional cerebral blood flow (rCBF) studies in patients suffering from migraine with aura between attacks using SPECT and ^{99m}Tc-hexamethyl-propylene-amide-oxime (HMPAO) (4).

MATERIAL AND METHODS

Thirty patients (9 men and 21 women, aged 17–61 years) suffering from migraine with aura and hemiplegic (n = 24) as well as exclusively ophthalmic (n = 6) symptoms ("scintillating scotoma") were investigated during the interictal phase. At the time of investigation all patients were headache-free and had not taken any medication for at least 2 weeks.

SPECT investigation of rCBF was performed under standardized environmental conditions (quiet room, dimmed light, eyes open). Fifteen min after intravenous (iv) administration of 400–600 MBq ^{99m}Tc-HMPAO 64 single images were obtained within a 360° circle using a rotating gamma camera (General Electric 400 ACT). Imaging time per projection was 30 sec, and 40 min per examination. Tomographic slices of 12.5 mm width were reconstructed in sagittal, coronal, and horizontal projections by filtered back projection employing a Butterworth filter with a cutoff frequency of 0.2 cycles/pixel. Interpretation was performed qualitatively and semiquantitatively by a specialist in nuclear medicine in a quasi-blinded way, as he knew only the diagnosis "migraine," but did not have any information on individual migraine subtype, neurologic symptoms, or pain localization.

By visual inspection, SPECT findings were divided into four categories:

1. symmetrical perfusion
2. inhomogeneous regional perfusion (bilateral)
3. slight hypoperfusion (regional side difference 2–4 of 16 steps on the color scale, representing a regional hypoperfusion of 14–28%)
4. marked hypoperfusion (regional side difference >4 of 16 steps on the color scale, representing a regional hypoperfusion of >28%).

According to ^{99m}Tc-HMPAO SPECT findings in healthy volunteers reported in literature (4), a regional difference of cerebral tracer uptake exceeding two steps ($\approx$14%) was considered to be significant.

RESULTS

Clinical neurological investigation revealed a normal result in all patients. There were no pathological findings in either computed tomography (CT; n = 23) or magnetic resonance imaging (MRI; n = 12) of the brain. Electroencephalographic patterns (n = 30) were normal in 18 patients whereas pathological alterations were obtained in 12 cases (focal changes: n = 4; unspecific dysrhythmic paroxysms: n = 6; dysrhythmic paroxysms with spike-/sharp-waves: n = 2). Table 1 summarizes ^{99m}Tc-HMPAO SPECT find-

TABLE 1. ^{99m}Tc-HMPAO SPECT findings in patients suffering from migraine with aura (n = 30)

| Results of ^{99m}Tc-HMPAO SPECT | Migraine with aura ||
	Ophthalmic subtype (n = 6)	Hemiplegic subtype (n = 24)
Normal perfusion	2	5
Bilaterally inhomogeneous or reduced perfusion	1	0
Slight hypoperfusion[a]	2	10 (8)[c]
Marked hypoperfusion[b]	1	9 (8)[c]
Cerebellar diaschisis	0	5

[a]Side difference of rCBF amounting to 2–4 steps on the color scale ($\approx$ 14–28%).
[b]Side difference of rCBF amounting to >4 steps on the color scale ($\approx$ >28%).
[c]Number of patients in whom site of hypoperfusion showed a relationship to the topography of transient neurologic symptoms during migraine attack.

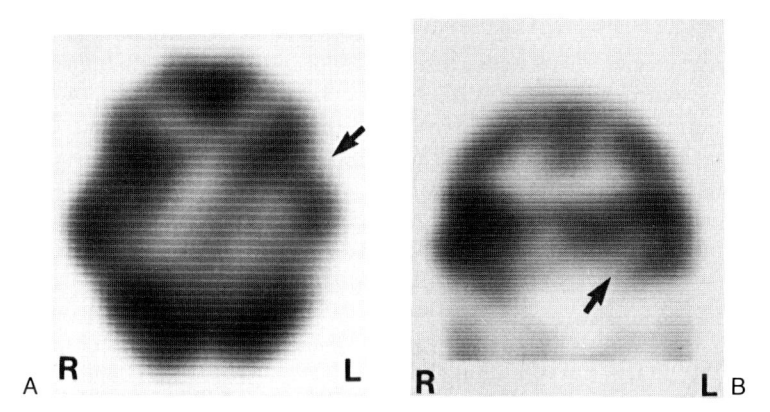

FIG. 1. Results of SPECT with ^{99m}Tc-HMPAO in a 26-year-old man suffering from migraine with aura for the past 3 years. See text for discussion.

ings in both subtypes of migraine with aura and their relation to transient neurologic symptoms during attacks.

In 19 of 24 patients with "hemiplegic migraine," a regional decrease of tracer uptake was observed, in whom 5 showed a corresponding hypoperfusion of the contralateral cerebellar hemisphere ("cerebellar diaschisis") (5). The areas of cerebral hypoperfusion corresponded to the topography of transient neurologic symptoms in 16 of these 19 cases. Three patients with "ophthalmic migraine" revealed a regional hypoperfusion, whereas in three cases no significant alterations of regional tracer uptake could be obtained.

Fig. 1 shows the results of SPECT with ^{99m}Tc-HMPAO in a 26-year-old man suffering from migraine with aura for the past 3 years. In this patient left-sided headache attacks were accompanied by scintillating scotoma, a transient sensorimotor paresis of the right upper limb, aphasic disturbances, and a transitory loss of orientation associated with an ill-defined alteration of consciousness. CT and MRI of the brain were normal. Between attacks, repeatedly performed electroencephalographic investigations showed dysrhythmic paroxysms with spike-waves and sharp-waves more pronounced over the left hemisphere.

^{99m}Tc-HMPAO SPECT in horizontal (Fig. 1A) and coronal (Fig. 1B) projections showed a marked hypoperfusion in the left-sided temporobasal region, corresponding to the side of pain as well as to the topography of neurologic symptoms and the electroencephalographic patterns.

DISCUSSION

In this chapter cerebral perfusion was investigated in 30 headache-free patients suffering from migraine with aura and hemiplegic (n = 24) as well as exclusively ophthalmic (n = 6) symptoms during migraine attack by means of SPECT and the flow tracer ^{99m}Tc-HMPAO. In contrast to our findings in migraine without aura, most patients suffering from migraine with aura showed a regional cerebral hypoperfusion—particularly those cases with the hemiplegic subtype. The observed areas of hypoperfusion could be more or less related to the topography of neurologic symptoms in 16 of 19 patients with "hemiplegic migraine."

Although the presented data are based on semiquantitative analysis, it is assumed that these ^{99m}Tc-HMPAO SPECT findings are less pronounced than those obtained with ^{123}I-IMP (1), suggesting that both tracers are not entirely comparable. Altogether, these observations confirm the view of permanent alterations of cerebral perfusion in migraine with aura—probably due to similar changes of brain metabolism.

REFERENCES

1. Schlake H-P, Grotemeyer K-H, Böttger IG, Husstedt IW, and Brune G. ^{123}I-amphetamine-SPECT in classical migraine and migraine accompagnée. *Neurosurg Rev* 1987; 10:191–196.
2. Lagréze HL, Dettmers C, and Hartmann A. Abnormalities of interictal perfusion in classic but not common migraine. *Stroke* 1988; 19:1108–1111.
3. Levine SR, Welch KMA, Ewing JR, and Robertson W. Cerebral blood flow asymmetries in headache-free migraineurs. *Stroke* 1987; 18:1164–1165.
4. Podreka E, Suess E, Goldenberg G, et al. Initial experience with Technetium-99m brain SPECT. *J Nucl Med* 1987; 28:1657–1666.
5. Baron JC, Bousser MG, and Comar D. "Crossed cerebellar diaschisis" in human supratentorial brain infarction. *Trans Am Neurol Assn* 1980;105:459–461.

11

^{99m}Tc-d,l-HMPAO SPECT in Migraine with Aura in the Headache-Free Interval

E. Suess, P. Wessely, G. Koch, and I. Podreka

Department of Headache, Neurological Clinic, University of Vienna, A-1090 Vienna, Austria

Several studies on the nature of cerebral blood flow alterations in migraine have been performed previously using ^{123}I-iodoamphetamine (IMP) single photon emission computed tomography (SPECT), and ^{133}Xe inhalation method, or Xe computed tomography–cerebral blood flow (CT-CBF) measurement (1,2). These studies reflect the properties of earlier stages of rCBF measurement techniques, but the use of newly developed tracer ^{99m}Tc-d,l-hexamethyl-propylene-amine-oxime (HMPAO) must be evaluated. This tracer freely crosses the blood-brain barrier with a high first pass extraction rate (>90%) and remains trapped within the brain without relevant washout during the investigation period (3). It therefore lacks the ability to demonstrate dynamic CBF changes during the investigation time but provides high quality images of regional CBF (rCBF) distribution at the time of tracer application. In this study ^{99m}Tc-d,l-HMPAO was used to demonstrate rCBF distribution patterns in migraineurs in the headache-free interval.

MATERIAL AND METHODS

A group of 18 patients (mean age 29.44 ± 11.1 years; 15 women, 3 men) suffering from *migraine with aura* were investigated in the headache-free interval using ^{99m}Tc-d,l-HMPAO SPECT. For control, a group of healthy young volunteers (n = 51; mean age 26.3 ± 4.6 years; 32 women, 19 men) were investigated after informed consent was given, following the same procedure as described below. Computed tomography (CT) was normal in all participants. Additional investigations (e.g., intraarterial angiography) were performed if clinically indicated. The patients were classified according to predominant side of headache, most frequent clinical symptoms during the attack, and electroencephalogram (EEG) findings in the interval. Eleven patients reported predominantly left-sided pain and two patients predominantly right-sided pain. In five patients diffuse or frequently changing locations of headache were reported. Although in most cases more than one isolated neurological deficit occurred during an attack, a dominant symptom could be named for classification. Unilateral or bilateral scintillating scotomas were described most frequently (nine patients). Transient unilateral motor and/or sensory deficits occurred in three patients on either side. In three patients the most pronounced neurological deficit was aphasialike speech disorders. SPECT was performed within 2–7 days after the last attack in three patients; in 15 cases the interval exceeded 2 or more weeks. The mean time since first onset of migraine was 9.9 years (ranging from 3 months to 30 years). At the time of the SPECT investigation eight patients were drug-free for several weeks. Seven patients were treated with Ca^+ antagonists, ergotamine derivates (n = 2), or other analgesic drugs (n = 6). Two patients took oral contraceptives.

SPECT was performed with a dual-head rotating scintillation camera (Siemens Dual Rota ZLC 37) under resting state conditions. The patients were placed in a supine position with eyes closed in a room with dim light and white background noise. Parallel-hole HIRES collimators (FWHM 12 mm) were used. Sodium perchlorate (500 mg) was given before tracer administration. Eighteen to 25 mCi (666–925MBq) of ^{99}mTc-d,l-HMPAO was injected intravenously immediately after formulation of the kit, 10 min before starting data acquisition. Sixty (2 × 30) projections were achieved within 30 min (60 sec/angle) with a linear sampling distance of 3.125 mm. Prereconstructional filtering of angle views, using a weighted filter of variable shape and size (4), and correction for tissue absorption were performed (5). For final evaluation, seven single slices (3.125 mm thick) were summed consecutively to obtain a set of 21.9 mm thick transverse sections covering the whole brain. For statistical data evaluation, 16 regions of interest (ROIs) per hemisphere were drawn in four representative cross-sections. The ROIs circumscribe visually discriminable anatomical structures in high resolution SPECT images (SF1, SF2, SF3: superior frontal gyrus; MF: mesofrontal gyrus; IF: inferior frontal gyrus; C1, C2: central regions; SP, IP: superior and inferior parietal regions; SO, IO: superior and inferior occipital region; ST, IT: superior and inferior temporal region; BG: anterior basal ganglia; TH: thalamus; HI: hippocampus). Finally, a regional index (RI = mean cts per voxel (ROI)/mean cts per voxel (all ROIs)) was calculated, indicating relative hyperperfused or hypoperfused areas.

RESULTS

When mean RIs ± 2× SD of controls were taken as normal range limits, a relative hyperperfusion was found in 21 regions (3.65% or 1.17 ROIs per

TABLE 1. *Comparison of left-sided versus right-sided RIs in migraine with aura in the symptom-free interval (paired t test, n = 16, df = 17).*

Hemispheric asymmetries

ROI	Left	Right	t =	p<	ROI	Left	Right	t =	p<
SF1	↓	↑	4.707	0.0002	SP	↓	↑	2.961	0.009
SF3	↓	↑	3.151	0.006	SO	↓	↑	3.447	0.003
MF	↓	↑	3.232	0.005	IO	↓	↑	2.144	0.05
IF	↓	↑	2.722	0.015	ST	↓	↑	3.987	0.001
C2	↓	↑	2.865	0.01	IT	↓	↑	4.733	0.0002

For abbreviations of ROIs see text.

patient) and a relative hypoperfusion in 24 regions (4.17% or 1.33 ROIs per patient) in the migraine group. Statistically significant hemispheric asymmetries were observed in 10 regions (paired t test). Relatively higher values were constantly seen in the right hemisphere (Table 1).

Statistical comparison of RIs between patients and normal controls (ANOVA $p<0.05$; $p<0.01$) revealed four left-sided and four right-sided abnormally perfused regions (Fig. 1). A significant regional hyperperfusion was found superior frontal (SF3) and in both central (C1,C2) regions of the left side as well as superior frontal (SF3) and superior occipital (SO) on the right side. A significant regional hypoperfusion was observed mesofrontal (MF)

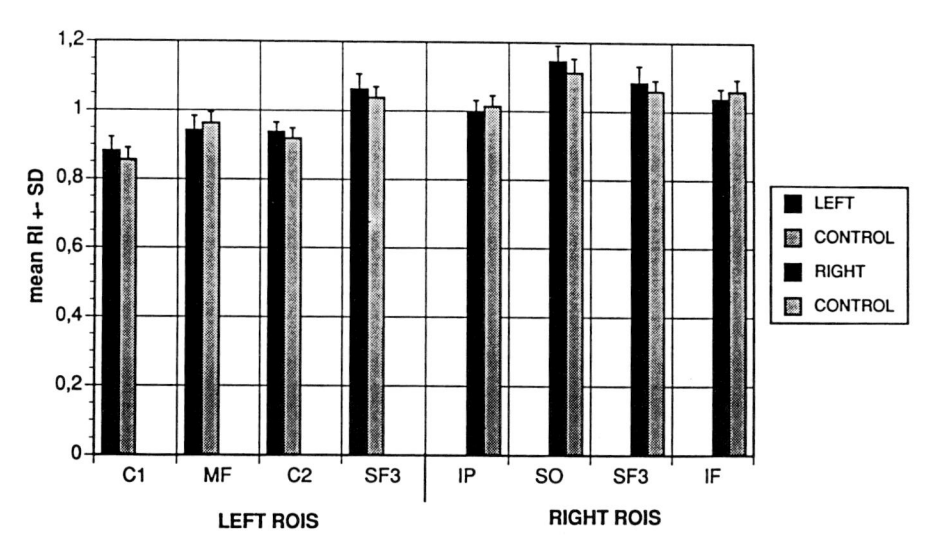

FIG. 1. Comparison (ANOVA $p<0.05$; (*)$p<0.01$) between RIs of patients with migraine with aura (n = 18) and normal controls (n = 51). (SF3: superior frontal; MF: mesofrontal; IF: inferior frontal; C1, C2: central; SO: superior occipital; IP: inferior parietal.)

TABLE 2. *Significant regional hyper- ($\uparrow$)/ hypoperfusion ($\downarrow$) in migraine with aura classified by symptoms, side of headache, and EEG findings when compared with normal controls.*

	Symptoms					Side			EEG	
	Hemi-right	Hemi-left	Speech	Scotoma	Left	Right	Diffuse	Left	Right
Left	MF ($\downarrow\downarrow$) IF ($\downarrow\downarrow$) IP ($\uparrow\uparrow$)	C1 ($\uparrow$)	SP ($\downarrow\downarrow$) IO ($\uparrow\uparrow$)	SF3 ($\uparrow\uparrow$) C2 ($\uparrow$)	MF ($\downarrow$) IF ($\downarrow\downarrow$) C1 ($\uparrow\uparrow$) C2 ($\uparrow\uparrow$)		SO ($\uparrow$)	IF ($\downarrow$) C1 ($\uparrow\uparrow$) SO ($\uparrow\uparrow$) IO ($\uparrow\uparrow$)	SF3 ($\uparrow\uparrow$) ST ($\uparrow\uparrow$)
Right	MF ($\downarrow\downarrow$) IF ($\downarrow\downarrow$) SO ($\uparrow\uparrow$) IO ($\uparrow\uparrow$)		BG ($\downarrow\downarrow$)	SF3 ($\uparrow\uparrow$)	SF3 ($\uparrow\uparrow$) IF ($\downarrow\downarrow$) SO ($\uparrow$)	C1 ($\downarrow$)	SO ($\uparrow\uparrow$)	SF3 ($\uparrow\uparrow$) MF ($\downarrow\downarrow$) IF ($\downarrow\downarrow\downarrow$) SO ($\uparrow\uparrow$) IO ($\uparrow\uparrow$)	

For abbreviations of ROIs see text.
ANOVA $p < 0.01$ indicated with double arrows.

left-sided and inferior frontal (IF) as well as inferior parietal (IP) in the right hemisphere. When classified by symptoms, comparison with normal controls [ANOVA ($p<0.05$)] reveals seven abnormally perfused regions in patients with right-sided hemisyndrome (n = 3), one region in left-sided hemisyndrome (n = 3), three in speech disorders (n = 3), and three in patients with scotoma (n = 9). When classified by side of headache, seven regions are affected in the left-side group (n = 11), one region in patients with right-sided pain (n = 2), and two in diffuse headache (n = 5). When classified by EEG findings, left-sided focal abnormalities (n = 7) correlate with nine abnormal regions and right-sided focal abnormalities (n = 1) with two regions. Diffuse abnormalities (n = 3) seen in EEG show no corresponding significant CBF differences between migraineurs and normal controls. EEG was normal in seven patients (Table 2).

DISCUSSION

Although it is a widely established observation that rCBF changes occur during migraine attacks, previous reports on CBF measurement in the headache-free interval provided complementary information. In an earlier study using ^{123}I-IMP-SPECT, a regional hypoperfusion was described in patients with complicated migraine in the symptom-free interval (6). Most recently, a study using the Xe CT-CBF method described regional hyperperfusion during the attack as well as in the interval (7). Disagreement also exists concerning observations on hemispheric asymmetries in migraine (7,8). In this study we have tried to evaluate the use of CBF imaging with ^{99m}Tc-d,l-HMPAO SPECT in migraineurs in the symptom-free interval. Although preliminary, our results demonstrate significant rCBF alterations including hemispheric asymmetries, regional hyperperfusion as well as hypoperfusion when compared with normal controls. When classified by predominant symptoms, side of headache, or EEG findings, distinct patterns of rCBF alterations can be shown. It must be considered, however, that ^{99m}Tc-d,l-HMPAO SPECT provides only a static, flow-related pattern, which per se supports the idea of altered rCBF related to the distribution area of intracerebral arteries but does not specifically support any theory concerning the pathogenesis of migraine. Furthermore, the statistical relevance of this study—like others—should be related to the classification problems inherent in the individual dynamics of migraine and its changing symptoms.

REFERENCES

1. Friberg L, Olsen T, Roland PE, et al. Focal ischemia caused by instability of cerebrovascular tone during attacks of hemiplegic migraine. *Brain* 1987; 110:917–934.
2. Sakai F and Meyer JS. Regional cerebral hemodynamics during migraine and cluster headaches measured by the ^{133}Xe inhalation method. *Headache* 1978; 18:122–132.

3. Ell PJ, Hocknell JML, Jarrizz PH, et al. A ^{99}Tcm-labelled radiotracer for the investigation of cerebral vascular disease. *Nucl Med Commun* 1985; 6:437–441.
4. Todd-Prokopek A and Di Paolo R. The use of computers for image processing in nuclear medicine. *IEEE Trans Nucl Sci* 1982; 21:1299–1309.
5. Bellini S, Piacentini M, Cafforio C, et al. Compensation of tissue absorption in emission tomography. *IEEE Trans Acous Speech Sign Proc ASSP* 1979; 27:213–218.
6. Schlake HP, Böttger IG, Grotemeyer KH, et al. Brain imaging with 123I-IMP-SPECT in migraine between attacks. *Headache* 1989; 29:344–349.
7. Kobari M, Meyer JS, and Kawamura J. Cortical and subcortical hyperperfusion during migraine and cluster headache measured by Xe CT-CBF. *Neuroradiology* 1990; 32:4–11.
8. Levine SR, Welch KMA, Ewing JR, et al. Cerebral blood flow asymmetries in headache-free migraineurs. *Stroke* 1987; 18:1164–1165.

12

The Effects of Aging on Cerebral Blood Flow in Patients with Migraine Equivalents

Wendy M. Robertson, Nabih M. Ramadan, Steven R. Levine, Lonni R. Schultz, and K. M. A. Welch

Center for Stroke Research, Department of Neurology, Henry Ford Hospital, Detroit, Michigan 48202

In a previous study, age-related changes in regional cerebral blood flow (rCBF) were found in patients with migraine (with and without aura) compared to controls (1). Migraine aura without headache (migraine equivalents) resembles migraine in symptomatology, but the pathophysiology is uncertain and often difficult to distinguish from transient ischemic attacks. The present study was performed to determine whether age-related changes in rCBF in patients with migraine equivalents (ME) resemble those in patients with migraine.

PATIENTS AND METHODS

We measured rCBF in 38 patients with migraine aura without headache (ME) defined according to the International Headache Society Classification (2). Results were compared to 49 patients with migraine with aura and 49 control subjects who had no history or physical examination findings suggestive of neurological disease (Table 1). All patients had normal neurological examinations and were symptom-free for at least 48 hours before the study. All were asked to discontinue headache medications 7–10 days before the study.

rCBF was studied by the ^{133}Xe inhalation technique (3). Measures were taken from 16 scintillation detectors arranged in a symmetrical array of eight probe pairs over each hemisphere. The initial slope index (ISI) was the measure of blood flow used in this study (4).

TABLE 1. *Patient population*

	N	Mean age	Age range (yrs)	% Female
Migraine aura without headache (ME)	38	57.8	23–83	84.0
Migraine with aura (M + A)	49	38.3	19–85	68.6
Controls	49	50.4	22–80	55.1

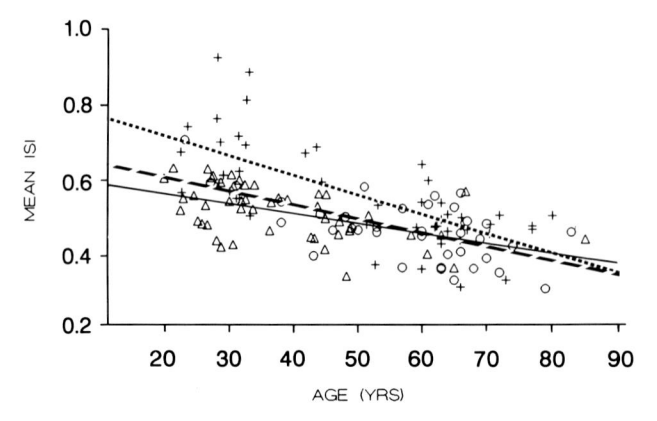

FIG. 1. Regression lines of mean ISI versus age for migraine equivalent patients (0 — — 0), migraine with aura patients (△——△), and controls (+ ----- +).

TABLE 2. *Mean ISI*

	Mean ISI ± SEM			
	N	<45 years	N	>45 years
Migraine aura without headache (ME)	7	54.71 ± 3.64[a]	31	45.05 ± 1.25
Migraine with aura (M + A)	37	53.67 ± 1.01[a]	12	45.40 ± 1.73
Controls	21	66.98 ± 2.42	28	47.71 ± 1.31

[a] $p < 0.02$ paired t test compared to controls.

TABLE 3. *Previous history of migraine*

	N	Mean ISI ± SEM
ME with migraine	14	46.97 ± 1.74[a]
ME without migraine	24	46.75 ± 1.90[a]
Controls	49	55.97 ± 1.87

[a] $p < 0.03$ age-adjusted analysis of covariance.

RESULTS

The slope of the regression line of mean ISI versus age (Fig. 1) was significantly less for ME patients than controls (-0.295 vs. -0.488; $p < 0.05$). Slope estimates for ME and migraine with aura (-0.263) did not differ significantly.

The mean ISI was significantly lower in the ME group as a whole (46.83 ± 1.34) compared to controls (55.97 ± 1.87; $p < 0.003$). The difference in mean ISI was pronounced in the younger age group (younger than 45 years) in both migraine groups compared to controls and was not significantly different in the older age group (Table 2). These differences were significant in ME patients regardless of whether there was a previous history of migraine headaches (Table 3).

Asymmetry of regional flow is considered significant if the ISI ratio,

$$\frac{|ISI_R - ISI_L|}{(ISI_R + ISI_L)/2} \times 100,$$

is greater than 7%. Young ME patients (younger than 45 years) have a higher percentage of subjects with at least one major asymmetric probe pair (57.1%) compared to controls (33.3%). This relationship changes with advancing years, when the percentage of controls with a major asymmetry increases to 75% (compared to 80.6% in the ME group).

DISCUSSION

There are few previous studies of cerebral blood flow in patients with migrainous symptoms without headache. One case studied acutely was reported to have "spreading oligemia" typical of migraine with aura (5). The interictal cerebral blood flow changes found in our study provide evidence of similarities with migraine with aura. Compared to controls, migraine with aura and migraine aura without headache groups were both found to have a lower mean ISI with more regional asymmetries of flow and a slower rate of decline of cerebral blood flow with age.

Clinical follow-up of patients with scintillating scotoma without headache has revealed a benign course (6), further evidence of a similarity to migraine as opposed to atherosclerotic cerebrovascular disease. Future studies comparing the age-related changes in blood flow in patients with known stroke risk factors may aid in the distinction of these two groups.

As suggested in an earlier paper (1), the lower mean ISI found in the young migraine population may render the brain more susceptible to spreading depression. The similar finding in the ME group, therefore, adds to the theory that the migraine aura is related to spreading depression. It is unlikely that we are seeing flow reduction secondary to an acute attack since patients were studied outside a 48-hr window. The possibility remains that the low flow, although not in an ischemic or oligemic range, is secondary to neuronal loss from repeated ME episodes in which ischemia might occur.

REFERENCES

1. Robertson WM, Welch KMA, Levine SR, and Schultz LR. The effects of aging on cerebral blood flow in migraine. *Neurology* 1989; 39:947–951.
2. Headache Classification Committee of the International Headache Society. Classification and diagnostic criteria for headache disorders, cranial neuralgias and facial pain. *Cephalalgia* 1988; 8[Suppl 7].
3. Obrist WD, Thompson HK, King CH, and Wang HS. Determination of regional cerebral blood flow by inhalation of ^{133}Xenon. *Circ Res* 1967; 20:124–135.
4. Risberg J, Ali Z, Wilson EM, Wills EL, and Halsey JH. Regional cerebral blood flow by ^{133}Xe inhalation: Preliminary evaluation of an initial slope index in patients with unstable flow compartments. *Stroke* 1975; 6:142–148.
5. Skyhøj Olsen T and Olesen J. Regional cerebral blood flow in migraine and cluster headache. In: Olesen J and Edvinsson L, eds. *Basic Mechanisms of Headache*. Amsterdam: Elsevier, 1988: 377–391.
6. Wiley RG. The scintillating scotoma without headache. *Ann Ophthalmol* 1979; 11:581–585.

13

Interictal Studies in Migraine with Aura: Discussion Summary

Olaf B. Paulson

Several studies demonstrated flow abnormalities in the interictal phase of migraine with aura. In some cases of severe hemiplegic migraine, changes are rather marked and correlate with the symptoms. In other cases of hemiplegic migraine, and in patients with typical aura, flow changes are minor and not correlated to type and location of symptoms. The significance of such minor flow changes is uncertain. One view is that they represent vascular instability or mild vascular dysregulation affecting the whole brain in migraineurs. Another view is that such changes, although statistically significant compared to control materials, are so small and often imperceptible by visual analysis that it is uncertain whether they are real. They may perhaps just reflect that the normal material has an especially low interregional variability. It is advocated to study the day-to-day variation of the described abnormalities and possibly to compare them to a second group of normal controls. The importance of standardized examination procedures and rigorous age and sex matching is emphasized. Further interictal studies using methods with high spatial resolution such as positron emission tomography and rigorous statistical analysis are recommended.

PART III

The Onset of Migraine Attacks with Aura

14

Migraine with Aura

Onset of the Attack: Intracarotid Xenon 133 Method

Tom Skyhøj Olsen

Department of Clinical Physiology and Nuclear Medicine, Bispebjerg Hospital, DK-2400 Copenhagen NV, Denmark

In the study of migraine with aura, the ^{133}Xe intracarotid injection method has been superior to all other cerebral blood flow (CBF) methods in one very important aspect. It has been possible, with this method, to study CBF in the same patient just before the onset of an attack, at the onset, during the aura, and even into the headache phase. The reason is quite simple: the procedure that involves puncture of the carotid artery (1,2) seems to provoke attacks in patients who suffer from migraine with aura (3,4). Carotid angiography is, likewise, known to provoke migraine with aura (5). Whether it is the puncture of the carotid itself or it is injection of contrast medium into the carotid circulation is not clarified. Unclarified also is the important fact that there is a delay of about 30–60 min between puncture of the carotid artery and onset of the aura symptoms (3,4). Undoubtedly, the process that causes or triggers the aura is running long before symptoms appear.

THE BLOOD FLOW CHANGES

CBF changes start to develop at least 5–15 min before the patient experiences the first symptom of the aura (3,4). A focal area of reduced flow develops posteriorly in the brain. When the CBF investigations are repeated at 5- to 15-min intervals, the low flow area enlarges and the patient experiences aura symptoms (3,4,6) (Fig. 1). This is the experience from two prospective studies comprising 9 and 11 patients, respectively (3,4). In a retrospective study comprising seven patients the blood flow reduction was preceded by a focal hyperemic area in two patients (6). Hence, as a rule,

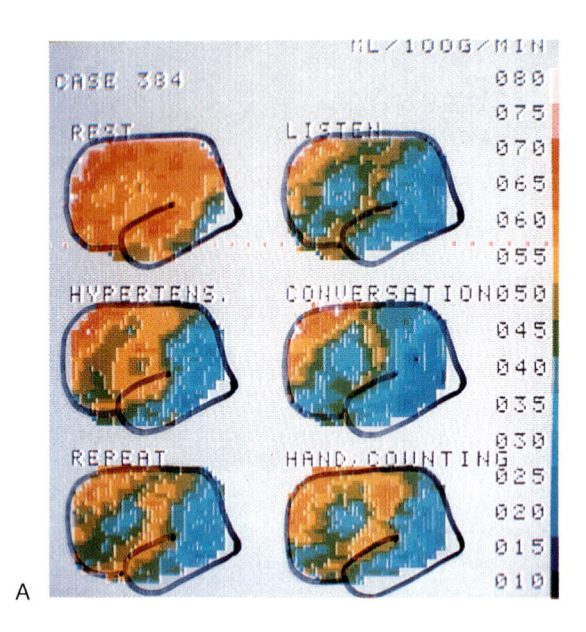

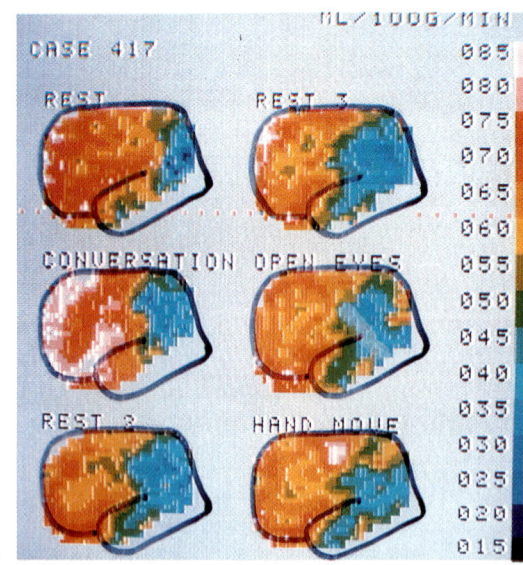

FIG. 1. Regional cerebral blood flow in two patients during the aura. Note the development of a low flow area in the posterior part of the brain. In one patient a low flow area develops also in the prefrontal area. [133]Xe intracarotid injection technique and a 254-multidetector camera. The absolute flow values in ml/100 g/min appear from the color scale.

start of the migraine attack is associated with focal hypoperfusion (3,4,6–9). Hyperemia seems to be more the exception than the rule.

When using the intracarotid injection method it is only the vascular territory of the carotid artery that can be investigated. Hence, it is impossible with this method to study if the flow reduction starts first in the occipital region. More or less gradually the low flow area appears to be larger and larger and may involve parietal, temporal, central, and frontal areas of the brain (3,4,6). When looking at the results of the flow studies performed with multidetector equipment (3,4,6), it appears that the territory of the anterior cerebral artery usually is spared—the process seems to go on in the middle cerebral artery territory (3,4,6).

At the same time or shortly after the appearance of the low flow area in the posterior part of the brain, a low flow area also may appear in the prefrontal area (3,4). Like the posterior low flow area, this prefrontal low flow area may also grow larger and larger and sometimes confluence with the posterior low flow area. It is well known from studies with single photon emission computed tomography that the low flow area changes into a hyperemic area a few hours after its appearance (10). With the intracarotid injection method it has not been possible to follow patients from the ischemic state into the hyperemic state. However, in the few studies performed with the intracarotid injection technique in the headache phase several hours after the aura symptoms have vanished, hyperemia has been reported (7).

BLOOD FLOW CHANGES AND SYMPTOMS

As mentioned, the blood flow changes precede the symptoms by at least 5–15 min or more (3,4). During CBF studies it is typical that the aura symptoms are in the mild end of the spectrum, that is, paresthesias, slight hypoesthesia/algesia, slight paresis of the face, arm, or leg, or discrete aphasia (3,4). This is in sharp contrast to the extensiveness of the areas involved. One patient had a fully developed and typical change of the blood flow involving parietal, temporal, and prefrontal areas of the brain but she did not report any symptoms (3). Typically, the symptoms disappear when the extension of the blood flow changes have reached a maximum (3,4). Headache is experienced in the low flow state of the aura (3,4,6,7,9).

INTERPRETATION OF THE BLOOD FLOW STUDIES

The results of the blood flow studies with the intracarotid injection technique have been interpreted in two ways. One interpretation may support the neuronal theory, especially spreading depression, whereas the other may support the vascular theory.

The Interpretation Supporting the Neuronal Theory

During the last 10 years possible neural causes of migraine with aura have been studied more intensively than ever. This development was inspired by the study of Olesen et al. (6). In a retrospective series of seven patients studied during migraine aura, they found, like others before them (7,8, 9,11,12), that the blood flow was focally reduced during the aura. The original and most important observation in this study was that the low flow area was not of constant size. It became larger and larger on repeated examinations and territories of major cerebral arteries were not respected. Olesen et al. (6) therefore considered arterial vasospasm unlikely as the cause of the blood flow reduction. They also noted that the blood flow reduction averaged 35%, which is not sufficient to cause ischemia. They termed, therefore, the blood flow alteration "spreading oligemia." The spreading character of the blood flow changes was even more evident in a prospective series of nine patients studied by Lauritzen et al. (3). They calculated the rate of spread to be 2.2 mm per min. Also in this series it was noted that the blood flow reduction was modest and well above ischemic thresholds (on average 40 ml/100 g/min); hence, a confirmation of Olesen et al.'s (6) findings and a further support of the neural theory. In this study the aura symptoms were carefully monitored and related to the blood flow changes. It was noted that the low flow area appeared before the neurological symptoms occurred and that the neurological symptoms had disappeared when the low flow area had reached its maximum of extension. This finding was taken to speak against a primary vascular cause of the symptoms that occur during the aura. Therefore, Olesen et al. (6) and Lauritzen et al. (3) use the term "spreading oligemia" instead of "spreading ischemia" to describe the blood flow changes that occur during the migraine aura. Such a relation between symptoms in remission despite persistence of a CBF reduction is present during spreading depression in the rat (13), in which electroencephalograms (EEGs) (14) and evoked responses (15) have returned to normal within 5 and 30 min, respectively, although CBF is still decreased at that time (13). Lauritzen et al. (16) also studied vascular reactivity in the brain during the aura. Autoregulation was found to be normal in the affected as well as in the nonaffected low flow area. CO_2 reactivity was reported to be normal in the nonaffected part of the brain but it was reduced by about 50% in the affected low flow areas. This is strikingly similar to the vascular reactivity observed in the rat brain after episodes of spreading depression, where autoregulation is normal while CO_2 reactivity is reduced but still preserved (17). Lauritzen et al. (3) also reported that the spreading oligemia usually stops before or upon reaching the central or lateral sulci. Similarly, spreading depression in the rat also stops where the cytoarchitecture undergoes abrupt changes (15)—as in the lateral and central sulci (3).

Lauritzen et al. (3) observed that in about half of their patients a prefrontal low flow area developed independently of the posterior low flow area during the migraine attack. They noted that this low flow area appeared some time after the appearance of the posterior low flow area. It was interpreted as a spreading oligemia circumventing the major macrostructural and microstructural changes (the central and lateral sulcus) by passing through the insula to the frontal lobe—as in spreading depression (3).

Thus, according to the interpretation by Olesen et al. (6) and Lauritzen et al. (3), the blood flow changes that occur during the migraine aura have the following characteristics: the blood flow reduction is modest and is not reduced to ischemic levels; the affected low flow area enlarges gradually and does not respect territories of supply of major cerebral arteries (spreading oligemia); the blood flow reduction occurs before the aura symptoms appear and is still present when they disappear and when the headache starts; the "spreading depression" stops before or upon reaching the central and lateral sulcus. When interpreting the results of the CBF studies in this way the similarity between migraine with aura in humans and spreading depression in the rat brain is evident.

The Interpretation Supporting the Vascular Theory

Skinhøj (7) presented the first series of patients studied during the migraine aura with the intracarotid injection technique. In four patients CBF decreased markedly in the aura and in two of these CBF had declined to critical levels. Skinhøj concluded that his results "indicate that a primary constriction in the carotid artery system plays an important role in the pathogenesis of migraine." Skinhøj (7) also observed that the decrease in cerebral blood flow during the migraine aura may continue into the headache phase. Simard and Paulson (8) studied one patient during the aura and measured a global CBF of 20 ml/100 g/min—a value just below the ischemic threshold. Hachinski et al. (10) studied two patients during the aura and recorded CBF values approaching or below the level for critical metabolism.

Skyhøj Olsen et al. (4) and Skyhøj Olsen and Lassen (18) criticized the studies of Olesen et al. (6) and Lauritzen et al. (3). They evaluated 11 consecutive patients studied during the aura and sometimes followed into the headache phase. All these patients developed a low flow area posteriorly in the brain that more or less gradually spread to involve parietal, temporal, and sometimes central and frontal areas of the brian, as also observed by Olesen et al. (6) and Lauritzen et al. (3). Their main observation was that mean CBF measured in the low flow areas was closely related to the CBF measured in the surrounding nonaffected part of the brain: if CBF was high in the surrounding areas CBF was also high in the low flow area and if CBF was low in the surrounding areas CBF was also low in the low flow area (Fig. 2). In the individual low flow areas, CBF was highest in the areas closest to the normally perfused areas, lower in the center of the area, and lowest in regions of the low flow areas that were located at the longest distance from the normally perfused part of the brain. They concluded that this finding might be caused by the phenomenon called Compton scattered radiation.

Because of this phenomenon, CBF values in low flow areas become overestimated (2). Compton scatter involves the interaction between an incident photon and an orbital electron. As the result of the interaction, the photon changes direction and loses energy. In practice this means that part of the radiation emerging from ^{133}Xe is recorded by detectors looking at areas at a distance from the place where the gamma radiation originates. This is demonstrated in Fig. 3. The detectors placed over a low flow area, as in migraine with aura, record not only radiation from isotope actually deposited in the areas. The washout curves obtained from low flow areas are the result of washout of isotope actually deposited in the low flow area (and representative of true flow) and of "washout" of Compton scattered radiation from the surrounding normally perfused areas, causing an overestimation proportional to flow in the surrounding areas and inversely proportional to true flow in the low flow area. It follows that the best estimate of flow in a low flow area is obtained where the influence of Compton scatter is lowest. This is the case if CBF in the surroundings is low and in regions of the low flow area located at the longest distance from the normally perfused area.

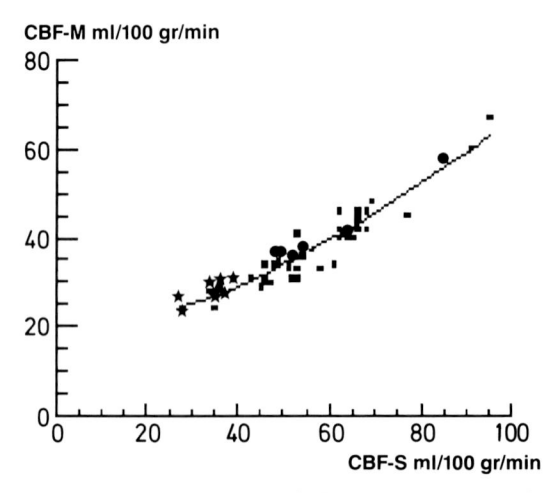

FIG. 2. CBF measured in 35 low flow areas (CBF-M) during attacks of migraine with aura related to CBF in the surrounding nonaffected part of the brain (CBF-S). ●, studies during induced hypertension (autoregulation); ■, studies during habitual paCO$_2$ and blood pressure; ★, studies during spontaneous hyperventillation (CO$_2$ reactivity). The curve seems to approach a level between 20 and 25 ml/100 g/min as an expression of true CBF in the low flow areas during the aura. (From Skyhøj Olsen and Lassen, ref. 18, with permission.)

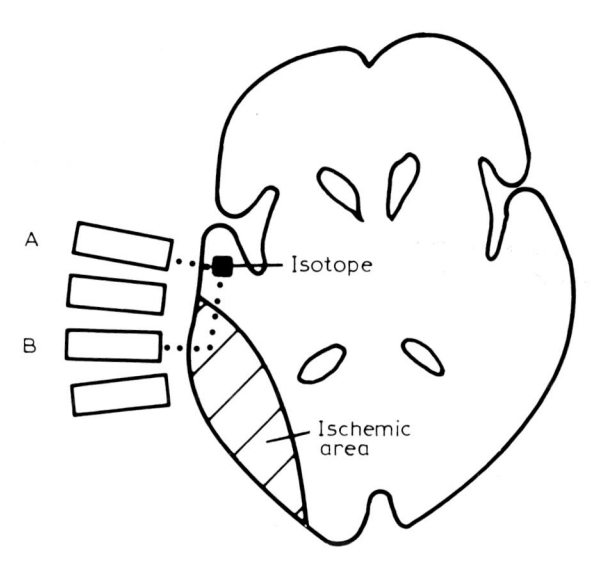

FIG. 3. Diagram demonstrating the effect of Compton scatter on rCBF recordings. Isotope from a normally perfused area is recorded by detector A reflecting true blood flow in the area. Other gamma rays from the same area are deflected and recorded by detector B. This radiation (Compton scatter) is washed out at a normal rate, since rCBF is normal at the site of its origin, but it is recorded as if it came from a low flow area. All detectors receive Compton scattered radiation. If rCBF beneath detector B was normal Compton scatter would not significantly influence the washout curves recorded by this detector. If, however, true rCBF beneath detector B is focally reduced as indicated on the figure, the contribution of Compton scatter to the washout curve gives rise to overestimation of rCBF in the low flow areas because Compton scatter comes from an area with a higher blood flow and therefore also a higher washout rate. (From Olesen and Edvinson, ref. 20, with permission.)

Considering the lowest CBF value measured in the areas at the longest distance to the normally perfused areas as representing true flow in the low flow area, CBF reductions averaging 52% were measured in the series by Skyhøj Olsen et al. (4). In 7 of the 11 patients CBF values ≤ 23 ml/100 g/min were measured, that is, values just around the ischemic threshold. The authors noted that the four patients in whom the ischemic threshold was not reached were characterized by having a high blood flow in the nonaffected surroundings. Therefore, they held open the possibility that in these four patients the effect of Compton scatter was so pronounced that ischemic flow values were masked by Compton scatter. Thus, their results were interpreted as if ischemic flow values were present in all their patients during the aura. Because the influence of Compton scatter is highest in the areas closest to the nonaffected area and lowest farthest away from this area, they suggested that CBF in these latter areas were representative of flow in the entire area. They suggested that CBF might be very low, approaching ischemic levels in the entire low flow area.

Spreading of the low flow area during the aura is undoubtedly Olesen et al.'s (6) most original observation. It was termed "spreading oligemia." Skyhøj Olsen and Lassen (18) suggested an alternative explanation of this phenomenon: if CBF gradually decreases in an area of constant size this gradual flow reduction will appear as a spreading oligemia—because of Compton scatter. The scattered radiation from nonaffected areas with normal flow will "cover up" the flow reduction, which will be apparent first in the areas farthest from the nonaffected area. The low flow area will gradually emerge at the same time as CBF decreases and in this way it will look as if the low flow area gradually enlarges even though the area, in fact, remains the same size. According to these investigators (18,19), the low flow area starts to appear on the flow map only when CBF is reduced by 20%. Half of the low flow area is seen when CBF is reduced by 35%, whereas the entire low flow area is seen only when CBF is decreased by more than 50%. Interpreting the CBF data in this way, Skyhøj Olsen and Lassen (18) explain why the flow reduction always precedes the symptoms: it takes some time before CBF is reduced to the ischemic level (about 50% or more). This interpretation may also explain why fully developed CBF changes may occur in patients who have no symptoms.

Skyhøj Olsen and Lassen (18) suggested that there might be a close relation between appearance of symptoms and CBF in the low flow area. When a low flow area is present while the patient has no symptoms, CBF in the low flow area may have not reached the ischemic level and therefore symptoms have not occurred. Skyhøj Olsen and Lassen (18) showed that CBF changes within the interval of 20–30 ml/100 g/min in the low flow area usually are impossible to register, especially if CBF in the surrounding normally perfused areas is normal, that is, 50–60 ml/100 g/min. Therefore, true CBF in the low flow area may increase from "ischemic values" to "nonischemic values" while the CBF that is measured remains the same. According to Skyhøj Olsen and Lassen (18), this could explain why the aura symptoms disappear despite the CBF changes (low flow) persist.

Lauritzen et al. (3) considered the appearance of a prefrontal low flow area as a continuation of spreading oligemia from the posterior part of the brain—the spreading oligemia had circumvented the lateral and central sulci by passing deep in the brain through the insula to the frontal lobe. Looking at the CBF changes in the way Skyhøj Olsen and Lassen (18) did, the posterior low flow area and the prefrontal low flow area might also start to develop independently of each other and at the same time. The reason why the prefrontal area appears some time after the posterior low flow area is that the influence of Compton scatter is much more pronounced in the prefrontal area than in the posterior part of the brain (2). CBF, therefore, has to decrease much more in the prefrontal area before being detectable.

According to the interpretation of Skyhøj Olsen and Lassen (18), CBF in migraine with aura may have the following characteristics: CBF decreases more or less gradually in an area of fixed size. The aura symptoms appear first when CBF in the low flow area decreases below the ischemic threshold (23 ml/100 g/min). Because of Compton scatter it looks like the low flow area becomes larger and larger but spreading is an artifact—CBF decreases in an area of fixed size. After the blood flow changes have reached their full extension, the blood flow increases in the low flow area to values above the ischemic threshold and the aura symptoms disappear. However, this increase cannot be recorded because of Compton scatter, giving the impression that the blood flow remains unchanged. Hence, the aura symptoms, according to this interpretation, are primarily caused by vascular changes, that is, ischemia.

CONCLUSION

The proponents of the neural theory and of the vascular theory may seem to be far apart in their view on CBF in migraine with aura. After all, however, there seems to be more agreement than disagreement.

There is agreement that ischemia may occur in the low flow areas during the aura and when present there seems to be agreement that ischemia usually is mild. The discussion is about frequency and extension of ischemia and whether ischemia is a primary or a secondary phenomenon. There is agreement that the blood flow changes usually precede the aura symptoms. The discussion turns to two points: Is it because CBF has not yet decreased below the ischemic level or is CBF not of primary importance for the development of aura symptoms? There is agreement that CBF is oligemic (i.e., low but not ischemic) when the aura symptoms have vanished and the headache sets in. There is agreement about the spreading character of the low flow area when looking at repeated CBF studies in the same patient during the aura. There is agreement that this is an expression of a process that takes time to develop to its full extent, as it also takes time to develop the aura symptoms to their full extent. The discussion is about interpretation of the phenomenon. Is a spreading process going on or is it an artifact caused by Compton scatter that in fact "covers up" a gradual decrease of CBF in an area of fixed size?

Correct recording of CBF with the intracarotid injection method presupposes a homogeneous blood flow and a stable blood flow in the brain during the measurement. Most of the disagreement between investigators in the field is probably because migraine does not suffice in these two conditions. The blood flow is not homogeneous and CBF is unstable and changes considerably during the attack. The intracarotid ^{133}Xe method has clarified important aspects of migraine with aura but has raised many more questions. These questions must be answered with alternative methods. Using isotope clearance methods it is, in particular, important to reduce or eliminate the effect of scattered radiation on the recordings.

REFERENCES

1. Olesen J, Paulson OB, and Lassen NA. Regional cerebral blood flow determined by the initial slope of the clearance of intra-arterially injected 133 Xe. *Stroke* 1971; 2:519–540.
2. Skyhøj Olsen T, Larsen B, Bech Skriver E, Enevoldsen E, and Lassen NA. Focal cerebral ischemia measured by the intraarterial 133-Xenon method. *Stroke* 1981; 12:736–744.
3. Lauritzen M, Skyhøj Olsen T, Lassen NA, and Paulson B. The changes of regional cerebral blood flow during the course of classical migraine attacks. *Ann Neurol* 1983; 13:633–641.
4. Skyhøj Olsen T, Friberg L, and Lassen NA. Ischemia may be the primary cause of the neurological deficits in classic migraine. *Arch Neurol* 1987; 44:156–161.
5. Janzen R, Tanzer A, Zschocke S, and Dieckmann H. Postangiographische spätreaktionen der hirngefässe bei migräne-kranken. *Z Neurol* 1972; 201:24–42.
6. Olesen J, Larsen B, and Lauritzen M. Focal hyperemia followed by spreading oligemia and impaired activation of rCBF in classic migraine. *Ann Neurol* 1981; 9:344–352.
7. Skinhøj E. Hemodynamic studies within the brain during migraine. *Arch Neurol* 1973; 29:95–98.
8. Simard D and Paulson OB. Cerebral vasomotor paralysis during migraine attack. *Arch Neurol* 1973; 29:95–98.
9. Hachinski VC, Olesen J, Norris JW, Larsen B, Enevoldsen E, and Lassen NA. Cerebral hemodynamics in migraine. *Can J Neurol Sci* 1977; 4:245–249.
10. Andersen AR, Friberg L, Skyhøj Olsen T, and Olesen J. Delayed hyperemia following hypoperfusion in classic migraine. *Arch Neurol* 1988; 45:154–159.
11. Skinhøj E and Paulson OB. Regional cerebral blood flow in internal carotid distribution during migraine attack. *Br Med J* 1969; 3:569–570.
12. Edmeas J. Cerebral blood flow in migraine. *Headache* 1977; 17:148–152.
13. Lauritzen M, Jørgensen MB, Diemer NH, Gjedde A, and Hansen AJ. Persisting oligemia of rat cerebral cortex in the wake of spreading depression. *Ann Neurol* 1982; 12:469–474.
14. Leao AAP. Spreading depression of activity in cerebral cortex. *J Neurophysiol* 1944; 7:359–390.
15. Bures J, Buresova O, and Krivanek J. *The mechanisms and applications of Leao's spreading depression of electroencephalographic activity.* New York: Academic Press, 1974.
16. Lauritzen M, Skyhøj Olsen T, Lassen NA, and Paulson OB. The regulation of regional cerebral blood flow during and between migraine attacks. *Ann Neurol* 1983; 14:569–570.
17. Lauritzen M. Long-lasting reduction of cortical blood flow in the rat brain after spreading depression with preserved autoregulation and impaired CO_2-response. *J Cerebr Blood Flow Metab* 1984; 4:546–554.
18. Skyhøj Olsen T and Lassen NA. Blood flow and vascular reactivity during attacks of classic migraine—Limitations of the Xe-133 intraarterial technique. *Headache* 1989; 29:15–20.
19. Skyhøj Olsen T. Migraine with and without aura: The same disease due to cerebral vasospasm of different intensity. A hypothesis based on CBF studies during migraine. *Headache* 1990; 30:269–272.
20. Olesen J and Edvinson L. *Basic mechanisms of headache.* Amsterdam: Elsevier Science Publishers, 1988.

15

Reversible Hemispheric Ischemia in a Patient with Migraine

*Ken Nagata, *Kazunari Fukushima, *Eriko Yokoyama,
*Yuichi Satoh, *Yasuhito Watahiki, *Yutaka Hirata,
†Fumio Shishido, and †Iwao Kanno

*Departments of Neurology and †Radiology and Nuclear Medicine, Research Institute for Brain and Blood Vessels, Akita 010, Japan

Although migraine is common in the general population, the coincidence of migraine and stroke (migrainous stroke) is a rare condition. Single or limited numbers of series of patients have been reported concerning their responsible mechanisms. The possible causes for migrainous stroke include cerebral vasospasm, impaired platelet aggregation, cerebral embolism caused by mitral prolapse, dissecting aneurysm, arteritis, hyperplasia, or multiple factors including some of these pathological processes. However, there has been controversy concerning the pathophysiological mechanisms of the migrainous stroke. In this chapter we present our study of hemodynamic pathophysiology in a patients with migrainous stroke using positron emission tomography (PET) and single photon emission computed tomography (SPECT).

ILLUSTRATIVE CASE REPORT

A 38-year-old right-handed woman was admitted to the hospital because of throbbing hemicranial headache and left hemiparesis. She had been well until 1 week before admission, when she developed a mild weakness in her left extremities, which followed a severe right-sided throbbing headache and blurred vision. History was remarkable for 20 years of recurrent hemicranial throbbing headache in the right side without aura. The headache occurred about twice a month but often improved spontaneously.

Upon admission she was alert and well oriented, but she did not pay serious attention to the weakness of her left extremities. The neurological examination revealed a mild left hemiparesis and left hemihypesthesia. No pathological reflex was elicited. Vital signs and physical examination were normal, and her neck was supple. The laboratory studies revealed an iron deficiency anemia; RBC count was 3,290,000, hemoglobin concentration was 8.3 g/dl, and hematocrit was 26.9%. The platelet aggregation was moderately accelerated to both ADP and collagen. Both bleeding time and prothrombin time were normal. Lumbar puncture yielded an opening pressure of 100 mm; the CSF was clear and colorless and contained two lymphocytes; protein content was 30 mg/dl and glucose content was 65 mg/dl. On day 7, the cortical sulci were obliterated in the right parietal lobe on x-ray CT. Cerebral angiography revealed a severe stenotic lesion in the right internal carotid artery (ICA) at the supraclinoid portion and the cortical perfusion was delayed to the right middle cerebral artery (MCA) territory. The persistent trigeminal artery was seen on the right side (Fig. 1).

When she had a recurrent severe right-sided headache on day 8, her left hemiparesis deteriorated and the right plantar response was extensor. During the headache attack, cerebral blood flow (CBF) was markedly reduced in the entire right hemisphere on CBF images of [123]-IMP SPECT. There was a rapid recovery from the hemiparesis. On day 14, CBF increased in the right hemisphere except for the right parietal region, which corresponded to the low density lesion on the follow-up x-ray CT (Fig. 2). The third SPECT on day 20 showed a symmetrical distribution of CBF except for the right parietal region (Fig. 2).

Vascular responses to hypocapnia and hypercapnia were evaluated by the CBF measurement according to the $H_2^{15}O$ intravenous injection method with PET. On day 15, the response to hypercapnia was severely impaired in the right hemisphere although there was a symmetrical distribution of CBF except for the right parietal region during the resting state (Fig. 3). On day

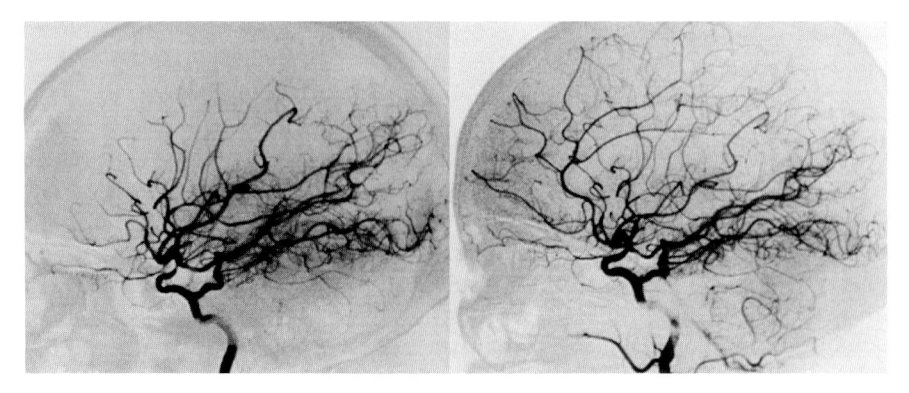

FIG. 1. Left: initial right carotid angiography revealed a segmental narrowing of the internal carotid artery at the supraclinoid portion. **Right:** Repeated right angiography 16 months later shows complete resolution of the stenosis previously demonstrated.

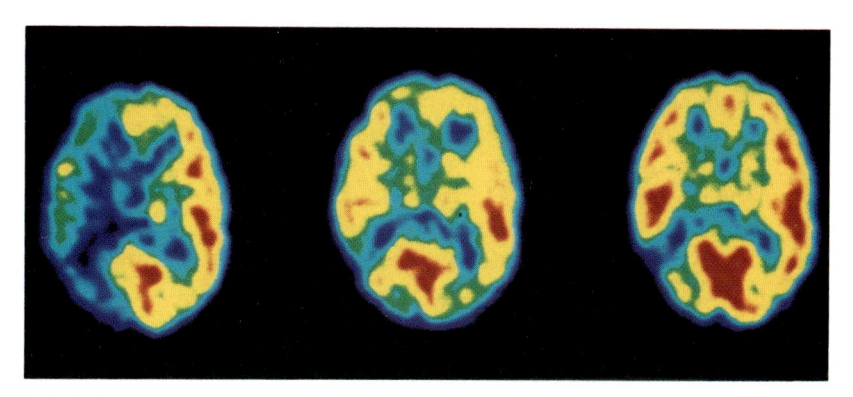

FIG. 2. Left: 123I-IMP SPECT shows right hemispheric reduction of CBF on day 8. **Center:** Hemispheric reduction of CBF was improved except for the focal lesions in the right parietal lobe on day 15. **Right:** CBF increased on the right hemisphere on day 20.

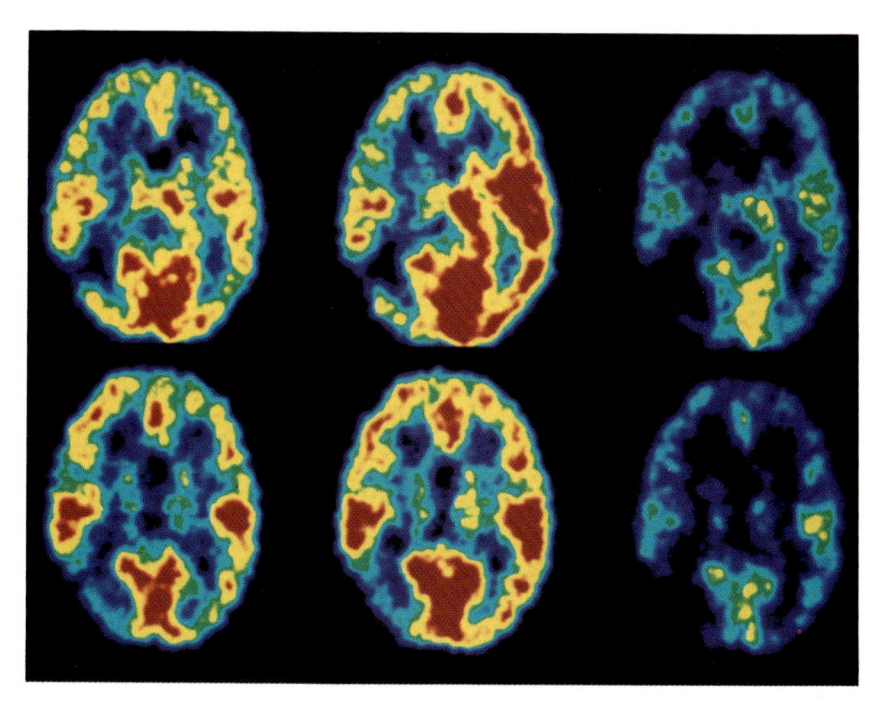

FIG. 3. Top: CBF measurement on day 15 by the H2^{15}O intravenous injection method with PET during resting state (*left*), hypercapnia by CO_2 inhalation (*center*), and hypocapnia by hyperventilation (*right*). Vascular response to hypercapnia was impaired in the right hemisphere. **Bottom:** CBF measurement on day 25 during resting state (*left*), hypercapnia (*center*), and hypocapnia (*right*). Vascular response to hypercapnia was improved in the right hemisphere except for the parietal lobe.

16, the circulation delay was improved in right MCA territory although the stenotic lesion of the right ICA was unchanged on angiogram. The vascular response to hypercapnia was improved in the right hemisphere except for the parietal region on day 25 (Fig. 3). The patient was discharged presenting with a trace weakness in her left hand on day 32. After the discharge, she never complained of severe headache. The stenotic lesion of the right ICA was completely restored in the follow-up angiogram that was performed 16 months after the onset. In the follow-up PET studies 19 months after the onset, similar results were obtained as on day 25.

COMMENT

Rapid recovery from the left hemiparesis seen in this patient could be closely associated with the reversible right hemispheric reduction of CBF that was caused by the segmental vasoconstriction of the right ICA. Reversible reduction of CBF has been reported in patients with classical migraine; the hypoperfusion in the prodrome phase is reversed to hyperperfusion during migraine attack. In the present case, however, the right hemispheric reduction in CBF was observed simultaneously with the attack of migraine when her neurological deficit worsened. This may indicate a coincidence of headache and hemispheric hypoperfusion in a patient with migrainous stroke even though that might be on the way of increasing CBF from the severe hypoperfusion.

Reduction of CBF during prodrome phase is thought to be responsible for the neurological deficits in classical migraine. In the present case, the right hemispheric severe reduction of CBF caused a permanent focal infarction in the right parietal lobe, and the impaired insight to her illness (anosognosia) seen in the acute stage could be related to this lesion. Except for this focal infarct, the right hemispheric ischemia was improved rapidly even when the right ICA lesion still remained severely stenotic in angiogram. It is suggested that the CBF increase occurred much earlier than the complete restoration of the segmental stenotic lesion of the ICA. Reversible stenotic vascular lesion has been reported in some of the patients with migrainous stroke and the relationship between the timing of recovery from neurological deficits and that of resolution of the vascular lesions on repeat angiogram is not consistent among patients. The underlying mechanisms of this reversible segmental vasoconstriction, often seen in patients with migrainous stroke, still remain unknown.

The impaired vascular response to hypercapnia seen in the right hemisphere could be explained by the reactive vasodilatation of small vessels following segmental vasoconstriction of the right ICA. Abnormal vascular responsiveness to $PaCO_2$ and blood pressure changes have been reported in migraine patients during and between the attacks, suggesting a permanent functional abnormality in the brain circulation of such patients. In the present case, however, the reactive vascular dilatation improved in about 1 month, save the right parietal focal lesion in which structural damage had been done to the brain tissue. This particular case demonstrated a reversibility of ischemia and vascular reserve in migraine-related stroke that might be caused by a reversible segmental vasoconstriction.

REFERENCES

1. Call GK, Flemming MC, Sealfon S, Levine H, Kistler JP, and Fisher CM. Reversible cerebral segmental vasoconstriction. *Stroke* 1988; 19:1159–1170.
2. Rothrock JF, Walicke P, Swenson MR, Lyden PD, and Logan WR. Migrainous stroke. *Arch Neurol* 1988; 45:63–67.
3. Lauritzen M, Skyhøj Olsen T, Lassen NA, and Paulson OB. Regulation of regional cerebral blood flow during and between migraine attacks. *Ann Neurol* 1983; 14:569–572.
4. Anderson AR, Friberg L, Skyhøj Olsen T, and Olesen J. Delayed hyperemia following hypoperfusion in classic migraine. *Arch Neurol* 1988: 254–259.
5. Skyhøj Olsen T, Friberg L, and Lassen NA. Ischemia may be the primary cause of the neurological deficits in classic migraine. *Arch Neurol* 1987; 44:156–161.

16

Onset of Migraine Attacks with Aura: Discussion Summary

Olaf B. Paulson

It was debated whether attacks induced by angiography represent spontaneous attacks. Careful comparison of the clinical features has indicated that this is so, and similar data may be found in the literature. One discussant reported patients who had an intraarterial study with an induced attack and who were restudied during a spontaneous attack using single photon emission computed tomography (SPECT). The findings were quite similar, apart from the fact that SPECT studies were not done in the very early phase of the attack. The fact that headache begins while blood flow is still depressed was not challenged during the discussion, since it has been observed by all investigators who have had a chance to measure blood flow at an early time during an attack. On the other hand, there was considerable disagreement about the magnitude of regional cerebral blood flow (rCBF) reduction and why it seems to spread. Based on correction procedures for Compton scatter, it seems that blood flow is reduced to the usual ischemic threshold or below. On the other hand, from several centers patients were presented who had a typical symptomatology and in whom no rCBF abnormalities were observed at all or changes had been very modest. It was suggested that blood flow changes may occur to a variable degree. Although ischemia is definitely present in some patients, it is just as definitively absent in other patients. The spread of hypoperfusion was similar to the spread observed in the animal model of cortical spreading depression, but calculations were presented whereby a similar phenomenon would be observed if blood flow was slowly reduced in a defined area of the brain. This would cause the observation of a spread of hypoperfusion due to Compton scatter. Although such a phenomenon may occur, it was pointed out that it is not compatible with the distinctive slow march of symptoms in migraine patients. Again, the necessity of further studies using positron emission tomography (PET) or other methods with less Compton scattered radiation and better spatial resolution was stressed. Finally, the regulation of cerebral blood flow in this phase of hypoperfusion was discussed. The observed finding has been a preserved autoregulation to blood pressure changes and a reduced reactivity during changes of arterial PCO_2. Because of Compton scatter problems, these findings might not be real, however, and it remains a possibility that blood vessels in the hypoperfused area are totally unresponsive to functional activation, blood pressure changes, and changes in arterial PCO_2.

PART IV
Spontaneous Attacks of Migraine with Aura

17

^{99m}Tc-HMPAO Studies in Migraine with Aura

Paul T. G. Davies and Tim J. Steiner

The Princess Margaret Migraine Clinic, Charing Cross Hospital, London W6 8RF, England

There is strong evidence that changes in cortical blood flow occur during acute migraine with aura. The degree to which regional cerebral blood flow (rCBF) is reduced, and how it changes with time, are key questions in migraine pathophysiology, reflecting the central issue of whether migraine is the clinical manifestation of a neural (1) or a vascular (2) disorder. The poor spatial resolution of ^{133}Xe, with the interference of Compton scatter, has ultimately defeated studies dependent on this technique as a means, on their own, to resolve this problem (3).

With the introduction of ^{99m}Tc-hexamethylpropylene-amine-oxime (HMPAO) and single photon emission computed tomography (SPECT) came a method for rCBF assessment offering good spatial resolution (9 mm at full width half maximum, using the Novo 810 SPECT scanner). The advantage of this technique is offset by its poor ability to follow rCBF changes with time because of intrinsic limitations on minimum intervals between serial scans. Consequently, HMPAO has its value more in complementing ^{133}Xe studies than in any greater likelihood of resolving issues on its own.

We have sought to study acute migraine with aura in different patients in its various stages, relying on increasing the number of attacks studied to provide a temporal sequence of images in onset, development, peak, and resolution.

METHODS

Patients (Table 1)

Patients were selected in two ways from those attending The Princess Margaret Migraine Clinic. Either they were first seen when reporting spontaneously for acute headache treatment or they were kept under follow-up in the routine clinic and encouraged to return, untreated, during a further attack. Migraine has been diagnosed largely according to Vahlquist's (4) criteria, but more recently by IHS criteria (5). Patients with abnormal neurological signs were excluded from the diagnosis of migraine and from this series. All migraine attacks were spontaneous: we have made no studies of induced attacks. Most were untreated before tracer injection. Patients with other types of headache were studied for comparison.

Preparation of ^{99m}Tc-HMPAO

HMPAO (Ceretec, Amersham) was mixed with freshly eluted technetium and 7–10 MBq/kg injected intravenously, within 30 min. Injections were given under standardized conditions of ambient light and noise levels.

Scanning of Cranial Tracer Distribution

Patients were scanned within 30 min of tracer injection, using the Novo 810 high-resolution single-slice acquisition SPET scanner (Table 2). Images were obtained at eight 12.5 mm transverse slices, parallel to the orbitomeatal line, at intervals of 1 cm, each being acquired over 5 min (total scan time: 35–45 min). Images were displayed by computer on a color monitor where regional coloration represented flow as a percentage of the maximum rCBF seen in that slice, according to a calibrated color scale depicted by the computer alongside the image. Quantification was thus relative per slice. Polaroid photographs were taken for easy reference. The analysis of images was

TABLE 1. *Characteristics of the patients studied*

Headache type	N (M:F)	Age range (yrs)	Aura	Headache	Asymptomatic
Migraine with aura	20 (6:14)	25–65	6	19	10
Migraine without aura	27 (4:23)	18–63		15	24
Tension-type	22 (5:17)	18–68		21	2
Cluster	10 (10:0)	36–62		5	10

(Symptoms at time of injection)

TABLE 2. *Novo 810 parameters for acquisition of data*

Energy window	110–170 keV
Number of slices	1–12 (8)
Time per slice	Limited only by computer memory (300 secs)
Slice thickness	1–25 mm (12.5)
Space between slices	5–15 mm (10)
Number of detectors	12
Pixel size	1.5 mm × 1.5 mm
Field of view	21 cm

( ) = Routine setting.

visual and performed by two independent reporters, one blinded to the patient's clinical details. No "abnormality" was regarded as significant unless there was agreement between both.

RESULTS

We have performed 35 scans in patients with migraine with aura (6 during aura, 19 during headache, 10 asymptomatic). Available for comparison were scans from patients with migraine without aura, chronic tension-type headache, and acute and asyptomatic cluster headache (Table 1). Differences between these series were not great, and none was consistent. In the series of patients with migraine with aura, only six scans (17%) indicated any abnormality of rCBF, in two cases during aura and in four with headache. The latter were all studied relatively early (30 min to 2 hr) after onset of the headache phase. The principal feature of abnormality was reduced tracer uptake in the posterior parietooccipital area, corresponding to the watershed between middle and posterior cerebral artery territories, affecting cortex and deep tissue, and not centered on primary visual cortex but in some cases including it (see Fig. 1). These association areas were not inappropriate to the visual aura experienced by patients, and in all cases were on the expected (contralateral) side, suggesting that they might reflect low rCBF and neuronal hypofunction. Nevertheless, cortical changes were inconstant whether observed in the aura or headache phases, and generally minor—not obviously a correlate of dense ischemia. Areas of cortical hyperemia were never imaged, not even at those times when ^{133}Xe studies had suggested they would occur. Deeper asymmetries of flow were of doubtful significance, being occasional and highly variable.

CASE STUDY

A 42-year-old physician had suffered from migraine with and without aura for many years. A few minutes before this SPECT study he had experienced

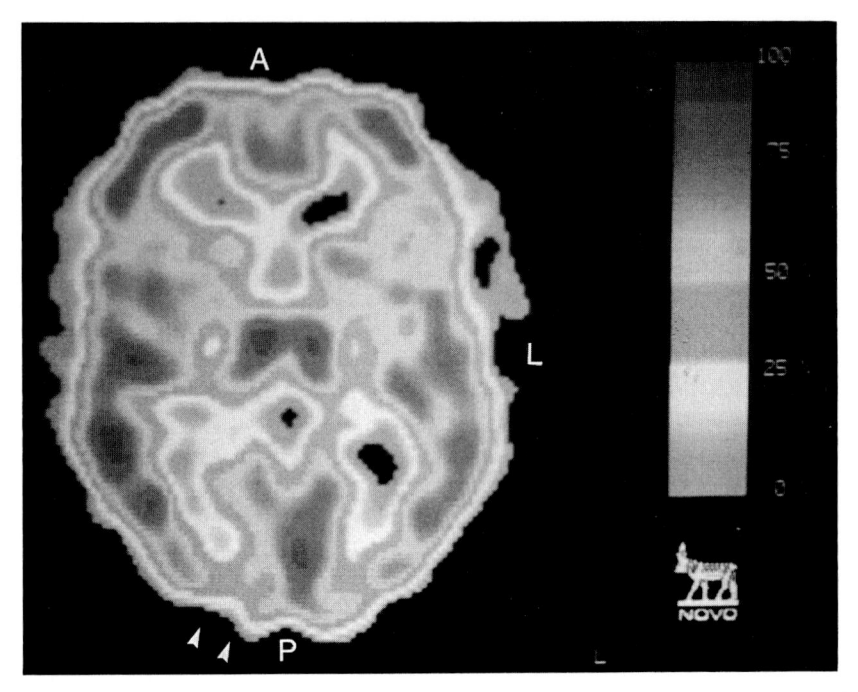

FIG. 1. Representative Novo 810 SPET image showing ^{99m}Tc-HMPAO distribution toward the end of a left-sided visual aura. The slice cuts the occipital and frontal lobes at the level of the thalami in a transverse plane 30 mm above the orbitomeatal line. Regional tracer distribution is expressed as a percentage of maximum according to the scale shown alongside. There is decreased tracer uptake in the right occipital area (arrows). A, anterior; P, posterior; R, right side; L, left side.

15 min of a spreading scintillation in his left visual field. Its cause appeared to be glare from a window in his upper left visual field. There was no headache at the time of the study. He was taking atenolol 100 mg/day as migraine prophylactic treatment.

The study showed a small area of decreased perfusion in the right parietooccipital area (Fig. 1). Increased frontal uptake of tracer was noted but the significance of this is uncertain. When symptom-free, the rCBF images were more symmetrical but not completely normal.

DISCUSSION

These findings give little support to a vascular hypothesis of migraine pathogenesis. Arguably, they are not incompatible with the moderate (25%) reductions in cortical blood flow reported by Olesen (1) in the same occipital area and also extending into the headache phase of the attack. Smaller reductions in tracer uptake may be impossible to identify on visual analysis, and are not excluded by our findings so far. Computerized analysis, under development at The Princess Margaret Migraine Clinic, may yet yield evidence of these.

Meanwhile, it might be remembered that HMPAO as a tracer will not readily reveal generalized hyperemia because of the lack of absolute quantification, rCBF being expressed as a relative distribution through the plane of the brain scanned. It is, furthermore, less than an ideal agent to show focal hyperemia, which its uptake characteristics tend to underestimate. It is best adapted to demonstrate focal areas of low flow which, especially if only of moderate degree, become easily masked in images of poorer spatial resolution. That such areas are seen uncommonly and inconsistently cannot be comfortably reconciled with a belief that ischemia is present invariably, as it must be if this is the process that underlies the whole migraine attack. Having made that point we return to the earlier argument that HMPAO studies, especially analyzed by visual inspection alone, should not be the sole basis for speculation upon pathophysiological issues in migraine: this should come from an overview including ^{133}Xe studies and other imaging modalities.

REFERENCES

1. Olesen J. Migraine and regional cerebral blood flow. *Trends Neurosci* 1985; 7:318–321.
2. Olsen TS, Friberg L, and Lassen NA. Ischaemia may be the primary cause of the neurologic deficits in classic migraine. *Arch Neurol* 1987; 44:156–161.
3. Olsen TS. Migraine with and without aura: the same disease due to cerebral vasospasm of different intensity. A hypothesis based on CBF studies during migraine. *Headache* 1990; 30:269–272.
4. Vahlquist B. Migraine in children. *Int Arch Allergy* 1955; 7:348–355.
5. Headache Classification Committee of the International Headache Society. *Cephalalgia* 1988; 8[Suppl 7]:1–96.

18

Stable Xenon CT-CBF Measurements in Migraine Patients with Aura

John Stirling Meyer, Jun Kawamura, and Yasuo Terayama

Cerebral Blood Flow Laboratory, Veterans Affairs Medical Center, and Department of Neurology, Baylor College of Medicine, Houston, Texas 77020

Fifty years ago, Wolff and coworkers concluded that prodromal symptoms, or aura of migraine, were caused by cerebral vasoconstriction, followed shortly by dilatation of the extracranial and intracranial vessels associated with the characteristic headache (1,2). Many studies have confirmed reductions of cerebral perfusion during the aura of classical migraine and cerebral hyperperfusion during the headache interval using ^{133}Xe intracarotid injection or inhalation methods for measuring cerebral blood flow (CBF), which have supported Wolff's vascular theory (3–13). Recently, based on observations of spreading oligemia, Olesen and colleagues proposed that spreading depression accounts for the pathophysiology of migraine using the ^{133}Xe intracarotid injection method and later single photon emission tomography (SPECT) (14–16), so that controversy still exists concerning the cerebral hemodynamic changes that occur during migraine with aura. Olesen and colleagues do agree, however, that scalp flow is increased on the side of the headache during migraine with aura (17).

The present investigation was designed to elucidate changes in cerebral perfusion during spontaneously occurring migraine with aura by measuring local CBF (LCBF) values using the xenon-enhanced computed tomography (Xe CT-CBF) method.

SUBJECTS

Twelve patients were selected with well established recurrent migraine with aura (Table 1) and results were compared to similar measurements in 22 age-matched normal volunteers. Diagnosis of migraine with aura met criteria required for Classification and Diagnostic Criteria for Headache Disorders, Cranial Neuralgias and Facial Pain (1988) recommended by the

TABLE 1.

Case no.	Age	Gender	Side	Aura
During attacks				
1	22	F	Bil	Photopsia, R-paresthesia
2	21	F	L	L-paresthesia, L-weakness
3	45	F	R	R-paresthesia
4	23	M	R	Photopsia
5	51	F	Bil	Photopsia
6	29	F	L	Photopsia, scotoma
7	45	F	Bil	Photopsia, R-paresthesia
Headache-free				
8	42	M		
9	41	F		
10	27	F		
11	59	F		
12	36	F		

Headache Classification Committee of the International Headache Society (18). The designation of "migraine with aura" corresponded to "classic migraine" as described in the recommendations of the Ad Hoc Committee on Classification of Headache (1962) (19). All patients were asked to discontinue any medications for 48 hr or longer before the measurements.

Patients were divided into two groups according to the presence or absence of headaches at the time of CBF measurements. Out of 12 patients with migraine with aura, 7 patients complained of moderate to severe migraine headache during the CBF examinations. None of the subjects complained of any aura symptoms or prodromes of migraine at the time of the CBF measurements.

Selection of normal volunteers required the following criteria: (a) normal neurological examination and normal Cognitive Capacity Screening Examination; (b) absence by history of any neurological or psychological disorder; (c) exclusion by CT or magnetic resonance imaging (MRI) of any intracranial abnormalities.

CBF MEASUREMENTS

LCBF was measured by CT scanning during inhalation of 27% stable xenon as the contrast agent (Xe CT-CBF method), details of which have been reported previously (20,21). Immediately before the CBF measurements, participants reclined on the CT table while inhaling 100% oxygen for 2 min. The CT levels were selected to include frontal, temporal, parietal, and occipital cortex and caudate nucleus, putamen, and thalamus. After two control CT scans, seven serial CT scans were obtained at 1-min intervals between the second and eighth min of inhalation of xenon gas. Two different high resolution, rapid CT scanners were used for the CBF measurements

(Somatom DR version H, Siemens Medical Systems, Inc., Iselin, New Jersey, or Picker Synerview SX 1200, Picker International, Inc., Ohio). End-tidal partial pressures of xenon gas (PEXe) and carbon dioxide (PECO$_2$) were recorded on a polygraph.

LCBF values were calculated and generated as color-coded images superimposed on each CT slice utilizing desk-top computer programs. Two control scans were used as baseline and seven postenhancement scans were used to define Xe tissue saturation curves according to Kety's formula. The original CT images (512 × 512 pixels) were compressed to 128 × 128 pixels before calculating LCBF values, with precalculation and postcalculation smoothing (3 × 3). By identifying specific anatomical locations on the plain CT images and using the cursor, LCBF values from 11 regions for each hemisphere (22 regions including frontal, temporal, parietal, and occipital cortex, caudate nucleus, putamen, and thalamus, frontal, parietal, and occipital white matter, and internal capsular white matter) were automatically computed.

RESULTS

Figure 1 illustrates the plain CT image and corresponding CBF map at the level of basal ganglia recorded from a 23-year-old man suffering from mi-

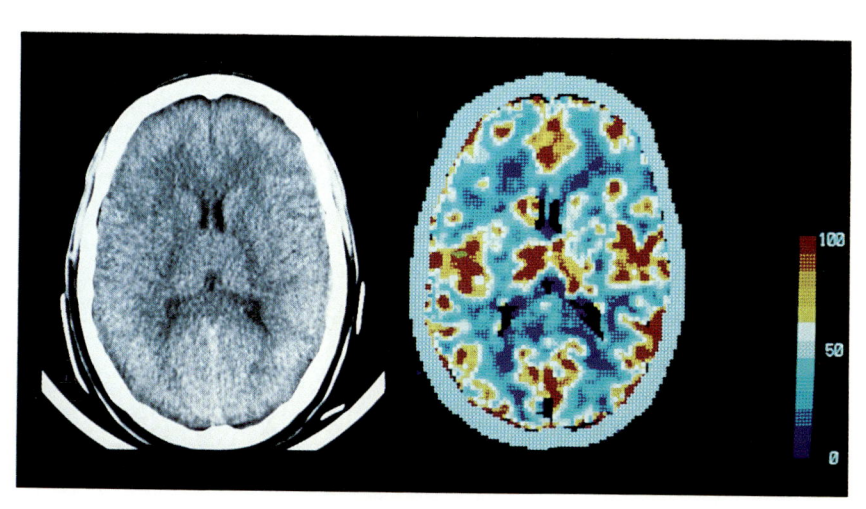

FIG. 1. Plain CT image of the brain at the level of basal ganglia and corresponding LCBF image recorded from a 23-year-old man suffering from migraine with aura. The patient complained of a severe headache predominantly over the right side of the head during the LCBF measurements. LCBF values are markedly increased not only in the cerebral cortex but also in the thalamus, putamen, and caudate nucleus of both hemispheres. No apparent right–left asymmetries are observed.

graine with aura during a typical headache interval (#S168). He complained of a severe migraine headache located predominantly to the right side of the head. LCBF values were markedly increased in the cerebral cortex as well as in the thalamus, putamen, and caudate nucleus of both hemispheres. No apparent right–left asymmetries were observed.

Figure 2 shows pooled mean LCBF values for nine representative cerebral regions in patients suffering from migraine with aura during their headaches compared to normal volunteers. LCBF values for each region are averaged values for both right and left hemispheres. There are significant increases in mean LCBF values for frontal and temporal cortex, putamen, thalamus, and frontal white matter in patients suffering from migraine with aura during the headache interval compared to those measured in normal volunteers.

Of the seven patients measured while suffering from migraine with aura during their headaches, four patients had clear-cut unilateral head pain. In Fig. 3, LCBF values for the nine cerebral regions are compared between the side with and without headaches. For all regions examined, cerebral hyperperfusion is present in the cerebral hemisphere ipsilateral to the head pain as well as in the contralateral hemisphere. There are no significant differences for LCBF values for either hemisphere ipsilateral or contralateral to the head pain.

Figure 4 illustrates mean LCBF values measured in patients suffering from

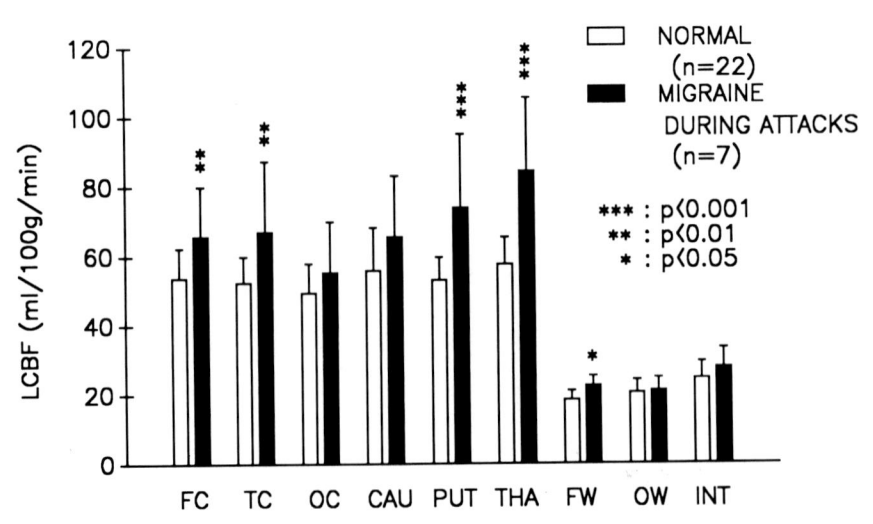

FIG. 2. Pooled mean LCBF values representing nine regions of the brain measured among normal volunteers (n = 22) compared with migraine with aura during attacks (n = 7). LCBF values are significantly increased for frontal and temporal cortex, putamen, thalamus, and frontal white matter in patients compared to normals. FC, frontal cortex; TC, temporal cortex; OC, occipital cortex; CAU, caudate nucleus; PUT, putamen; THA, thalamus; FW, frontal white matter; OW, occipital white matter; INT, internal capsule.

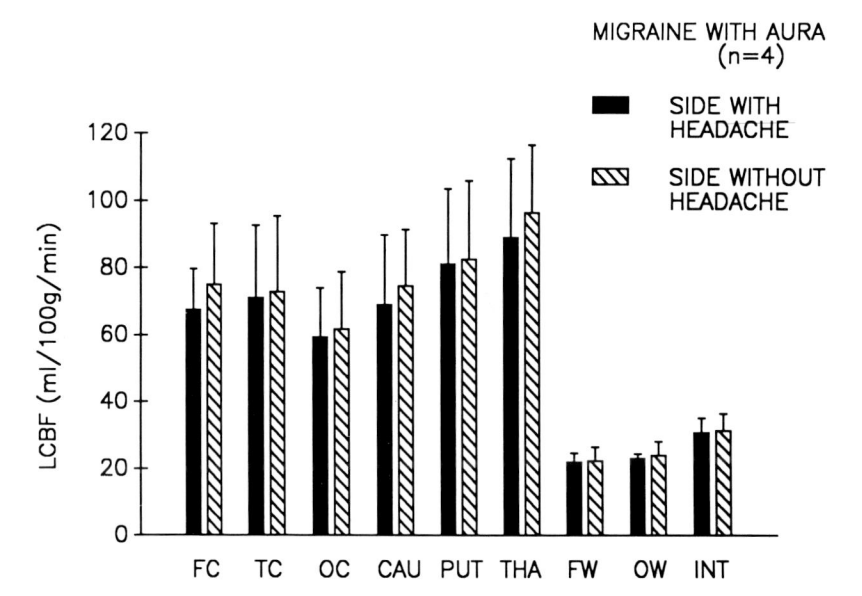

FIG. 3. LCBF values for nine cerebral regions are compared between the side with and without headaches in patients suffering from migraine with aura during attacks of unilateral head pain (n = 4). For all regions examined, cerebral hyperperfusion is present not only in the cerebral hemisphere ipsilateral to the headache but also in the contralateral hemisphere. There are no significant differences for LCBF values between ipsilateral and contralateral hemispheres to the head pain. Abbreviations are as Fig. 2.

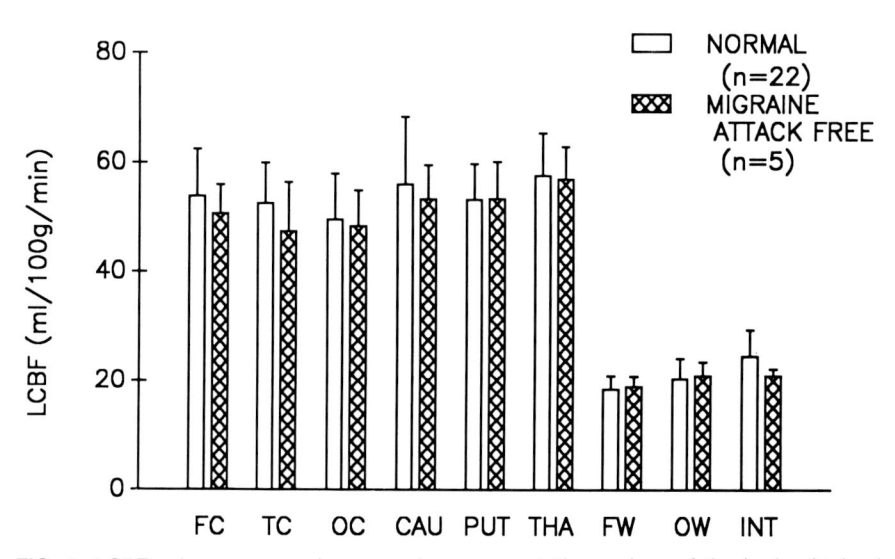

FIG. 4. LCBF values measured among nine representative regions of the brain obtained from patients suffering from migraine with aura when headache-free (n = 5) compared with normals. No statistically significant differences were observed for LCBF values compared for any regions between normals and patients when headache-free. Abbreviations are as for Fig. 2.

migraine with aura during their headache-free intervals compared to similar measures in normal volunteers. There are no significant differences in LCBF values for all cerebral regions between migraineurs when headache-free compared to normal volunteers.

DISCUSSION

Relevant observations noted in the present study can be summarized as follows: (a) in patients measured during their typical migraine headaches, LCBF increases in the cerebral cortex and in subcortical gray matter and white matter; (b) no consistent asymmetries for LCBF increases are noted that can be correlated with the preponderant side of the head pain; (c) there are no differences in LCBF values between patients suffering from migraine with aura when they are headache-free compared with normal volunteers.

There have been many studies reporting CBF changes in patients with migraine during their headache using ^{133}Xe intraarterial or inhalation methods. Skinhøj and Paulson measured rCBF in two patients with migraine and reported that CBF in the entire internal carotid arterial territory was decreased during the aura or the prodromal period of migraine (3). These rCBF reductions were most prominent in cerebral locations, which could be responsible for the prodromal neurological symptoms of patients during their auras. By contrast, marked increases in rCBF were observed throughout the entire internal carotid arterial system during the interval of migraine headache. Likewise, O'Brien, using the ^{133}Xe inhalation method, also reported that cortical perfusion rates were increasing during migraine headache whereas they were decreased during aura (4). Consonant observations have been reported by numerous investigators (5–13).

Sakai and Meyer examined sequential changes of rCBF among patients with different types of headache and among 32 neurologically normal controls using the ^{133}Xe inhalation method (11,12). Significant regional reductions in gray matter blood flow, which correlated with the neurological deficits, were measured during the aura of patients suffering from migraine with aura (classic migraine). In the head pain interval, gray matter flow became increased in direct proportion to the severity of headache. Increases of cephalic blood flow continued for 48 hr after the headache had ceased and gradually subsided to normal values within 6 days. The hyperperfusion during migraine was attributed to either postischemic reactive hyperemia or possibly to functional hyperemia related to the head pain itself, although this was less likely since the hyperemia was diffuse and bilateral.

Later, Olesen et al. reported different observations using the ^{133}Xe intracarotid injection method for measuring rCBF and later utilizing single photon emission computed tomography (SPECT) (14–16). Among patients suffering from migraine with aura, these authors describe a spreading cortical oligemia that began during the aura from posterior portions of the brain and proceeded anteriorly at a speed of 2 mm/min. Cortical oligemia continues during the headache phase. This phenomenon of spreading oligemia was considered to be similar to the spreading cortical depression reported by Leao in rabbit brain (22). It should be mentioned that because at least 15 min are required for clearance of ^{133}Xe, it is technically difficult to measure the evolution of CBF changes over intervals of a few minutes. This becomes even more difficult to assess with SPECT where the isotope remains in the brain for even longer intervals.

The increases in LCBF values of 25% noted in the cerebral cortex in the present study agree with previously reported results. However, this study reports for the first time marked and consistent increases noted during classic migraine headaches with aura that involve not only cerebral cortex but also subcortical structures, including basal ganglia and frontal deep white matter. Previous studies using ^{133}Xe clearance methods were unable to measure LCBF changes in deep subcortical brain structures.

The present observations of bihemispheric increases of LCBF involving subcortical as well as cortical structures during migraine headache do not support the results reported by Olesen et al., who described cortical hypoperfusion during migraine headache with aura (14–16). Although spreading depression is easy to provoke in the cerebral cortex of rabbits, it is difficult to elicit in cats and extremely difficult in the monkey (23). After extensive experience with electrophysiological recordings of the exposed human brain in nearly 1,000 conscious patients undergoing neurosurgical exploration and excision for epilepsy, Gloor stated that the electrical changes typical of spreading depression were never seen in human subjects (24). Local glucose utilization of the cerebral cortex of rats increase during and after recovery from spreading cortical depression; however, cerebral glucose use becomes decreased in thalamus, putamen, and caudate nucleus during spreading depression, confirming the cortical nature of this phenomenon (26). Recently, Andersen, working with Olesen, conceded that delayed cerebral hyperemia does follow the cortical hypoperfusion observed among their patients with migraine with aura during the head pain (26).

A number of theories have been advanced to account for the pathogenesis of migraine. These attempt to explain the characteristic headache and the increase in CBF that accompany them. The fact that the LCBF increases reported here were observed bilaterally, and were not clearly related to the side opposite the preponderant head pain, suggests that they are not functional increases secondary to the head pain alone nor can they be the primary cause of the head pain. It is possible, therefore, that distention of the extracranial arteries may play an important part in the localization of the head pain during migraine with aura, as originally proposed by Wolff et al. (1,2).

In summary, present observations support those previously reported by many others that cerebral perfusion becomes increased during headaches of patients suffering from migraine with aura. Because of improved spatial resolution of the method used, it is clear that these LCBF increases during migraine involve not only the cerebral cortex but also subcortical brain structures including basal ganglia and white matter. These new observations are not consistent with spreading oligemia during headache nor with the theory of spreading cortical depression as a cause of migraine. Observed bilateral hemispheric increases of cortical and subcortical blood flow accompanying migraine headaches are more likely related to altered neurogenic and chemical control of cephalic vasomotor regulation.

REFERENCES

1. Graham JR and Wolff HG. Mechanism of migraine headache and action of ergotamine tartrate. *Arch Neurol Psychiat* 1938; 39:737–763.
2. Schumacher GA and Wolff HG. Experimental studies on headache. A. Contrast of histamine headache with the headache of migraine and that associated with hypertension. B. Contrast of vascular mechanism in preheadache and in headache phenomena of migraine. *Arch Neurol Psychiat* 1941; 45:199–214.
3. Skinhøj E and Paulson OB. Regional blood flow in internal carotid distribution during migraine attack. *Br Med J* 1969; 3:569–570.
4. O'Brien MD (1971): Cerebral blood changes in migraine. *Headache* 1971; 10:139–143.
5. Skinhøj E. Hemodynamic studies within the brain during migraine. *Arch Neurol* 1973; 29:95–98.
6. Simard D and Paulson OB. Cerebral vasomotor paralysis during migraine attack. *Arch Neurol* 1973; 29:207–209.
7. Norris JW, Hachinski VC, and Cooper PW. Changes in cerebral blood flow during a migraine attack. *Br Med J* 1975; 3:676–677.
8. Mathew NT, Hrastnik F, and Meyer JS. Regional cerebral blood flow in the diagnosis of vascular headache. *Headache* 1976; 15:252–260.
9. Edmeads J. Cerebral blood flow in migraine. *Headache* 1977; 17:148–152.
10. Hachinski VC, Olesen J, Norris JW, Larsen B, Enevoldsen E, and Lassen NA. Cerebral hemodynamics in migraine. *Can J Neurol Sci* 1977; 4:245–249.
11. Sakai F and Meyer JS. Regional cerebral hemodynamics during migraine and cluster headaches measured by the ^{133}Xe inhalation method. *Headache* 1978; 18:122–132.
12. Sakai F and Meyer JS. Abnormal cerebrovascular reactivity in patients with migraine and cluster headache. *Headache* 1979; 19:257–266.
13. Meyer JS, Zetusky W, Jonsdottir M, and Mortel K. Cephalic hyperemia during migraine headache. A prospective study. *Headache* 1986; 26:388–397.
14. Olesen J, Larsen B, and Lauritzen M. Focal hyperemia followed by spreading oligemia and impaired activation of rCBF in classic migraine. *Ann Neurol* 1981; 9:344–352.
15. Lauritzen M, Olsen TS, Lassen NA, and Paulson OB. Changes in regional cerebral blood flow during the course of classic migraine attacks. *Ann Neurol* 1983; 13:633–641.
16. Lauritzen M and Olesen J. Regional cerebral blood flow during migraine attacks by xenon-^{133} inhalation and emission tomography. *Brain* 1984; 107:447–461.
17. Iversen HK, Nielsen TH, Olesen J, and Tfelt-Hansen P. Arterial responses during migraine headache. *Lancet* 1990; 336:837–839.
18. Headache Classification Committee of the International Headache Society. Classification and diagnostic criteria for headache disorders, cranial neuralgia and facial pain. *Cephalagia* 1988; 8 [Suppl 7]:1–96.
19. Ad Hoc Committee on Classification of Headache. Classification of headache. *JAMA* 1962; 179:127–128.
20. Meyer JS, Shinohara T, Imai A, et al. Imaging local cerebral blood flow by xenon-

enhanced computed tomography—Technical optimization procedures. *Neuroradiology* 1988; 30:283–292.
21. Imai A, Meyer JS, Kobari M, Ichijo M, Shinohara T, and Oravez WT. LCBF values decline while Lλ values increase during normal human aging measured by stable xenon-enhanced computed tomography. *Neuroradiology* 1988; 30:463–472.
22. Leao AAP. Spreading depression of activity in the cerebral cortex. *J Neurophysiol* 1944; 7:359–390.
23. O'Leary JL and Goldring S. Changes associated with forebrain excitation processes: D.C. potentials of the cerebral cortex. In: Magoun HW, ed. *Handbook of Physiology*. Section 1: neurophysiology. Washington, DC: American Physiological Society, 1959; 1:315–328.
24. Gloor P. Migraine and regional cerebral blood flow. *Trends Neurosci* 1986; 9:21.
25. Shinohara M, Rapoport S, and Sokoloff L. Cerebral glucose utilization: Local changes during and after recovery from spreading cortical depression. *Science* 1979; 203:188–190.
26. Andersen AR, Friberg L, Olsen TS, and Olesen J. Delayed hypermemia following hypoperfusion in classic migraine: Single photon emission computed tomography demonstration. *Arch Neurol* 1988; 45:154–159.

# 19

Xenon 133 Cerebral Blood Flow Measurements in Migraine with Aura

John Stirling Meyer, Jun Kawamura, and Yasuo Terayama

Cerebral Blood Flow Laboratory, Department of Veterans Affairs Medical Center, and Department of Neurology, Baylor College of Medicine, Houston, Texas 77020

The nature of cerebrovascular hemodynamic changes seen in migraineurs with aura and their relation to headache remains controversial. The present study was designed to clarify cerebrovascular mechanisms in patients suffering from migraine with aura by measuring regional cerebral blood flow and cerebral vasomotor responsiveness during headache, during the aura, and during headache-free intervals. The present study, limited to migraine patients with aura, has not been reported previously.

PATIENTS AND METHODS

Regional cerebral blood flow (rCBF) was measured by a modification of the ^{133}Xe inhalation method described by Obrist et al. (1).

Serial measurements of noninvasive rCBF were made in 24 patients with migraine with aura (mean age 33 ± 9 years; 2 men, 22 women) and compared with age-matched normal volunteers (n = 32; mean age 35 ± 12 years, 17 men, 15 women). Attempts were made to obtain rCBF measurements during the headache, during the immediate postheadache interval (2–48 hr after headache had subsided), during aura, and during headache-free intervals.

Cerebral autoregulation was tested by decreasing cerebral perfusion pressure during orthostatic hypotension by tilting the patient 30° head-up by means of a tilt table in six patients with migraine during either the headache, postheadache, or headache-free intervals. Quantitative analyses of impairments of cerebral autoregulation were made by means of the Autoregulation Index (AI) (2).

Cerebral vasomotor responsiveness to either 5% CO_2 in air or 100% O_2 inhalation or to hyperventilation was expressed as Δ%Fg (Δgray matter blood flow) per Δmm Hg $PECO_2$ (Δend-tidal CO_2 tension), and these were tested during the headache (n = 5), postheadache (n = 3), or headache-free (n = 6) intervals.

Normal CO_2 responsiveness was tested by hypercapnia (5% CO_2 inhalation) in 21 patients (53 ± 17 years) and hypocapnia (voluntary hyperventilation) in 17 patients (45 ± 15 years) for purposes of comparison.

RESULTS

During the headache interval, mean Fg values in a group of five patients with migraine with aura (31 ± 9 years old; five women) was significantly higher than those measured during the headache-free interval (headache absent for 5 days or longer) in a group of 13 migraineurs (35 ± 9 years old; 2 men, 11 women: $p < 0.01$). In six patients (32 ± 7 years old; six women) with severe migraine studied 2–24 hr after the headache subsided, mean Fg values remained significantly increased ($p < 0.01$) during the immediate postheadache interval compared with patients who had remained headache-free for 6 days or longer and with normal volunteers. In contrast to the significant increase in rCBF during the headache and immediate postheadache intervals, reduction in rCBF was demonstrated in three patients (32 ± 7; three women) during the prodromal interval (Fig. 1).

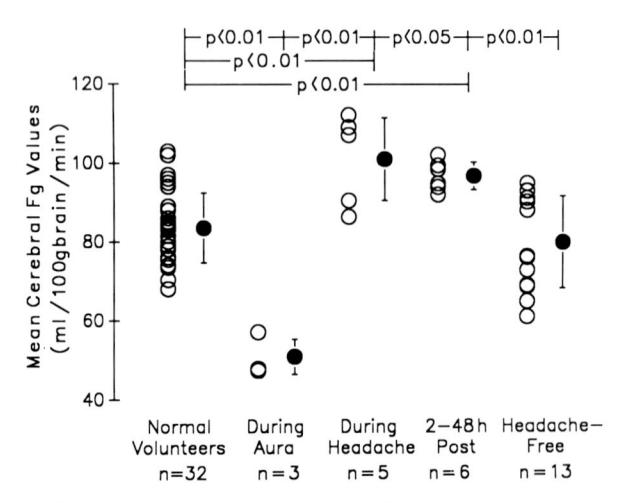

FIG. 1. Mean cerebral Fg values in patients suffering from migraine with aura compared with normal volunteers. During headache in a group of five patients, mean Fg values were significantly higher (100.9 ± 10.5 ml/100 g brain/min) than those measured during the headache-free interval (headache absent for 5 days or longer) in a group of 13 migraineurs (79.8 ± 11.7 ml/100 g brain/min; $p < 0.01$). In six patients with severe migraine, headache preceded by aura and studied 2–24 hr after the headache subsided, mean Fg values remained significantly increased (91.6 ± 12.9 ml/100 g brain/min) compared with patients who were headache-free for 6 days or longer or with normal volunteers ($p < 0.01$).

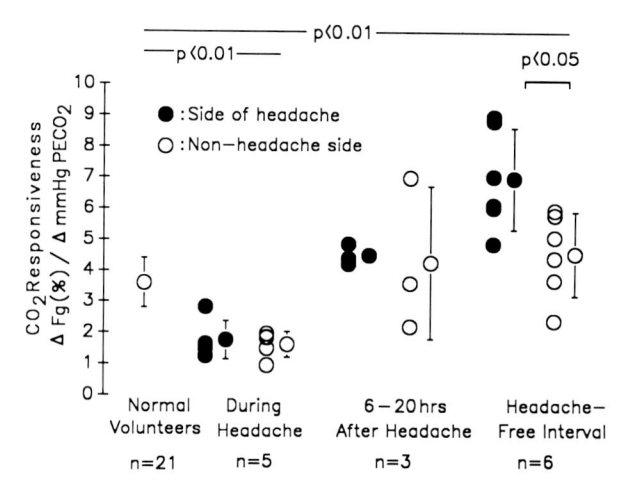

FIG. 2. Mean hemispheric vasodilator responsiveness to 5% CO_2 in patients with migraine with aura comparing the side of the most recent headache with nonheadache side. CO_2 responsiveness in patients during headache was impaired throughout both hemispheres (mean value: 1.25 ± 1.21 △Fg(%)/△mm Hg $PECO_2$; $p < 0.01$) compared with normal volunteers. During headache-free intervals (n = 6), CO_2 responsiveness was excessive (5.8 ± 1.1), with greatest increases in CO_2 responsiveness noted on the side of the usual headache (7.0 ± 1.5 △%Fg/△mm Hg $PECO_2$) and compared with the opposite side (4.6 ± 1.3) ($p < 0.01$).

Dysautoregulation was present in three patients during either the headache phase or during the interval up to 36 hr after subsidence of headache (AI = 2.3 ± 0.8), but dysautoregulation was no longer present after the second day in three patients.

As shown in Fig. 2, CO_2 responsiveness among patients during headache was significantly impaired throughout both hemispheres compared with similar testing in age-matched normal volunteers ($p < 0.01$). However, during the headache-free interval among migraineurs with aura (n = 6), there was excessive cerebrovasodilator responsiveness to 5% CO_2 inhalation with significantly greater CBF increases on the side of the headache compared with the nonheadache side ($p < 0.05$).

The effects of 100% oxygen inhalation on rCBF (3) were measured in six patients with migraine with aura and results indicated similar cerebral vasoconstrictive responsiveness to 100% oxygen inhalation (6.8 ± 3.6%) as was observed in age-matched normal volunteers (n = 10; 6.0 ± 5.6%).

DISCUSSION

During headache among patients suffering from migraine with aura, CBF is increased and remains so for 48 hr after headache has subsided. During the aura, CBF is decreased in regions corresponding to the symptoms of the aura. Cerebrovascular reactivity among patients with migraine with aura during the headache-free interval is characterized by excessive and asymmetric cerebral vasodilator responses to hypercapnia with greater responses on the side of the predominant head pain, despite the fact that cerebral vasodilator responses to hypercapnia are lost or impaired during headache intervals.

While cerebral lactic acidosis, secondary to cerebral ischemia during the interval of aura, has been logically invoked as a contributory cause for impaired cerebral vasomotor responsiveness to changes in end-tidal CO_2 during the prodrome or headache phase of migraine (4,5), excessive CO_2 responsiveness during the headache-free intervals cannot be attributed to this mechanism. Increased cerebral vasomotor CO_2 responsiveness during headache-free intervals among patients with migraine with aura is best attributed to abnormalities of neurotransmitter receptor sites, including both alpha- and beta-adrenergic receptors.

This hypothesis for abnormal cerebrovascular hemodynamic changes among migraineurs is consonant with reports in the literature citing excessive vasomotor responsivity elsewhere in the body among migraineurs (6,7), with abnormalities of innervation and pharmacological response of receptor sites in the iris as indicated by pupillary responses (8) and with increased norepinephrine release (5). These data from numerous sources are adduced to indicate disorders of the autonomic nervous system and vascular receptor sites among migraineurs. The fact that CO_2 responsiveness is exaggerated to a greater degree on the side of the head pain, as observed in the present study, implies that cerebrovascular receptor sites become abnormally activated and may be disordered more in one cephalic region than another. The observation that orthostatic cerebral dysautoregulation is present during the headache among patients with migraine preceded by aura explains their complaints of postural light-headedness and ataxia on standing and worsening of the headache when the head is suddenly lowered.

In conclusion, the evidence provides for the presence of cephalic sympathetic hypofunction with denervation hypersensitivity among migraineurs with aura. Derangements of sympathetic innervation of the cranial arteries are believed to account for the instability of CBF observed in migraineurs when headache-free and to contribute to hemodynamic changes and symptoms during the aura and headache interval.

REFERENCES

1. Obrist WD, Thompson HK, Wang HS, and Wilkinson WE. Regional cerebral blood flow estimated by ^{133}Xe inhalation. *Stroke* 1975; 6:245–256.
2. Meyer JS, Shimazu K, Fukuuchi Y, et al. Impaired cerebrovascular control and dysautoregulation after stroke. *Stroke* 1973; 4:169–186.

3. Deshmukh VD and Meyer JS. Non-invasive measurement of regional cerebral blood flow in man. New York: Spectrum Publications, 1978.
4. Skinhøj E. Hemodynamic studies within the brain during migraine. *Arch Neurol* 1973; 29:95–98.
5. O'Brien MD. Cerebral cortex perfusion rates in migraine. *Lancet* 1967; 1:1036.
6. Appenzeller O, Davidson K, and Marshall J. Reflex vasomotor abnormalities in the hands of migrainous subjects. *J Neurol Neurosurg Psychiat* 1963; 26:447–450.
7. Price RP and Tursky B. Vascular reactivity of migraineurs and non-migraineurs: A comparison of responses to self control procedures. *Headache* 1976; 16:210–217.
8. Fanciullacci M. Iris adrenergic impairment in idiopathic headache. *Headache* 1979; 19:8–13.

20

Xenon 133 SPECT Studies in Migraine with Aura

*Jes Olesen and †Lars Friberg

*Department of Neurology, Gentofte Hospital, University of Copenhagen, DK-2900 Hellerup, and †Department of Clinical Physiology and Nuclear Medicine, Bispebjerg Hospital, DK-2400 Copenhagen NV, Denmark

There is no reliable way (except for carotid angiography) to provoke a migraine attack with aura. All single photon emission computed tomography (SPECT) studies have therefore been done on spontaneous attacks. This poses the problem that it is rare for patients to be able to reach the regional cerebral blood flow (rCBF) laboratory less than 1 hr after onset of aura symptoms. Visual auras, which usually last for 20 min, have thus disappeared half an hour before the patient arrives. Even with longer lasting auras such as those involving both the visual and sensory systems, the aura symptoms have spread to their largest extent and are usually in the resolution phase or have terminated before the first measurement. As discussed by Skyhøj Olsen earlier in this book, focal rCBF reduction, as a rule, persists into the headache phase and outlasts the aura symptoms by minutes or hours. This is the reason why it has been possible to demonstrate focal low flow areas in spontaneous attacks.

REVIEW OF PUBLISHED STUDIES

The first SPECT studies were those of Lauritzen and Olesen (1); theirs was also the first study to follow rCBF changes with repeated measurements before and after treatment as well as outside of attacks. A detailed account of the clinical symptoms of the 11 patients was given, and these data were compared to the actual clinical symptoms on the day of study. The studied attacks were representative. Timing of studies, clinical characteristics, and blood flow results are given in Table 1. Of 11 patients, 3 exhibited a completely normal rCBF. They were studied ⅔–4 hr after onset and again 4 hr later when rCBF was still normal. Two patients had visual symptoms only,

TABLE 1. ^{133}Xe SPECT studies in migraine with aura compared to clinical symptoms

Case no.	Time since onset of attack (hr)	Symptoms during investigation	Blood flow distribution
1	2	Bilateral scintillations terminated 1 hr before, then right hemiparesis/hemianesthesia and rhythmic 10–20 Hz tremor of the right hand, discrete aphasia, and pain on top of head. Symptoms and blood flow unchanged during two following investigations (2½ and 3 hr after onset of attack).	Hypoperfusion of lateral left temporal lobe.
	6½	After treatment (no symptoms).	Hyperperfusion of lateral left temporal lobe.
2	1	Right scintillations, right arm, tongue, and facial paresthesias/hypesthesia terminated 15 min before, then only right hand paresthesias and bifrontal headache. Symptoms and blood flow unchanged in two following investigations (1½ and 2 hr after onset of attack).	Symmetrical perfusion.
	4½	No symptoms.	Symmetrical perfusion.
3	½	Discrete left scintillations, mild bifrontal headache.	Hypoperfusion of mesial and lateral right occipital and lateral posterior temporal lobes.
	1	Mild to moderate right headache.	Hypoperfusion unchanged.
	1½	Moderate right frontal headache, nausea, and photophobia.	Hypoperfusion unchanged.
	7	After treatment (no symptoms).	Symmetrical perfusion.
4	1	Right scintillations, hemiparesis/paresthesias and aphasia at start of attack, then only paresthesias of right arm, photophobia.	Hypoperfusion of lateral left temporal, parietal, and frontal lobes.
	1½	Paresthesias of right arm, left headache, photophobia, nausea. Symptoms and blood flow unchanged in one additional investigation (2 hr after onset of attack).	Hypoperfusion unchanged.
	7	After treatment (no symptoms).	Hypoperfusion of left insula region.
5	⅔	Left scintillations terminated ½ hr before. Then, right headache, nausea, photophobia. Symptoms unchanged in two following investigations (1 and 1½ hr after onset of attack).	Symmetrical perfusion.
	5½	After treatment (no symptoms).	Symmetrical perfusion.
6	3	Bilateral scintillations terminated 2 hr before. Then, left headache, nausea, photo/phonophobia. Symptoms unchanged in the following measurement (3½ hr after onset of attack).	Symmetrical perfusion.

TABLE 1. Continued.

Case no.	Time since onset of attack (hr)	Symptoms during investigation	Blood flow distribution
7	7½ 3½	After treatment (no symptoms). Left scintillations, tongue, throat, and facial paresthesias terminated 1–2 hr before. Then only left hand par/hypesthesias, light right headache. Symptoms and blood flow unchanged in one additional investigation (4 hr after onset of attack).	Symmetrical perfusion. Hypoperfusion of lateral right frontal lobe.
8	6½ 3	After treatment (no symptoms). Left scintillations, mild hemiparesis/paresthesias, right headache, and photo/phonophobia.	Symmetrical perfusion. Hypoperfusion of lateral right occipital temporal and parietal lobes.
9	4½ 2¼	After treatment (no symptoms). Predominantly right scintillations terminated 1½ hr before, right hand paresthesias and aphasia in remission, slight left pressing headache.	Hypoperfusion of lateral right temporal pole. Hypoperfusion of lateral left temporal lobe.
10	5 3	After spontaneous recovery. Bilateral scintillations terminated 2½ hr before, then diffuse, bilateral pressing headache, nausea, and photophobia.	Symmetrical perfusion. Hypoperfusion of left temporal lobe.
11	5 1½	After treatment (no symptoms). Right scintillations terminated 1 hr before, left arm paresthesias and slight bilateral pressing headache.	Hypoperfusion unchanged. Hypoperfusion of lateral left parietal cortex and right temporal pole.
	2	Left arm paresthesias in remission, bilateral pressing headache, phono/photophobia.	Hypoperfusion unchanged.
	6	After spontaneous recovery.	Hyperperfusion of left occipital and right temporal and frontal lobes.

The terms hypoperfusion and hyperperfusion refer to statistically significant differences in flow between the two hemispheres, i.e., a difference of 10% or more between symmetrical brain regions.
From Lauritzen and Olesen, ref. 1, with permission.

but the last patient had scintillations as well as paresthesias involving the right arm, face, and tongue. Eight cases displayed focal low flow areas in the hemisphere giving rise to the aura symptoms. They were studied ½–3½ hr after their first symptom, that is, roughly at the same time as the patients with a normal blood flow. One patient had a low flow area in the right frontal lobe, but the other seven patients had low flow areas in the posterior half of the hemisphere. The flow reduction was largely confined to the cortex and no asymmetries of deeper structures could be demonstrated. The measured average blood flow decrease in the focal region was 17 ± 7% compared with the corresponding contralateral region. When first studied, six patients had headache as their main symptom; two other patients, who were studied during aura symptoms, were restudied in the early phase of headache and still had low flows. The patients were restudied after treatment or after spontaneous recovery 3–7 hr after onset of attack when symptom-free. Blood flow distribution had then normalized in three of the seven patients who previously exhibited a hypoperfusion. In two patients the size of the hypoperfused region had decreased considerably and in one the size and intensity of hypoperfusion was unchanged, whereas in two patients regions of hyperperfusion appeared in either or both hemispheres. It was concluded that the usual duration of hypoperfusion in treated migraine with aura was in the order of 6 hr. A typical example is shown in Fig. 1. There was no change in blood flow on the unaffected side after treatment with ergotamine and metoclopramide, indicating that these drugs do not affect rCBF. At reexamination at least 1 week after attack all but one patient displayed a normal symmetrical blood flow distribution. In a severe hemiplegic case the left insula still showed some degree of hypoperfusion. Comparing global flows at onset of attack, after treatment and outside of attack, there was no significant difference.

In two patients Lauritzen and Olesen (1) observed the development of increased focal perfusion at 6 hr. This and the studies of Sakai and Meyer (2) and Gullichsen and Enevoldsen (3) led to a further investigation with emphasis on the later phases of attacks (4). The study involved 12 patients studied during attacks of migraine with aura. Three had normal rCBF and nine initially displayed focal low flow regions. These patients were then studied repeatedly. In two patients the low flow area disappeared and rCBF became normal. Detailed results of the seven remaining patients are given in Table 2. A typical case is shown in Fig. 2. The first study was done between 0.5 and 2.5 hr after onset and patients were then restudied after another 2–7 hr and after approximately 24 hr. Three patients had only visual aura, whereas four also had sensory and/or other symptoms. A common pattern was seen in all patients: a focal low flow region transforming after hours into hyperperfusion. The low flow area was present at the first examination in all patients. At the second measurement it was still present in one patient 3 hr after onset, whereas the other patients 3–9 hr after onset already had hyperperfusion. The one patient with hypoperfusion at 3 hr had hyperperfusion at 6 hr after onset. Of five patients studied between 20 and 31 hr after onset, three had normal symmetrical perfusion and two still displayed some hyperperfusion. The delayed hyperperfusion was focal and always located to the previously hypoperfused area. It usually occurred at a time when the headache was beginning to regress and was changing from throbbing to pressurelike (4). Hyperperfusion outlasted headache in two patients and head-

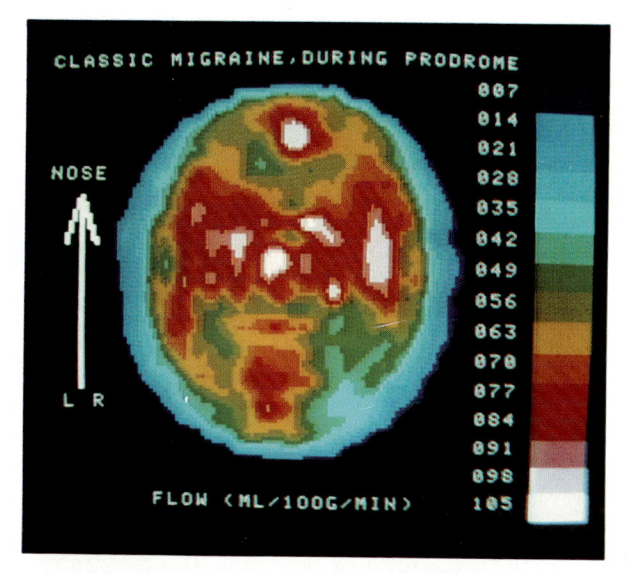

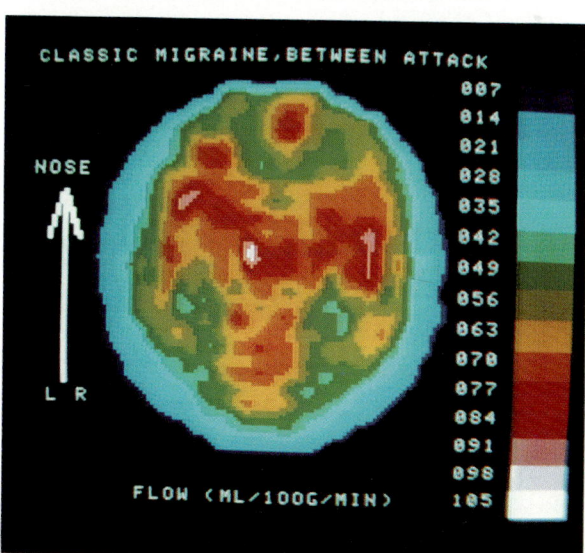

FIG. 1. rCBF tomograms in a migraineur studied when his visual aura symptoms had almost ended. **A:** The patient had a mild right frontal headache. The tomogram 5 cm above the orbitomeatal line showed hypoperfusion in the right occipital and temporal cortex (the picture is viewed from above, right being right, anterior being up). Blood flow values in ml/100 g/min are translated into colors on the scale to the right. **B:** The patient was studied outside of an attack and the rCBF map is normal and symmetrical. (From Lauritzen and Olesen, ref. 1, with permission.)

TABLE 2. ^{133}Xe SPECT studies of the later phases of migraine attacks with aura compared to clinical symptoms rCBF in Classic Migraine[a]

Case	Time since onset of attack	Symptoms during investigation	rCBF
1	2 hr	Left hemianopia, right headache	Right occipital hypoperfusion
	6 hr	Right headache	Right occipital hyperperfusion
	1 wk	Interval headache	Symmetrical perfusion
2	0.7 hr	Left-sided fortifications	Right occipital hypoperfusion
	4 hr	Slight bilateral headache	Right occipital hyperperfusion
	1 wk	No symptoms	Symmetrical perfusion
3	0–1 hr	Aphasia, right hemianopia, right hemiplegia, right hemiparesthesia	—
	2.5 hr	Bilateral headache, photophobia	Left temporal pole and left frontal lobe hypoperfusion
	25 hr	Slight bilateral headache	Left temporal pole and left frontal lobe hyperfusion
	1 wk	No symptoms	Normal symmetrical perfusion
4	1 hr	Left hemiparesthesia, left hemianopia	Right occipital hypoperfusion
	3 hr	Bilateral headache	Right occipital hyperperfusion
	31 hr	No symptoms	Almost normal perfusion
	1 wk	No symptoms	Normal symmetrical perfusion
5	0.5 hr	Left hemiplegia, left hemiparesthesia, right unilateral headache	Right occipital, temporal, frontal, and basal ganglia hypoperfusion
	3 hr	Slight left, weakness, bilateral headache	Hypoperfusion in same areas
	6 hr	Slight interval headache	Hyperperfusion in same areas
	22 hr	No symptoms	Less hyperemia in same areas
	1 wk	No symptoms	Normal symmetrical perfusion
6	0–1 hr	Left hemianopia, left hemiparesthesia	—
	1.5 hr	Bilateral headache	Right occipital and parietal hypoperfusion
	9.5 hr	Slight throbbing headache	Right occipital and parietal hyperperfusion
	20 hr	No symptoms	Symmetrical perfusion
	1 wk	No symptoms	Symmetrical perfusion
7	0.33 hr	Right hemianopia	—
	1.3 hr	Bilateral headache	Right occipital and parietal hypoperfusion
	4 hr	Bioccipital headache	Right occipital and parietal hyperperfusion
	5 hr	Bioccipital headache	Symmetrical perfusion
	1 wk	No symptoms	Symmetrical perfusion

[a] Time of relation of blood flow distribution to symptoms. Left- and right-sided hemispheric changes are related to contralateral neurologic deficits.
From Andersen et al., ref. 4, with permission.

ache outlasted hyperperfusion in one patient whose hyperperfusion has disappeared by 5 hr.

A few results from a large new series of patients studied by our group have been presented in abstract form (5). Of 29 patients studied during an attack, focal low flow areas were discovered in 24. In some patients we have observed a focal hyperperfusion similar to the observations of Andersen et

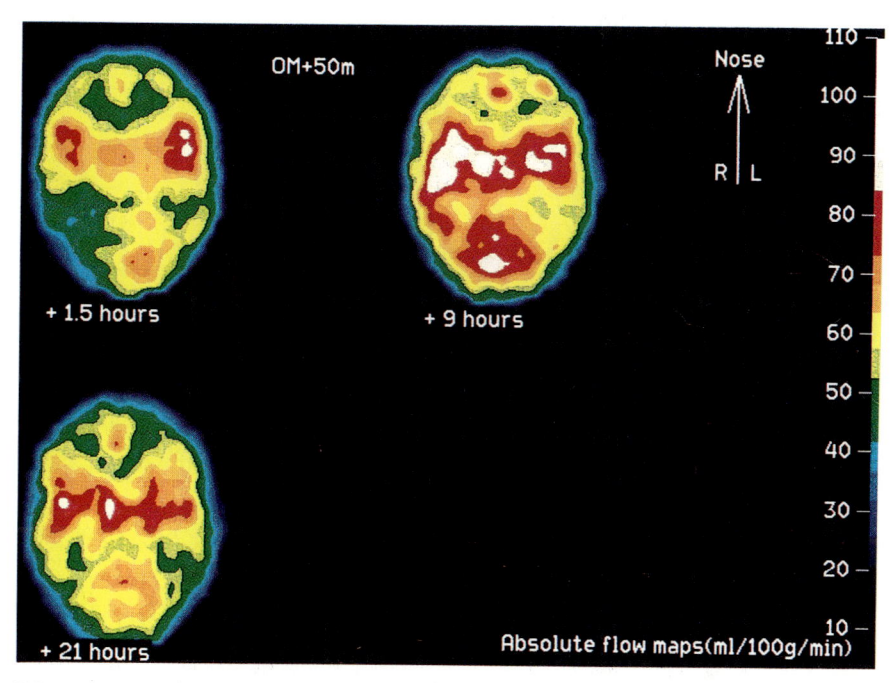

FIG. 2. ^{133}Xe SPECT study of a man studied 1.5 hr after onset of a left homonymous negative scotoma and numbness as well as paresthesias in the left hand spreading to the tongue. There is a low flow area in the right occipital region. In the same area blood flow has increased to above normal at 9.5 hr and, finally, at 20 hr the blood flow map is normal and symmetrical. (From Andersen et al., ref. 4, with permission.)

al. (4), but no patient has demonstrated a marked global flow increase such as those reported by Sakai and Meyer (2) and Juge (6).

Most recently, Olesen et al. (7) combined this new series of patients with some previous studies to obtain a more coherent picture of temporal and topographical events during migraine with aura. In analyzing the early phase of the attacks, intracarotid studies were also included. The material totalled 63. The aura symptoms occurred before headache in 56 patients and simultaneously with the headache in 1 patient, but headache was never present before hypoperfusion. In the early headache phase rCBF was focally reduced in 34 patients, normal in 7, and increased in 2. At later stages of the attack, hyperperfusion or normal rCBF was observed. Hyperperfusion outlasted headache in 11 patients, occurred before headache in 2 patients and, in one patient, headache outlasted the hyperperfusion. The temporal relationships between blood flow, aura symptoms, and headache are schematically shown in Fig. 3.

rCBF was studied with SPECT in 43 patients. Abnormalities were unilat-

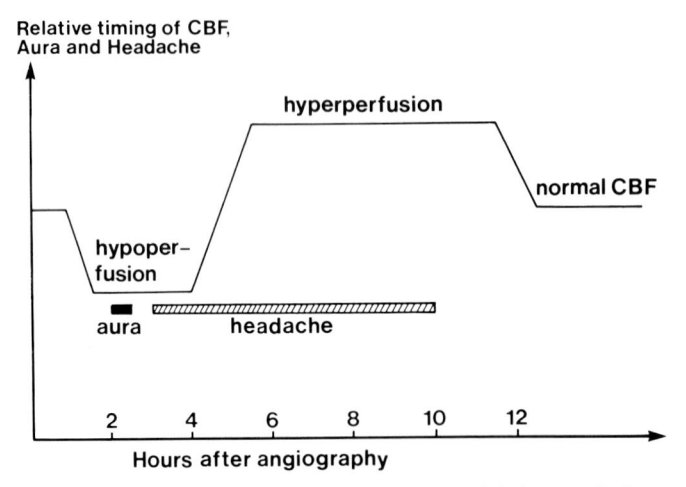

FIG. 3. The temporal relation between angiography (time 0 hr), hypoperfusion, aura, headache, hyperperfusion, disappearance of headache, and disappearance of hyperperfusion. The time axis is chosen to illustrate what is typical. The angulation of the flow curve is to show that we do not know details about how fast flow changes. The real course of rCBF changes is probably smooth. (From Olesen et al., ref. 7, with permission.)

eral in 36 and bilateral in 3 whereas rCBF was normal in 4. Only one patient displayed bilateral somatosensory disturbances, whereas all other patients with somatosensory motor or speech auras had unilateral symptoms. Three patients had pure bilateral visual aura. Another five patients had bilateral visual aura and unilateral symptoms in the extremities. In patients with unilateral abnormalities of rCBF, the aura symptoms originated from the same hemisphere in 53 patients and from the other hemisphere in 1 patient. They were bilateral in two patients. The headache was unilateral in 40 patients, bilateral in 19, absent in 3, and not described in 1. Of 38 patients in whom both headache and aura were unilateral, 35 perceived headache and aura symptoms as contralateral to each other, that is, the headache was located over the affected hemisphere. In only three patients were the aura symptoms and headache perceived as ipsilateral, that is, the headache was over the nonaffected hemisphere ($p < 0.01$). Of 19 patients with bilateral headache, 6 had bilateral symptoms of aura, 8 had left-sided, and 5 right-sided aura symptoms. In these 19 patients, rCBF changes were bilateral in 2, right-sided in 8, and left-sided in 8; normal flow was observed in 1 patient. Of 10 patients with bilateral aura (including 5 with the bilateral visual aura but unilateral aura in the extremities) 6 had bilateral and 4 unilateral headache; changes in rCBF were bilateral in 2 patients, unilateral in 7, and absent in 1 patient. Thus, the migrainous cerebral process, as reflected by abnormalities in the rCBF, was usually unilateral. Aura symptoms originated from the same hemisphere and, when it was unilateral, headache was located over the same hemisphere.

CONCLUSION

Results of the three published studies and our unpublished series are in agreement. The picture that emerges is the following: In the aura phase and early headache phase of migraine, a focal hypoperfusion is observed corresponding to the location expected from the nature of the aura symptoms. It is unilateral in the great majority of cases. Headache is also located over this area but, not infrequently, it may be bilateral despite unilateral aura symptoms and/or unilateral rCBF reduction. Via a transitional phase with normal rCBF, hypoperfusion is followed by hyperperfusion in the same region. There is a wide variation in the timing of these events. We have observed hypoperfusion to disappear earlier than 2 hr after onset of aura. An even earlier change has been observed in intracarotid studies (8). On the other hand, we have observed hypoperfusion at 5 hr, indicating that it may last longer. Hyperperfusion has been observed already at 3 hr and, in some, is still present after 24 hr. In others hyperperfusion was gone already at 5 hr (4). As best we can tell from our scattered observations, with pure visual aura hypoperfusion is located at the occipital or occipitoparietal lobes. When patients had sensory symptoms, hypoperfusion was located in the parietal lobe and sometimes the temporal lobe. Aura symptoms of hemiparesis or aphasia were associated with hypoperfusion further anteriorly. Variability pertains not only to the size of the brain regions affected and to the timing of events but also to their intensity. This again seems to reflect the severity and duration of the aura symptoms. A further variable is the drug treatment of attacks. Lauritzen and Olesen (1) gave ergotamine and observed hyperemia in only 2 of 11 patients. Anderson et al. (4) gave aspirin and metoclopramide, which have no known vascular effects, and observed hyperemia in 7 of 12 patients. Perhaps constriction of large arteries caused by ergotamine (9) partially inhibits the development of hyperemia.

Despite the extreme variability in symptoms and rCBF findings, careful correlation between symptoms and repeated rCBF measurements in the individual patient have demonstrated a coherent picture of rCBF abnormalities in migraine with aura. There is little doubt that headache is a reflection of the pathological process in one hemisphere, which causes focal hypoperfusion. It is also clear that hyperperfusion is not related to headache, neither at its onset nor at its termination. Hyperperfusion must be viewed as an epiphenomenon secondary to the initial process.

REFERENCES

1. Lauritzen M and Olesen J. Regional cerebral blood flow during migraine attacks by Xenon-133 inhalation and emission tomography. *Brain* 1984; 107:447–461.
2. Sakai F and Meyer JS. Regional cerebral hemodynamics during migraine and cluster headache measured by the 133-Xe inhalation method. *Headache* 1978; 18:122–132.
3. Gullichsen G and Enevoldsen E. Prolonged changes in rCBF following attacks of migraine accompagnee. *Acta Neurol Scand* 1984; 69[Suppl 98]:270–271.
4. Andersen AR, Friberg L, Olsen TS, and Olesen J. SPECT demonstration of delayed hyperemia following hypoperfusion in classic migraine. *Arch Neurol* 1988; 45:154–159.
5. Friberg L, Olesen J, and Iversen H. Regional cerebral blood flow during attacks and when free of symptoms in a large group of migraine patients. *Cephalalgia* 1989; 9[Suppl 10]:29–30.
6. Juge O. Regional cerebral blood flow in the different clinical types of migraine. *Headache* 1988; 28:537–549.
7. Olesen J, Friberg L, Olsen TS, et al. Timing and topography of cerebral blood flow, aura and headache during migraine attacks. *Ann Neurol* (in press).
8. Norris JW, Hachinski VC, and Cooper PW. Changes in cerebral blood flow during a migraine attack. *Br Med J* 1975; 3:676–677.
9. Tfelt-Hansen P. The effect of ergotamine on the arterial system in man. *Acta Pharmacol Toxicol* 1986; 59[Suppl 3]:1–29.

21

Migraine with Aura: Discussion Summary

T.J. Steiner

In this section three presentations of different methods for blood flow measurement and imaging have raised many issues. To keep the correct perspective on these, we should avoid overspecified questions arising from individual cases or atypical attacks, and series concentrating on particularly severe migraine. We know everyone shows their most dramatic images.

We need to concentrate on three issues. First, what do the different techniques actually show? Second, do the different studies all show the same thing, or, if they do not because they are looking at different aspects of the problem, are they showing findings compatible with each other? Third, although this discussion may be better left for later sessions concerned more specifically with pathophysiology, how do we interpret the various findings in line with what we understand of the mechanisms of the migraine symptom complex, especially aura?

Taking an overview first, the technetium-labeled hexamethyl-propylene-amine-oxime (HMPAO) studies from the Charing Cross Group show principally, perhaps only, changes indicative of hypoperfusion in the occipital cortex and deeper tissue, affecting association areas more than primary visual cortex, but certainly extending sometimes to involve the latter. These changes are inconsistent and variable, and seen in a minority of cases, more during the aura phase than during headache, and more during headache than during the asymptomatic period. When they are seen they appear to be real. No hyperemic changes have been imaged with HMPAO in any stage of the attack. In contrast, the Houston studies with stable Xenon feature a diffuse cortical and subcortical hyperemia as the principal finding. This is of a magnitude 25–30% over normal flow and is seen during the headache phase, from 6–12 hr after its onset and persisting for up to 48 hr. These hyperemic changes are never characterized by asymmetry even when the headache is noticeably unilateral. They normalize during the attack-free period. In the studies from Copenhagen with xenon 133 and single photon emission computed tomography (SPECT), the significant features first have been a 20–25% focal reduction in flow affecting the occipital area on the neurologically symptomatic side and, second, in the same area, reversal to hyperemia. This later phase may be imaged after 3–8 hr and may still be seen after some 20 hr, being 15–20% over normal flow.

Can we establish consensus views on these separate issues: generalized hyperemia occurring as an aftermath to the attack, focal hyperemia in the brain area presumed to give rise to the neurological symptoms of the aura, and preceding focal oligemia in this same area? Diffuse hyperemia shown convincingly by stable xenon has not been described in the ^{133}Xe SPECT series presented here, nor in the HMPAO series. Yet, review of some of Olesen's studies suggests that similar appearances—a bilateral hyperemia affecting both cortex and deep gray matter—may be visualized during approximately the same time period. The difficulty with HMPAO studies is that, through lack of ability to quantify absolute flow, they cannot reliably demonstrate a *generalized* increase in blood flow. Some possibility is afforded by images corrected by standardizing cerebellar flow, assuming that cerebellar flow is not affected by the migraine process, but the technique for this is not well agreed. It should also be remembered that HMPAO is not an ideal tracer for imaging hyperemia, which it tends to underestimate. But from the xenon studies there appears to be consensus that in some cases at least there is a late diffuse hyperemia, and this is to be regarded in some way as part of the migrainous process.

Turning to the issue of focal hyperemia, it has been argued on simple physiological grounds that if focal ischemia is a feature of migraine with aura then we must expect focal hyperemia in the same area subsequently. Do we see it? Xenon studies certainly show it in some cases, and it is particularly evident in some of the SPECT studies of Olesen. Again with HMPAO, it has not been seen in the series of Davies, nor has it been seen by the Italian group of De Benedittis. There needs to be more studies using HMPAO with careful assessment of the possibility of focal hyperemia, which is better visualized with this technique than generalized changes, and in terms of spatial resolution HMPAO and SPECT may be the preferred method. The main problem may be timing. Patients with acute migraine must be imaged as and when they appear, but of course the emphasis has been on imaging as early as possible to see changes related to the aura, and it is possible that later changes are being overlooked because of this. Meanwhile, further consensus has been reached that focal hyperemia is a feature of many xenon studies and we should believe that these changes are a reflection of the pathophysiology of the migraine attack with aura.

This leads to perhaps the most important issue—that of focal oligemia, which has been seen with all methods. The area affected is the parietooccipital watershed area, which has already been referred to as the "migraine area," involving gray and white matter, and this is agreed by all groups. The focus may therefore be in association areas rather than in the primary visual cortex, which may cause difficulty in relating the precise site of these oligemic changes to the neurological symptoms of the typical migraine aura.

But even with xenon these changes have not been constant, and some patients with marked aura symptoms have been imaged with blood flow appearing to remain normal throughout.

So, we come to the crux of the whole discussion. We agree that low flows occur in this area but, remembering that it is not always imaged at all, how low is this low flow? Is it sufficient to be interpreted as ischemia rather than merely oligemia, compatible with a process that underlies pathophysiologically the whole migraine attack? It is certainly difficult to take this view from the HMPAO studies where the changes do not appear to be so severe, but the lack of quantification with this technique makes this a difficult conclusion to be sure about. The changes with xenon are of greater magnitude at least in some cases, and may well be compatible with ischemia. Dr. Moskowitz, on the basis of his experimental studies of postischemic hyperemia in animals, has suggested that the focal migraine hyperemia is more indicative of a response to prolonged minor oligemia rather than intense ischemia, which would inevitably give rise to a hyperemic phase occurring sooner. The way in which lactic acidosis in this area may alter the underlying vasoconstrictor tone is uncertain. Dr. Meyer has observed that there is no threshold for the development of lactic acidosis, which will begin as soon as there is any element of ischemia and may transform images to give the appearance of normal flow. There are, however, limited data from positron emission tomography (PET) studies, some of which suggest a high oxygen extraction ratio in the area concerned, clearly indicating ischemia if this is the case. However, the great logistic problems with PET have meant these studies are few. As a final consensus, we agree that it would not fit the data so far available from all of these imaging modalities to say that in all cases the symptoms of aura are caused by dense ischemia. It may not yet be possible to rule this out as an explanation, but those who hold this view of migraine pathophysiology are in the position of needing to produce the evidence to substantiate it.

In summary, therefore, we have agreed over a number of points and future studies will determine whether or not we are correct in these conclusions. At the beginning of the attack of migraine with aura there is commonly a focal oligemia in the so-called migraine area at the watershed of middle cerebral and posterior cerebral artery territories in the parietooccipital area.

Evidence does not support the proposal that in all cases, or even any, these changes amount to ischemia, but this possibility is not so far excluded. Subsequently, in this same area there is a reversal to focal hyperemia, seen 3–8 hr after the onset of symptoms, which may persist for many hours. Over a similar or longer time course there is reasonable evidence of a more diffuse hyperemia more anteriorly, which is bilateral and affects cortex and deep tissues at the level of the basal ganglia. These changes may persist until perhaps 48 hr after the onset of the attack.

Future studies should emphasize longitudinal investigation of the same patients, with serial scanning with imaging modalities that allow this. Studies with xenon are most likely to clarify the hyperemic changes, unless groups using HMPAO find that techniques of standardization can be employed to reveal assymetrical or focal hyperemic areas. There is a pressing need to look more carefully at the initial oligemic changes and to resolve once and for all the question of whether these are ischemic. Of the modalities available, PET is potentially most able to answer this question, but the severe logistic problems inherent in PET throw doubt on whether it will do so with isotopes that are available at present. It is perhaps worrisome that HMPAO, which is well suited to the imaging of focally reduced blood flow, fails to see such changes in the majority of cases. However, in all studies timing is a problem with spontaneous attacks, and the occasions of access to patients at the very onset of the aura are inevitably few. Although oligemic changes have been seen many hours later, even in the headache phase, there is no reason to assume that they have persisted in the same degree. Therefore we need emphasis on very early studies as well as serial scans taken later in the attack when the hyperemic stages develop. Given the time scale of the latter—up to 48 hr—serial scanning is clearly possible even with the technetium-labeled HMPAO.

PART V
Mechanisms of Migraine with Aura

Migraine and Other Headaches:
The Vascular Mechanisms,
edited by Jes Olesen.
Raven Press, Ltd., New York © 1991.

22

Mechanisms of Migraine with Aura

Primary Ischemia

Tom Skyhøj Olsen

The Department of Clinical Physiology and Nuclear Medicine, Bispebjerg Hospital, DK-2400 Copenhagen NV, Denmark

Focal brain ischemia leads to neurological deficits. The concept that the neurological deficits in the migraine aura are caused by ischemia is therefore not unreasonable. However, the presentation of the neurological deficits most often is quite different from that of transient ischemic attacks. Characteristically, the patient experiences "marching" symptoms. Because the rate of speed of the "march" is much like that of a spreading depression (1), this process has been suggested as the cause of the aura symptoms (i.e., a neural cause) (2). During spreading depression, the blood flow is only modestly reduced, and values consistent with ischemia are not measured (3). During the 1970s early investigators of cerebral blood flow (CBF) in migraine with aura, however, reported markedly reduced flow during the aura with flow values below or approaching the ischemic threshold (3–6). In the early 1980s these reports were challenged in CBF studies performed with multidetector equipment (7,8). On average, CBF was found to be only modestly reduced. The focal hypoperfusion exhibited a spreading character as the low flow area became larger and larger during the aura. No consistent relation between CBF and the appearance/disappearance of symptoms was seen. In fact, hypoperfusion was present some time before the patient experienced symptoms and the symptoms disappeared at a time when the CBF changes had reached a maximum (8). Focal hypoperfusion might even persist for hours after the symptoms had disappeared (9). During recent years a neural mechanism in particular spreading depression has been considered the most likely cause of migraine with aura (10). However, the blood flow studies on which this neural theory have found support can also be interpreted in the opposite direction (11–13)—supporting the vascular theory that enjoyed popularity in the 1960s and 1970s (14). Making use of this interpretation, this chapter attempts to explain migraine with aura as being primarily the result of vascular changes that give rise to ischemia.

THE BLOOD FLOW REDUCTION DURING THE AURA

CBF decreases focally in the brain during the aura. Using the ^{133}Xe intracarotid injection technique, Skinhøj (4), Simard and Paulson (5), and Hachinski et al. (6) recorded marked blood flow reductions to the ischemic threshold. Olesen et al. (7) and Lauritzen et al. (8), proponents of the neural theory, also recorded CBF values around the ischemic threshold. Olesen et al. (7) reported ischemic flow values to be present in one of seven patients and Lauritzen et al. (8) reported small areas of ischemia within the low flow areas in six of nine patients studied during the aura. There is general agreement, therefore, that CBF may be reduced to ischemic values in at least small regions of the hypoperfused areas. Olesen et al. (7), however, stressed that mean CBF in the low flow areas usually (six of seven patients) was far above the ischemic threshold and calculated the reduction to average 35%. It was concluded, therefore, that the CBF reduction was not of a sufficient magnitude to explain the symptoms except in one of seven patients. Lauritzen et al. (8) stressed that the mean regional perfusion in nine oligemic areas was close to or above 40 ml/100 g/min and, thus, well above the threshold for producing ischemia. This quantitative consideration supported their conclusion that ischemia was not of primary importance in the development of focal migraine symptoms. Thus, according to these two studies there was no substantial evidence to support the idea that ischemia was present during migraine with aura. Therefore, they found no evidence to support the vascular theory of migraine with aura.

Skyhøj Olsen et al. (11) and Skyhøj Olsen and Lassen (12) studied 11 patients with the ^{133}Xe intracarotid injection technique. In their evaluation they stressed the importance of Compton scatter on the results of the blood flow studies. This phenomenon is accounted for in details elsewhere in this book. In short, Compton scatter gives rise to an overestimation of CBF in low flow areas (11,12,15). The effect is most pronounced in the areas closest to the nonaffected surroundings and the influence decreases with the distance to the normally perfused surroundings. Thus, the influence is least pronounced in the areas farthest from the normally perfused part of the brain. If true CBF is the same in the entire low flow area, the best estimate of CBF is found in the areas farthest from the normally perfused surroundings. The effect of Compton scatter is also directly related to CBF in the nonaffected part of the brain. The higher the CBF in this part of the brain the higher the overestimation of CBF in the low flow area.

When evaluating the CBF studies in light of the Compton scatter, it was concluded that the CBF reduction was at the level of 50% (11,12). When this phenomenon was not taken into account the CBF reduction was only at the level of 25% (8). They concluded, therefore, that CBF most likely decreases to the ischemic level in all their cases and that this degree of blood flow reduction is present in the entire low flow area, that is, the entire low flow area is ischemic. This is in contrast to the reports of Olesen et al. (7) and Lauritzen et al. (8), but these investigators did not account for Compton scatter in their studies.

ISCHEMIA DURING THE AURA?

Although the blood flow is decreased below the ischemic threshold it does not mean that ischemia is present in the low flow areas. In ischemia the blood flow is so low that normal energy metabolism cannot be maintained. In migraine the neurones might be conditioned in one way or the other, so that they could be more resistant to ischemia during the attack. Positron emission tomography (PET) might answer the question whether ischemia is present or not during migraine with aura. PET has, however, only been performed in two patients during migraine aura (16). The results were inconclusive. In one patient CBF was focally reduced and the oxygen extraction fraction was increased, but the cerebral oxygen consumption was normal. According to the authors this finding could be taken as evidence of ischemia during the aura. However, in the other patient, CBF, oxygen extraction, and oxygen metabolism were normal.

What speaks in favor of ischemia? First, the fact that neurological deficits occur during the aura. Second, that the neurological deficits that occur during the aura sometimes persist. Persisting abnormalities has been reported on electroencephalography (EEG) (17,18), computed tomography (CT) (19,20), and CBF studies with single photon emission computed tomography (SPECT) (21). Spreading depression is, however, a fully reversible process that does not damage the neurones (22). The EEG abnormalities accompanying spreading depression are normalized within 10 min (10) and evoked potentials are normalized within about 15 min after the start of the depression (23). Spreading depression, therefore, cannot explain persistent neurological deficits or persistent abnormalities on EEG, CT, or SPECT. It is now well documented that the low flow area that occurs during the aura changes into a hyperemic area 3–6 hr after onset of the attack (24). It is not known whether the low flow area that follows spreading depression also changes into a hyperemia. However, in stroke it is well known that focal ischemia due to arterial occlusion changes into focal hyperemia after removal of the occluding material—postischemic hyperemia (25). In migraine with aura the change of the low flow area into a hyperemia might be considered as reactive postischemic hyperemia and, thus, evidence of ischemia during the aura.

THE RELATION BETWEEN APPEARANCE/DISAPPEARANCE OF AURA SYMPTOMS AND BLOOD FLOW CHANGES

The focal blood flow reduction in migraine typically precedes the aura symptoms by 5–15 min or more (8,11). Lauritzen (10) states that this dissociation in time between reduced CBF and focal symptoms suggests that the neurological deficits are not caused by reduced CBF. On the other hand, this finding hardly suggests that a neuronal mechanism such as spreading depression is the cause of the migraine aura. If that were the case, a spreading depression might run without giving rise to any symptoms. Of course, the areas in question could be silent areas. But if they were silent in relation to spreading depression they should also be silent in relation to ischemia. In one patient fully developed CBF changes were observed with a large low flow area involving parietal, temporal, and frontal areas of the brain, but the patient did not experience symptoms (8). This cannot be explained by spreading depression. The vascular theory might, however, explain why this patient did not experience aura symptoms. Skyhøj Olsen and Lassen (12) point out that the blood flow during the aura seems to be reduced only to a level just around the ischemic threshold and if ischemia occurs it is only in the mild end of the "ischemic spectrum." This is in accordance with the fact that the neurological deficits during the aura usually are mild and that persistent deficits occur only on rare occasions. CBF in this patient was probably not reduced below the ischemic threshold and symptoms, therefore, did not occur. How can spreading depression give rise to only mild neurological deficits when the neurones involved are depolarized? Unless depolarization does not involve all neurones in the wave front one would expect a maximal functional deficit.

The aura symptoms typically disappear when the extension of the blood flow changes have reached a maximum (8,11). The low flow state may persist for 3–6 hr without accompanying neurological deficits. This has been taken to speak against a vascular cause of the aura symptoms (8). Skyhøj Olsen and Lassen (12), however, showed that because of Compton scatter CBF may increase considerably in focal low flow areas without being measurable with the ^{133}Xe method. Hence, CBF may appear to be unchanged although increase of flow from ischemic to nonischemic levels has occurred. Such a development might explain the persistence of the blood flow changes despite disappearance of the aura symptoms. It can be concluded, therefore, that the dissociation in time between reduced CBF and focal symptoms does not rule out a vascular cause of the aura symptoms.

GRADUAL FOCAL DECREASE OF CBF IN AN AREA THAT DOES NOT SPREAD: THE CAUSE OF THE "MARCHING" SYMPTOMS DURING THE AURA?

Olesen et al. (7) and Lauritzen et al. (8) described spreading oligemia in the aura and suggested that this process was caused by spreading depression. Spreading oligemia and, hence, spreading depression were taken to explain the characteristic "march" of the symptoms during the aura. Skyhøj Olsen and Lassen (12) proposed an alternative explanation of the phenomenon termed "spreading oligemia." The phenomenon might be an artifact caused by Compton scatter. The effect of Compton scatter decreases with increasing distance from the radiation source. If CBF gradually decreases in an area of fixed size this gradual flow reduction will appear as a "spreading oligemia." The scattered radiation from nonaffected areas will "cover up" the flow reduction that will be apparent first in the areas farthest from the nonaffected part of the brain. The low flow area will gradually enlarge at the same time as CBF decreases and in this way it will look as if the low flow area gradually enlarges, although the area remains the same size. According to this interpretation the blood flow decrease takes place more or less gradually in an area of constant size—spreading may be artifact.

The characteristic "march" of the symptoms has found no correlate in ischemic stroke. How can a gradual decrease of flow in an area of constant size give rise to "march" of the symptoms? Skyhøj Olsen (13) offered this explanation. It is well known that there are differences in vulnerability among various neurones. Some neurones discontinue their spontaneous activity at flow values of 22 ml/100 g/min whereas others keep firing down to values of 6 ml/100 g/min (25). The "march" of the aura symptoms might then be caused by dysfunction of increasing neurones as the blood flow gradually decreases. In that case neurones of the visual cortex should be the most vulnerable, as visual symptoms usually are the first to appear, more vulnerable than neurones of the somatosensory cortex, that again are more vulnerable than neurones of the motor cortex. Within the individual areas of the brain the vulnerability to ischemia may also be different (i.e., the ischemic threshold is varying). In this way "march" of paresthesias from the fingers up the arm and to the face could be explained. This is of course a hypothesis that remains to be proven. However, spreading depression has never been demonstrated in humans during migraine. Nevertheless, it has found widespread acceptance as the cause of migraine with aura.

CONCLUSION

During the last 10 years neural causes of migraine with aura, especially "spreading depression," have enjoyed popularity. However, in the author's opinion it is premature to reject the possibility of vascular factors as being the cause of migraine with aura. In retrospect it seems that methodological sources of errors, in particular Compton scatter, have not been sufficiently taken into account when evaluating the results of CBF studies during migraine with aura. Our analysis of CBF during migraine with aura (11–13) has produced many more questions than answers and we do not pretend to know whether migraine with aura is caused by neural or vascular causes. We are convinced, however, that both possibilities should still be kept open.

REFERENCES

1. Leao AP and Morrison RS. Propagation of spreading cortical depression. *J Neurophysiol* 1945; 8:33–45.
2. Milner PM. Note on a possible correspondence between the migraine scotoma and cortical spreading depression. *EEG Clin Neurophysiol* 1958; 10:705.
3. Lauritzen M, Jørgensen MB, Diemer NH, Gjedde A, and Hansen AJ. Persisting oligemia of rat cerebral cortex in the wake of spreading depression. *Ann Neurol* 1982; 12:469–474.
4. Skinhøj E. Hemodynamic studies within the brain during migraine. *Arch Neurol* 1973; 29:95–98.
5. Simard D and Paulson OB. Cerebral vasomotor paralysis during migraine attack. *Arch Neurol* 1973; 29:95–98.
6. Hachinski VC, Olesen J, Norris JW, Larsen B, Enevoldsen E, and Lassen NA. Cerebral hemodynamics in migraine. *Can J Neurol Sci* 1977; 4:245–249.
7. Olesen J, Larsen B, and Lauritzen M. Focal hyperemia followed by spreading oligemia and impaired activation of rCBF in classic migraine. *Ann Neurol* 1981; 9:344–352.
8. Lauritzen M, Skyhøj Olsen T, Lassen NA, and Paulson B. The changes of regional cerebral blood flow during the course of classical migraine attacks. *Ann Neurol* 1983; 13:633–641.
9. Lauritzen M and Olesen J. Regional cerebral blood flow during migraine attacks by Xenon-133 inhalation and emission tomography. *Brain* 1984; 107:447–461.
10. Lauritzen M. Cerebral blood flow in migraine and cortical spreading depression. *Acta Neurol Scand* 1987; 76[Suppl 113]:1–40.
11. Skyhøj Olsen T, Friberg L, and Lassen NA. Ischemia may be the primary cause of the neurological deficits in classic migraine. *Arch Neurol* 1987; 44:156–161.
12. Skyhøj Olsen T and Lassen NA. Blood flow and vascular reactivity during attacks of classic migraine—Limitations of the Xe-133 intraarterial technique. *Headache* 1989; 29:15–20.
13. Skyhøj Olsen T. Migraine with and without aura: The same disease due to cerebral vasospasm of different intensity. A hypothesis based on CBF studies during migraine. *Headache* 1990; 30:269–272.
14. Wolf HG. Headache and other head pain. New York: Oxford University Press, 1963.
15. Skyhøj Olsen T, Larsen B, Bech Skriver E, Enevoldsen E, and Lassen NA: Focal cerebral ischemia measured by the intraarterial 133-Xenon method. *Stroke* 1981; 12:736–744.
16. Herold S, Gibbs JM, Jones AKP, Brooks DJ, Frackowiack RSJ, and Legg NJ. Oxygen metabolism in migraine. *J Cereb Blood Flow Metab* 1985; 5[Suppl 1]445–446.
17. Bradshaw P and Parsons M. Hemiplegic migraine, a clinical study. *Q J Med* 1965; 34:65–68.
18. Harding GFA, Debney LM, and Maheshwari M. EEG changes associated with hemiplegic migraine in childhood. *J Electrophysiol Technol* 1977; 3:90–101.
19. Dorfman LJ, Marshall WH, and Enzmann DR. Cerebral infarction and migraine: Clinical and radiological correlations. *Neurology* 1979; 29:317–322.
20. Bickerstaff ER: Complicated migraine. The 1982 Sandoz foundation lecture. In: Clifford Rose F ed. *Progress in migraine research* 2. London: Pitman, 1984; 83–101.
21. Schlacke H-P, Bottger IG, Grotemeyer K-H, and Husstedt IW: Brain imaging with ^{123}I-IMP-SPECT in migraine between attacks. *Headache* 1989; 29:344–349.
22. Hansen AJ and Lauritzen M. Spreading depression of Leao. In: Olesen J, Edvinsson L, eds. *Basic mechanisms of headache*. Amsterdam: Elsevier, 1988; 99–107.
23. Bures J, Buresova O, and Krivanek J. *The mechanisms and applications of Leao's spreading depression of electroencephalographic activity*. New York: Academic Press, 1974.
24. Andersen AR, Friberg L, Skyhøj Olsen T, and Olesen J. Delayed hyperemia following hypoperfusion in classic migraine. *Arch Neurol* 1988; 45:154–159.
25. Skyhøj Olsen T. Regional cerebral blood flow after occlusion of the middle cerebral artery. *Acta Neurol Scand* 1986; 73:321–337.

23

Links Between Cortical Spreading Depression and Migraine: Clinical and Experimental Aspects

Martin Lauritzen

Department of General Physiology and Biophysics, University of Copenhagen, DK-2200 Copenhagen N, Denmark

THEORIES

Migraine with aura (MA) is a common disorder characterized by paroxysmal headaches associated with focal neurological symptoms and signs. MA attacks have a characteristic course: At first the patient experiences transient focal neurological symptoms with a characteristic pattern of evolution (see below), spontaneously remitting within 30–60 min. At the same time as the focal symptoms, or after they have disappeared, the headache, most often unilateral and throbbing, ensues.

To explain this characteristic sequence of events there are two theories. One is the vascular theory, which assigns the primary event in migraine to a disturbance of cerebral vascular function. The focal symptoms are supposed to be causally related to transient constriction of a cerebral artery, and the headache to a sterile inflammatory reaction around the walls of dilated cephalic vessels (1).

Several arguments are in favor of a vascular concept. First, the throbbing pain quality in migraine suggests vasodilatation. Second, headache is a common accompaniment of other diseases involving blood vessels such as stroke, subarachnoid hemorrhage, arterial hypertension, and temporal arteritis. Third, the brain itself is insensitive to pain while pain-sensitive fibers have been identified at its ventral surface corresponding to the larger vessels and associated structures. Fourth, the peripheral vasoconstrictor ergotamine is a potent drug in the alleviation of the headaches (1). The vascular theory has dominated the migraine field for decades.

The second theory assigns the primary event in migraine to a disturbance of nerve cell function (2). First, the stereotyped recurrence of an unprovoked, transient disturbance of brain function is reminiscent of epilepsy more than of any known disorder of the peripheral vasculature. Second, the focal symptoms in migraine develop in a characteristic creeping fashion. The regular march of symptoms is commonly used to differentiate migraine and epilepsy. For example, many patients with MA have a characteristic disturbance of vision, a scintillation-scotoma that develops symmetrically in the visual fields, starting at the center of the field of vision and propagating to the peripheral (temporal) parts within about 10–15 min. Visual function returns to normal within another 10–15 min. The symmetrical development suggests a cortical localization of the underlying disturbance. The slow progression indicates a wave of excitation in the primary visual cortex moving at the speed of 3 mm/min, followed by a longer period of inhibition (Fig. 1) (3). Similar considerations and calculations can be made if somatosensory or somatomotor symptoms develop instead of visual. The orderly development of symptoms makes a vascular origin a remote possibility (2), whereas a primary disturbance of cortical nerve cell function, probably cortical spreading depression, is a more attractive explanation (4).

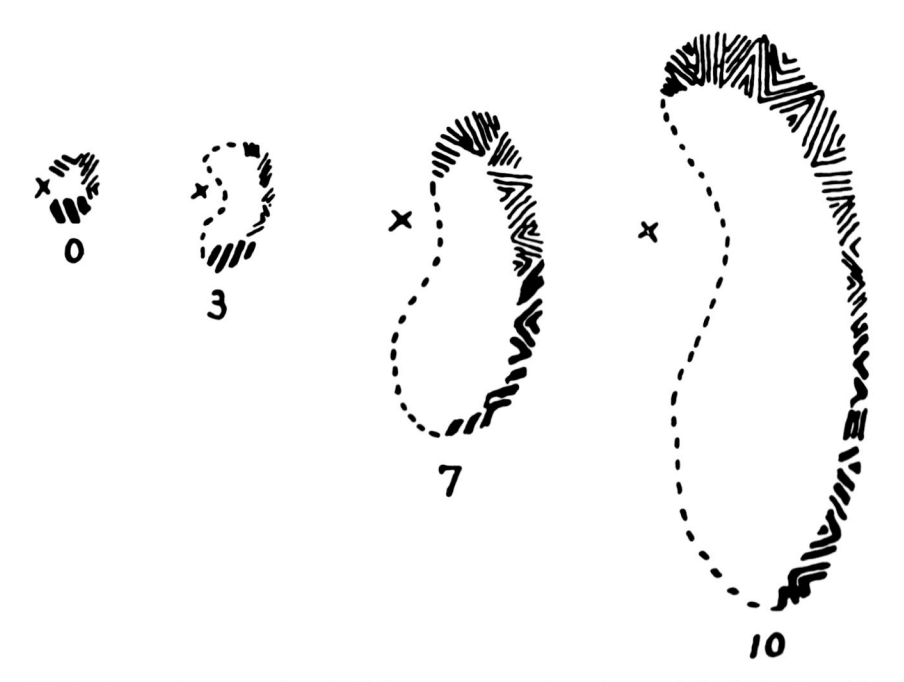

FIG. 1. Successive maps of a scintillation-scotoma to show characteristic distribution of the fortification figures. In each case the asterisk indicates the fixation point. Knowledge of the retinotopic organization of the visual cortex allowed Lashley (3) to calculate the speed of propagation of the excitation-depression wave as approximately 3 mm/min. (From Lashley, ref. 3, with permission.)

The two theories may be unified if on one hand a cortical spreading depression (CSD) develops during the onset of the migraine attack, and if on the other hand CSD causes changes of the perivascular microenvironment, which activates pain-sensitive fibers, in turn causing pain (5,6). This chapter presents data in favor of this possibility.

BRAIN BLOOD FLOW IN HUMANS

Regional cerebral blood flow (rCBF) studies during acute attacks of MA have revealed (reviewed in ref. 5):

1. rCBF decreases during the initial part of the attack in the posterior part of the brain. Subsequently, the low flow region expands in an irregular fashion and to different extent in individual patients at a rate of 2–3 mm/min.

2. Spread of the hypoperfusion does not respect supply territories of the large arteries, but follows the cortical surface. Major cytoarchitectonic boundaries, for example, the central sulcus, and larger foldings, for example, the lateral sulcus, remain uncrossed. The hypoperfusion propagates from temporal and parietal cortices to frontal regions along the insular region and the parietal operculum, respectively.

3. The rCBF reduction is localized mainly to the cortex, but it cannot be excluded that rCBF is reduced in the underlying white matter as well.

4. Blood pressure autoregulation is preserved. This indicates cortical arterioles as the site of increased resistance with residual capacity to constrict and dilate in response to changes of perfusion pressure. Vasospasm of a large artery would cause compensatory dilatation of the arterioles if severe enough to reduce rCBF. Hence, increased blood pressure would lead to rCBF increases in a pressure-passive arteriolar bed. Since the systemic factors (blood gases, hematocrit) remain constant, local factors are suspected to cause the increased vascular tone.

5. Vascular reactivity to mental tasks, metabolic autoregulation, and the CO_2 reactivity is impaired in hypoperfused parts, but present in neighboring noninvaded tissue, suggesting decreased vascular responsiveness to local chemical stimuli in affected regions.

6. Focal symptoms appear at some point during the (early) spread of the hypoperfusion, but ceases while the hypoperfusion continues to spread. From closely spaced studies it has become clear that the reduced rCBF persists for some time during the headache period. After about 5–6 hr and lasting for up to 24 hr a hyperperfusion develops in the brain regions that were previously hypoperfused (5,7).

7. The rCBF reduction amounts to about 20–25%. Recently it has been claimed that the reduction of rCBF is larger than originally believed because of errors of measurement inherent in our technique (8). In brief, the reduced rCBF in the hypoperfused regions may be overestimated because of Comp-

tom scattered radiation from the neighboring normoperfused regions (8). However, it is still unclear whether this source of error plays any significant role for the conclusions reached previously (9,10).

In conclusion, the time base of the focal symptoms and the reduced rCBF is clearly different. This is a strong argument against the vascular theory of migraine. The vascular changes are consistent with a slowly propagating, extinguishable cortical process: spreading at a rate of 2–3 mm/min, constricting cortical arterioles, and causing focal neurological symptoms while expanding. The reduced rCBF appears to be an epiphenomenon, but may under certain (unknown) conditions contribute to the persistence of neurological deficits. The headache in turn is not associated with increased rCBF. It is possible that the spreading cortical disturbance, which has sufficient impact to constrict the arterioles, also activates the pain-sensitive nerve fibers around the larger arteries, but this remains to be shown.

There is only one known cortical disturbance that fits into the above description of rCBF changes during migraine attacks: the cortical spreading depression of Leao (11).

BRAIN BLOOD FLOW IN RATS

rCBF changes during CSD occur in a regular fashion (reviewed in ref. 5). There is probably no blood flow change before the nerve cells depolarize or during the onset of depolarization. During return to normal of the ionic changes a flow rise is sometimes observed, especially if the basic flow level is depressed because of the use of anesthetics or other blood flow lowering drugs. When present, the flow rise lasts for about 1–2 min, being rapidly succeeded by a 20–30% flow reduction. The rCBF reduction is cortical, thus corresponding to the site of the large-scaled ionic changes, whereas noninvaded tissues have a normal flow. Arteriolar vasoconstriction is clearly observed in the rat, but the chloralose-anesthetized cat displays a continued arteriolar vasodilation. Thus, there are species differences with respect to the vascular reaction (12).

The hypoperfusion in rats persists for 1–2 hr. Blood pressure autoregulation is preserved in the entire brain while the responsiveness to changes of $PaCO_2$ and locally applied chemical stimuli is markedly impaired in hypoperfused regions. The cerebral metabolic rate of glucose remains normal despite the low flow. Thus, the rCBF reduction is not severe enough to impede cortical glucose consumption (13).

In summary, CSD in rats is associated with a brief initial flow rise under certain conditions. After CSD, rCBF declines and remains reduced for about 2 hr. The reduced rCBF is caused by arteriolar vasoconstriction and is associated with preserved autoregulation and diminished chemical responsiveness. This pattern of rCBF changes replicates almost point by point the rCBF changes associated with migraine.

ENERGY METABOLISM

Our knowledge of the changes of energy-rich phosphate compounds and oxygen and glucose metabolism during migraine attacks is minimal. This is because of the inherent difficulties in investigating short-lasting paroxysmal disorders, in which the disturbance of metabolic function may have disappeared at the time the patient is referred to or applies to the clinic. Furthermore, the use of the positron emission tomography (PET) scanner requires preparatory procedures and the relevant radiochemical compound may not be available when the patient is at location. Nevertheless, one PET study has been carried out and the results showed normal cerebral metabolic rate of oxygen in the hypoperfused regions of a patient with MA at the time of neurological deficits (14). This result is incompatible with cerebral ischemia. Therefore, the PET data support the theory that cerebral ischemia is not causally linked to the existence of focal deficits in migraine.

Magnetic resonance imaging (MRI) techniques have been applied to migraine patients at 3–48 hr after the beginning of the attack using a surface coil to obtain signals from a 4-cm spherical source of the cerebrum. The preliminary results showed a decrease of the phosphocreatine (PCr) concentration and an increase of inorganic phosphate, but a constant adenosine triphosphate (ATP) and intracellular pH. The absence of pH changes was taken as argument against the vascular theory since pH was found to be reduced in the affected region in almost all patients with a stroke or transient ischemic attack (15).

The intracellular pH during and after CSD is unknown. We do know, however, that the concentration of energy metabolites changes markedly at the wave front, lasting for a few minutes: PCr decreases by about 38% while ATP remains constant (16). Thus, the changes of PCr and ATP during CSD and MA attacks are similar, suggesting an increased turnover rate of these compounds, but no evidence of ischemia!

THE MAGNETOENCEPHALOGRAM

The magnetoencephalogram (MEG) signal associated with CSD was obtained for the first time under *in vitro* conditions using the isolated turtle cerebellum and a one-channel DC-coupled SQUID (17,18). The results revealed a well-defined signal in the picotesla range, raising the possibility of noninvasively detecting CSD in the human cerebral cortex in association with migraine attacks. Thus, the field appeared to be strong enough to be measured outside the head in single trials, provided that the strength of the magnetic field generated by the human neocortex was within the same order of magnitude as the field recorded from the turtle cerebellum.

The results obtained with a seven-channel AC-coupled MEG system in a group of migraine patients are promising (19). The MEG signals share important features with the signals recorded with the same equipment during CSD in rabbits (20). However, we are still ignorant of the specificity of these signals, and further confirmation of the results is needed. No doubt the MEG technique has the potential of contributing to the discussion with respect to the vascular versus the CSD theory of migraine. But, also, there is no doubt that a regularly propagated, highly specific signal is required if we are to be convinced that a wave of CSD has been recorded.

BEHAVIOR AND SYMPTOMS

Single unilateral waves of CSD induce remarkably modest signs of cortical dysfunction in rats. Contralateral sensory neglect and motor impairment of the contralateral forepaw are the most reliable neurological signs lasting for about 15–30 min, that is, a much shorter time than the blood flow reduction. It is unknown whether CSD is an aversive or a pleasant stimulus. It is also unknown if CSD causes headache in rats, nor can it be judged whether the rat has headache or not (21,22).

Behavioral changes due to remote effects of CSD on subcortical centers are usually longer lasting than the cortical deficits. Signs of possible hypothalamic origin include abnormal thermoregulation and feeding behavior, water retention, and ovarian hormone secretion.

In conclusion, CSD in rats is accompanied by transient contralateral somatosensory and motor deficits, and signs of involvement of the hypothalamus. Attacks of MA display a similar time course and symptomatology. The analysis can hardly be driven more rigorously since a major discrepancy between the animal experiments and the human condition is the involvement of the whole hemicortex in the rat, while during the MA attack most often only regions located in the posterior parts of the brain are involved (5,6).

PERSPECTIVES

In conclusion, it appears likely that CSD is involved in the sequence of events that leads to acute migraine episodes. This changes our view of migraine from that of episodic changes of blood vessel function to a well-defined disturbance of cortical neuronal function, the cortical spreading depression (Fig. 2).

Although our understanding of CSD is still incomplete, the recent development and application of drugs directed against glutamate receptors have

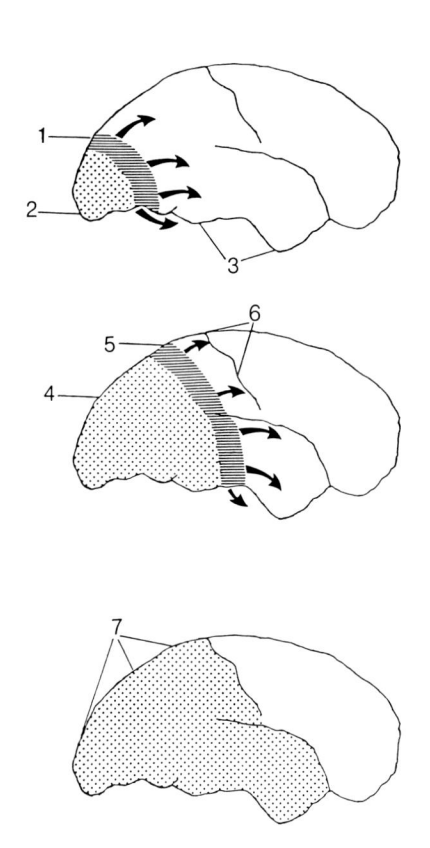

FIG. 2. Hypothesis of development of a MA attack based on aspects of CSD and migraine summarized in the text. The figures represent lateral views of the human brain at different time intervals after beginning of the attack, spaced by approximately 30 min. The dotted area represents the region of reduced rCBF, the striped area the region of neuronal depolarization during the first minutes of CSD. The arrows represent the direction of progression of CSD. 1, Initially during a MA attack a CSD is elicited at the occipital pole, spreading anteriorly at the lateral, mesial, and ventral sides of the brain. At the CSD wave front, transient ionic and metabolic disequilibria trigger perturbed neuronal function, rCBF changes, and neurological symptoms. 2, After CSD, cortical rCBF decreases by 20–30% for 2–6 hr. 3, rCBF in regions not invaded by CSD remains normal until encountered by CSD. 4, The region of reduced rCBF expands as the CSD move anteriorly. 5, Somatosensory symptoms from the extremities appear when the CSD invades the primary sensory cortex at the postcentral gyrus. 6, CSD usually stops on reaching the central sulcus, but in many patients it does not even propagate this far. The ventral spread of CSD causes activation of pain-sensitive fibers, and headache. 7, Full-scale attack. The CSD has stopped and is now detectable as a persistent reduction of cortical rCBF. At this time the patient suffers from headache, but has no focal deficits. (From Lauritzen, ref. 6, with permission.)

given us important clues to events at the synaptic level, which are presumed to be important in the production of CSD.

Van Harreveld (23) was the first to propose that glutamate had an active role in CSD. A few years later it was shown that N-methyl-D-aspartate (NMDA) was 100 times more potent than glutamate in triggering CSD (24). In another series of experiments it was found that glutamate is released during CSD and that various glutamate antagonists block CSD in the chicken retina (25–27). Recently it has been shown that:

1. Hippocampal and cerebellar CSD occur spontaneously in Mg-free medium. This condition is supposed to facilitate the entrance of calcium ions through the NMDA-operated membrane channel and suggests a role for this receptor channel complex in CSD (28,29).

2. CSD is blocked by D-a-aminoadipate, ketamine, MK-801, amino-5-phosphonovaleate (APV), and amino-7-phosphonoheptanoate (APH), that is, competitive and noncompetitive NMDA antagonists (27,29–32).

3. Antagonists of non-NMDA glutamate subtype receptors are ineffective as blockers of CSD (Lauritzen & Hansen, unpublished observations).

The results indicate that NMDA receptor activity is of crucial importance for the production of CSD. If indeed CSD proves to be the causative mechanism of migraine, NMDA antagonists could be the next bid of a rational migraine therapy.

REFERENCES

1. Wolff HG. *Headache and other head pain.* Oxford University Press, 1963; 1–688.
2. Gowers WR. *The borderland of epilepsy.* London: Churchill, 1907.
3. Lashley KS. Patterns of cerebral integration indicated by the scotomas of migraine. *Arch Neurol Psychiat* 1941; 46:331–339.
4. Milner B. Note on a possible correspondence between the migraine scotomata and spreading depression. *Electroenceph Clin Neurophysiol* 1958; 10:705.
5. Lauritzen M. Cerebral blood flow in migraine and cortical spreading depression. *Acta Neurol Scand* 1987; 113 [Suppl 76]:9–40.
6. Lauritzen M. Cortical spreading depression as a putative migraine mechanism. *Trends Neurosci* 1987; 10:8–13.
7. Andersen AR, Friberg L, Skyhøj Olsen T, and Olesen J. Delayed hyperemia following hypoperfusion in classic migraine. *Arch Neurol* 1987; 44:156–161.
8. Skyhøj Olsen T, Friberg L, and Lassen NA. Ischemia may be the primary cause of neurological deficits in classic migraine. *Arch Neurol* 1987; 44:156–161.
9. Kronborg D, Dalgaard P, and Lauritzen M. Letter to the editor. *Arch Neurol* 1990; 47:124–125.
10. Dalgaard P, Kronborg D, and Lauritzen M. Migraine with aura, cerebral ischemia, cortical spreading depression, and the importance of Comptom scattered radiation for the evaluation of data obtained with the intracarotid ^{133}Xenon method. *Headache* 1991; (in press).
11. Leao AAP. Spreading depression of activity in the cerebral cortex. *J Neurophysiol* 1944; 7:359–390.
12. Wahl M, Lauritzen M, and Schilling L. The influence of cortical spreading depression upon pial arterial reactions to various vasoactive stimuli in cats and rats. *Brain Res* 1987; 411:72–80.
13. Lauritzen M and Diemer NH. Uncoupling of cerebral blood flow and metabolism after single episodes of cortical spreading depression in the rat brain. *Brain Res* 1986; 370:405–408.
14. Herold S, Gibbs JM, Jones AKP, Brooks DJ, Frachiowak RSJ, and Legg NJ. Oxygen metabolism in migraine. *J Cereb Blood Flow Metab* 1985; 5 [Suppl 1]:S445–446.
15. Welch KMA, Levine SR, D'Andrea G, Schultz LR, Helpern JA. Preliminary observations on brain energy metabolism in migraine studied by in vivo phosphorus 31 NMR spectroscopy. *Neurology* 1989; 39:538–541.
16. Lauritzen M, Hansen AJ, Kronborg D, and Wieloch T. Cortical spreading depression is associated with arachidonic acid accumulation and preservation of energy charge. *J Cereb Blood Flow Metab* 1990; 10:115–122.
17. Okada Y, Lauritzen M, and Nicholson C. MEG source models and physiology. *Phys Med Biol* 1988; 32:43–51.
18. Okada Y, Lauritzen M, and Nicholson M. Magnetic field associated with spreading depression: A model for the detection of migraine. *Brain Res* 1988; 442:185–190.
19. Tepley N, Barkley GL, Moran JE, Simkins RT, and Welch KMA. Observation of cortical spreading depression in migraine patients. In: Williamson S, Kaufmann L, et al., eds. *Biomagnetism.* New York: Plenum Press, 1990; 327–330.
20. Gardner-Medwin AR, Tepley N, Barkley GL, et al. Magnetic observation of spreading cortical depression in anesthetized rabbits. In: Williamson S, Kaufmann L, et al., eds. *Biomagnetism.* New York: Plenum Press, 1990; 323–326.

21. Bures J, Buresova O, and Krivanek J. *The mechanism and applications of Leao's spreading depression of electroencephalographic activity*. New York: Academic Press, 1974.
22. Bures J, Buresova O, and Krivanek J. The meaning and significance of Leao's spreading depression. *An Acad Bras Cienc* 1984;56:385–400.
23. Van Harreveld A. Compounds in brain extracts causing spreading depression of cerebral cortical activity and contraction of crustacean muscle. *J Neurochem*, 1959; 3:300–315.
24. Curtis DR and Watkins JC. Analogues of glutamic acid and gamma-amino-n-butyric acids having potent actions on mammalian neurones. *Nature* 1961; 191:1010–1011.
25. Van Harreveld A and Fifkova E. Glutamate release from the retina during spreading depression. *J Neurobiol* 1970; 2:13–29.
26. Van Harreveld A and Fifkova E. Effects of glutamate and other amino acids on the retina. *J Neurochem* 1971; 18:2145–2154.
27. Van Harreveld A. The nature of the chick's magnesium-sensitive retinal spreading depression. *J Neurobiol* 1984; 15:333–344.
28. Mody I, Lambert JDC, and Heinemann U. Low extracellular magnesium induces epileptiform activity and spreading depression in rat hippocampal slices. *J Neurophysiol*, 1987; 57:869–888.
29. Lauritzen M, Rice M, Okada Y, and Nicholson C. Spreading depression by activation of glutamate receptors in turtle cerebellum *in vitro*. *Brain Res* 1988; 475:317–327.
30. Goroleva NA, Koroleva VI, Amemori T, Pavlik V, and Bures J. Ketamine blockade of cortical spreading depression in rats. *Electroencephal and Clin Neurophysiol* 1987; 66:440–447.
31. Marannes R, Willems R, De Prins E, and Wauquier A. Evidence for a role of the *N*-methyl-D-aspartate receptor in cortical spreading depression in the rat. *Brain Res* 1988; 457:226–240.
32. Hansen AJ, Lauritzen M, and Wieloch T. NMDA antagonists inhibit cortical spreading depression, but not anoxic depolarization. In: EA Cavalheiro, J Lehmann, and L Turski, eds. *Frontiers in excitatory amino acid research*. New York: Alan R. Liss, 1988; 661–666.

24

Receptors on Sensory Fibers Provide a Locus for Antimigraine Drug Action

Michael A. Moskowitz

Department of Neurosurgery and Neurology, Massachusetts General Hospital, Harvard Medical School, Boston, Massachusetts 02114

This chapter summarizes the results from recent studies examining the mechanism of action of drugs useful in the acute treatment of migraine headaches and considers the potential sources of nociceptive molecules relevant to headache. The topic is fundamental to the study of pain mechanisms from cephalic blood vessels, and is therefore important to consider in this forum. The data suggest that specific populations of serotonin receptors reside on sensory fibers surrounding cephalic blood vessels and that these receptors are coupled to inhibition of neuropeptide release and the development of neurogenic inflammation within the dura mater. The binding of ergot alkaloids or sumatriptan to these receptors may provide the mechanism for their action and appears to be independent of their vasoconstrictor functions.

METHODS

For detailed methods, the reader is referred to the original publications (1–4) and several relevant reviews (5,6). In brief, male Sprague-Dawley rats (150–200 g) and male Hartley guinea pigs (250–300 g) were used in all experiments. Electrical stimulation of the rat trigeminal ganglion was accomplished in pentobarbital-anesthetized rats placed in a stereotaxic frame. A 2-mm diameter hole was drilled on each side of the sagittal suture for electrode placement. ^{125}I-BSA, 50 µCi/Kg was injected as a bolus. After 5 min, bipolar electrodes were lowered into both trigeminal ganglion. A shock stimulus (1.2 mA, 5 Hz, 5 msec duration) was delivered for 5 min to the right trigeminal ganglion. These parameters were sufficient (by electrophysiological criteria) to discharge small unmyelinated C fibers (unpublished data). Animals were perfused for 3 min immediately after stimulation. The dura mater, conjunctiva, eyelid, and lip were dissected. Samples were weighed and counted for radioactivity. Radioactivity (cpm/mg wt) was compared between the stimulated and the unstimulated sides. Data are expressed as the ratio between the two sides.

Pretreatment

The following drugs were administered intravenously 10 min before electrical trigeminal stimulation or systemic capsaicin: sumatriptan, dihydroergotamine (DHE), ergotamine tartrate, 5-carboxamidotryptamine (5-CT), methysergide, ketanserin, pizotifen, MDL72222, and ICS 205-930. Sumatriptan and DHE were also administered 10 min before SP, NKA, and BK.

RESULTS AND DISCUSSION

Leakage of plasma proteins from dural blood vessels develops shortly after electrical trigeminal ganglion stimulation or capsaicin pretreatment. Extravasation was not observed in animals lacking C fibers (i.e., adult animals treated with capsaicin during the neonatal period) (3). However, protein leakage was observed in response to infusions of substance P or neurokinin A in both normal animals and in animals depleted of C fibers. Release of vasoactive neuropeptides probably mediated this response since trigeminal ganglia stimulation elevated levels of immunoreactive CGRP within sagittal sinus blood within one minute of stimulation (Buzzi et al., in preparation).

The blood vessels of the dura mater contain fenestrated capillary endothelium and lack a blood-brain barrier. After trigeminal stimulation, the endothelium within postcapillary venules exhibited an increase in the number of cytoplasmic vesicles and adherent platelets. Some vessels demonstrated subintimal edema and the tendency to damage during tissue fixation (Dimitriadou et al., in preparation). Arterioles do not show these changes as frequently. Similar findings are observed within ipsilateral postcapillary venules in the tongue, another tissue innervated by trigeminal fibers. By contrast, vessels on the contralateral side do not show any of these changes. Adult animals treated with capsaicin during the neonatal period do not show endothelium and platelet changes after electrical trigeminal stimulation.

The Effects of Antimigraine Drugs

The ability of ergot alkaloids (ergotamine tartrate, dihydroergotamine, chronic methysergide) to block neurogenic plasma extravasation in the rat dura mater was reported in 1988 by our group (4). The fact that the ergot alkaloids have been used to treat classic, common, and cluster headaches suggests that they may work at a mechanism common to all headache. Methysergide, a third ergot derivative, is useful for prophylaxis when chronically administered, but not for the acute attack. A single injection of ergotamine or dihydroergotamine, but only chronic administration of methysergide, blocked neurogenic inflammation in dura mater induced either by trigeminal electrical stimulation or by capsaicin. Therapeutically relevant doses were sufficient. Since the ergot alkaloids did not block SP- or NKA-induced extravasation, and since the vasoconstrictors angiotensin or phenylephrine did not block the effects of trigeminal stimulation (4), ergotamine-induced vasoconstriction (by decreasing luminal surface area) was not the apparent mechanism responsible for drug activity. We concluded from these findings that ergots decrease neurogenic plasma extravasation by a C fiber-dependent mechanism, perhaps by blocking tachykinin release from perivascular fibers via prejunctional serotonin receptor mechanisms (e.g., a prejunctional mechanism). Consistent with this observation are recent data showing that dihydroergotamine decreases levels of CGRP within the sagittal sinus during electrical trigeminal stimulation (Buzzi et al., in preparation). The possibility remains that the ergot alkaloids block neurotransmitter release from primary afferent terminals within the brain stem as well (Lambert et al., personal communication). Hence, a neuronal action of the ergots on sensory transmission has been suggested.

The ergot alkaloids are $5-HT_1$ receptor agonists, but are not selective for the type 1 receptor or for the serotonin receptor itself (7). Sumatriptan, however, is selective for the $5-HT_1$ receptor (8) and aborts the pain of migraine headaches (9–12). Sumatriptan passes the blood-brain barrier poorly and like the ergot alkaloids, exhibits vasoconstrictor actions on cephalic blood vessels. Sumatriptan blocks plasma extravasation selectively within the dura mater of experimental animals when administered before electrical or chemical stimulation of the trigeminovascular system (1). Like the ergot alkaloids, the compound does not reduce the extravasation caused by systemic SP or NKA, thereby suggesting the possibility of a prejunctional action. Not shared by the ergot alkaloids, sumatriptan blocks the plasma extravasation caused by the systemic administration of the nociceptor bradykinin. A $5-HT_1$ receptor mechanism is also suggested by the observation that 5-carboxyamidotryptamine ($5-HT_1$ agonist) inhibits extravasation whereas ketanserin or pizotifen ($5-HT_2$ antagonists) and MDL 72222 or ICS 203950 ($5-HT_3$ antagonists) do not exacerbate or inhibit extravasation after electrical trigeminal stimulation.

Nonsteroidal antiinflammatory drugs block neurogenic inflammation in the dura mater as well (2). Drugs such as aspirin and indomethacin are useful in treating migraine. Clinical studies report the high efficacy of aspirin in common migraine, and indomethacin in common migraine, "hemicrania continua," and cluster headache. Indomethacin and high-dose aspirin markedly reduced plasma protein extravasation in rat dura mater induced by electrical trigeminal stimulation. The mechanism of action is less clear for these agents than for the ergots. High dose but not low dose indomethacin and aspirin blocked SP-induced protein extravasation, suggesting a direct action on blood vessels (postjunctional mechanism). Low dose indomethacin does not block the effects of SP but does attenuate the leakage of albumin after electrical trigeminal stimulation. Hence, an effect on the nerve fiber seems plausible as well. Since platelet adhesion and aggregation recently has been identified within postcapillary venules after electrical trigeminal stimulation, an antiplatelet action could also underlie this inhibitory activity.

In summary, serotonin type 1 receptors modulate neurogenic plasma extravasation within the dura mater induced by trigeminal nerve stimulation or capsaicin administration. Whether the serotonin receptors of interest exist on unmyelinated perivascular fibers or are present on other tissue elements within the vessel requires further study.

SOURCES OF NOCICEPTIVE MOLECULES AND SITES OF DRUG ACTIVITY

The Blood Vessel Wall

Most clinicians and patients believe that cephalic blood vessels cause migraine headaches. This assumption is not unreasonable because blood vessels possess the densest sensory innervation within the cranium, and the throbbing or pulsating pain is reproduced by faradic or mechanical stimulation applied directly over dural arteries, sinuses, and large arteries of the circle of Willis; it is not reproduced by stimulating other tissues (13). However, the inference that blood vessels cause all headaches is probably incorrect because the blood vessel wall, the blood and its component elements, and the brain parenchyma have the potential to modulate activity within visceral afferent axons.

Cephalic blood vessels are also potent generators of nociceptive molecules. They probably possess the enzymes responsible for synthesizing bradykinin (by cleaving the precursor kininogens found in the circulation). Endothelial cells contain mechanisms for deacylating phospholipids leading to the release of arachidonic acid and formation of prostaglandins (14). Smooth muscle cells also possess receptor mechanisms (e.g., serotonin type 2) that are coupled to arachidonate release in response to the addition of this biogenic amine (15). Mast cells located within the adventitial layer contain histamine and other biogenic amines that can be released by chemical or mechanical stimulation. Serotonin, present within nerve fibers, is also in abundance within circulating platelets and probably within the endothelium as well. Along with mechanisms for synthesizing "pain-promoting chemicals," blood vessels and their attendant nerve fibers also possess receptors for their detection. As suggested above, recent work in the dura mater suggests that vascular smooth muscle and perivascular afferents possess receptors not shared with the vasculature in other organs.

Specific receptor populations expressed exclusively on cephalic blood vessels could explain why headaches (and not other vascular pains) develop as a consequence of certain provocative stimuli. Similarly, the binding of antimigraine drugs to specific receptor populations on cephalic vessels (and not peripheral tissues) might explain why migraine headaches and not other painful conditions are relieved by these drugs. These receptors are not present on extracranial vascular tissues innervated by the trigeminal nerve. As noted, 5-HT-like agonists block the development of neurogenic inflammation selectively within dura mater after trigeminal antidromic stimulation.

To what extent vasoconstriction contributes to headache relief is somewhat uncertain at this point. The fact that intense headaches accompany subarachnoid hemorrhage, a condition marked by vasoconstriction, contradicts the dogma that dilation equals headache and constriction equals headache relief. Severe dilatation has not been documented during migraine headaches and vessel caliber (as assessed by carotid angiography) is normal; focal narrowing is sometimes present. Furthermore, blood flow most commonly is decreased during the headache phase of classical migraine and normal in common migraine and cluster headache (16). (Of course blood flow reflects more precisely the caliber of the small, relatively pain-insensitive resistance vessels.) Under some circumstances, dilatation may be painful, as, for example, during angioplasty or balloon catheterization (17). However, the relevance of this type of vessel injury to migraine headaches is somewhat obscure. Less marked dilatation, if present, could be consistent with axon reflex mechanisms and develop pari passu with depolarization of trigeminal perivascular axons and neuropeptide release (18). Vasodilators such as nitroglycerine are associated with headaches, but alternative mechanisms for pain generation must be considered. For example, nitrates cause dilation in vascular smooth muscle upon their conversion to nitric oxide (see ref. 19). This, in turn, stimulates cyclic guanosine monophosphate to promote phosphorylation of contractile proteins and relaxation of vascular smooth muscle. Under certain conditions, however, nitric oxide can also be converted to the hydroxyl radical, a potent free oxygen radical and mediator of tissue injury. Headache then may not be caused by vessel distension *per se*, but by a biochemical mechanism related to relaxation of vascular smooth muscle.

Although it is unlikely that vasoconstriction explains the actions of ergot alkaloids in the dura mater model, the merits in favor of a vasoconstrictor drug mechanism should be considered independently of the mechanism responsible for the pain. Vasoconstriction certainly modifies the geometry of perivascular axons and by so doing may modify the electrophysiological properties of these axons. Nevertheless, the evidence that ergot alkaloids and sumatriptan relieve two types of headaches that are clinically very different and develop by distinct pathophysiological mechanisms favors a neurogenic mechanism.

The Brain

The brain, of course, contains many of the above chemicals that function normally as neurotransmitter substances (e.g., serotonin and histamine). Since neurotransmitters are released into brain tissue during the course of normal synaptic events, it seems obvious that the brain has evolved by necessity a sparse sensory innervation and a primitive pain-generating system. A more extensive network might not be compatible with a headache-free existence. During organ dysfunction, however, both endogenous and newly generated molecules diffuse away from synapses to the perivascular space in cortical gray matter to approximate visceral afferent fibers. It has been suggested that cortical gray matter is an important source of nociceptive molecules during cerebral ischemia, classical migraine, or seizures. Trigeminovascular activation occurs during ischemia and seizures as evidenced by the hyperemia that develops in cortical gray matter by axon reflex mechanisms (18,20,21). Mild–moderate blood flow reductions during classical migraine (or an electrophysiological event such as spreading depression) may provoke through similar mechanisms activation of this nerve and cause headache (and sometimes delayed hyperemia). It is noteworthy that conditions associated with involvement of deep gray or white matter are less commonly accompanied by headache.

Excitotoxic mechanisms involving the N-methyl-D-aspartate (NMDA) receptor suggest more subtle mechanisms for initiating neuronal injury (real or threatened), and do not by necessity implicate triggering events within the cerebral circulation (see ref. 22). Excitotoxic theories may have special relevance to migraine pathogenesis because nociceptor molecules may be a product of synaptic events within cortical gray matter. Of note, arachidonic acid release accompanies activation of the NMDA receptor (23). It is proposed that altered physiological states (stress, fatigue), bright lights, and sleep deprivation (migraine precipitating events) modulate neuronal activity and synaptic events within cortical gray matter and by so doing may modulate activity within innervating trigeminovascular fibers. Precisely how this coupling is accomplished remains for further study. Regardless, neurophysiologically induced events mediate local increases in cortical blood flow in order to facilitate removal of potentially noxious chemicals and hence to restore cortex to its premorbid state. Gray matter structures deep within the brain must condition this activity as well, as evidenced by the disturbances in limbic function, which may anticipate the headache of common migraine by hours or days (24).

More information is known about the origin and triggers of pain from the heart, urinary, and gall bladder, for example, than about pain emanating from the brain and its coverings. Since knowledge about the physiology of the nervous system is more primitive, this is not unexpected. Classical teachings hold that ischemia, inflammation, smooth muscle spasm, hollow organ distension, or traction are most pain-provoking (25). Although some may be related to the origin of migraine headaches, it seems doubtful that distension of a hollow viscus (and by analogy, blood vessel dilatation) will continue to merit the attention that it has in the past. Stimuli demonstrated to activate visceral afferents experimentally include electrical or chemical (bradykinin, potassium, prostaglandins, histamine, serotonin) stimulation, ischemia, and extreme mechanical distension. Electrical stimulation, bradykinin, potassium, ischemia, and severe mechanical distension (e.g., angioplasty) (all are noxious stimuli) activate the trigeminovascular system in humans as well as in experimental animals (26–28).

REFERENCES

1. Buzzi MG and Moskowitz MA. The antimigraine drug, sumatriptan (GR43175), selectively blocks neurogenic plasma extravasation from blood vessels in dura mater. *Br J Pharmacol* 1990;99:202–206.
2. Buzzi MG, Sakas DE, and Moskowitz MA. Indomethacin and acetylsalicylic acid block neurogenic plasma protein extravasation in rat dura mater. *Eur J Pharmacol* 1989; 165:252–258.
3. Markowitz S, Saito K, and Moskowitz MA. Neurogenically mediated leakage of plasma protein occurs from blood vessels in dura mater but not brain. *J Neurosci* 1987; 7:4129–4136.
4. Saito K, Markowitz S, and Moskowitz MA. Ergot alkaloids block neurogenic extravasation in dura mater: Proposed mechanism for vascular headache. *Ann Neurol* 1988; 24:732–737.
5. Moskowitz MA. The neurobiology of vascular head pain. *Ann Neurol* 1984; 16:157–168.
6. Moskowitz MA. Basic mechanisms of headache. Neurol Clin North Am (in press).
7. McCarthy BG and Peroutka SJ. Comparative neuropharmacology of dihydroergotamine and sumatriptan (GR43175). *Headache* 1989; 29:420–422.
8. Feniuk W, Humphrey PPA, and Perren MJ. The selective carotid arterial vasoconstrictor action of GR43175 in anesthetized dogs. *Br J Pharmacol* 1989; 96:83–90.
9. Byer J, Gutterman DL, Plachetka JR, and Bhattacharyya H. Dose response study for subcutaneous GR43175 in the treatment of acute migraine. *Cephalalgia* 1989; 9 [Suppl 10]:349–350.
10. Dahlof C, Winter P, and Ludlow S. Oral GR43175, a 5HT1-like agonist, for treatment of the acute migraine attack: An international study—preliminary results. *Cephalalgia* 1989;9 [Suppl 10]:351–352.
11. Doenicke A, Brand J, and Perrin VL. Possible benefit of GR43175, a novel 5-HT$_1$-like receptor agonist, for the acute treatment of severe migraine. *Lancet* 1988;i:1309–1311.
12. Ferrari M, Bayliss EM, Ludlow S, and Pilgrim AJ. Subcutaneous GR43175 in the treatment of acute migraine: An international study. *Cephalalgia* 1989; 9 [Suppl 10]:348.
13. Ray BS and Wolff HG. Experimental studies on headache: Pain sensitive structures of the head and their significance in headache. *Arch Surg* 1940; 41:813–856.
14. Weksler BB, Marcus AJ, and Jaffe EA. Synthesis of PGI$_2$ by cultured human and bovine endothelial cells. *Proc Nat Acad Sci USA* 1976; 72:2994–2998.
15. Coughlin SR, Moskowitz MA, Antoniades H, and Levine L. Serotonin receptor-mediated stimulation of smooth muscle cell prostacyclin synthesis and its modulation by platelet-derived growth factor. *Proc Natl Acad Sci USA* 1981; 78:7134–7138.

16. Andersen AR, Friberg L, Skyhoj Olsen T, and Olesen J. Delayed hyperemia following hypoperfusion in classic migraine. *Arch Neurol* 1988; 45:154–160.
17. Nichols FT III, Mawad M, Mohr JP, et al. Focal headache during balloon inflation in the internal carotid and middle cerebral arteries. *Stroke* 1990; 21:555–559.
18. Moskowitz MA, Sakas D, Wei EP, et al. Post occlusive hyperemia in cortical grey matter is markedly attenuated by trigeminalectomy. *Am J Physiol* 1989; 257:H1736–1739.
19. Marletta MA. Nitric oxide: Biosynthesis and biological significance. *Trends Biol Sci* 1989; 14:488–492.
20. Sakas, DE, Moskowitz MA, Wei EP, et al. Trigeminovascular fibers increase blood flow in cortical gray matter by axon reflex-like mechanisms during acute severe hypertension or seizures. *Proc Nat Acad Sci USA* 1989; 86:1401–1405.
21. Moskowitz MA, Wei E, Saito K, and Kontos HA. Trigeminalectomy modifies pial arteriolar responses to hypertension or norepinephrine. *Am J Physiol* 1988; 255:H1-6.
22. Choi DW. Glutamate neurotoxicity and diseases of the nervous system. *Neuron* 1988; 1:623–634.
23. Dumuis A, Sebben M, Haynes L, Pin J-P, and Bockaert J. NMDA receptors activate the arachidonic acid cascade in striatal neurons. *Nature* 1988; 336:68–70.
24. Blau N. Migraine prodromes separated from the aura: Complete migraine. *Br Med J* 1980; 281:658–660.
25. Ayala M. Douleur sympathetique et douleur viscerale. *Rev Neurol* 1937; 68:222–242.
26. Davis KD and Dostrovsky JO. Activation of trigeminal brain-stem nociceptive neurons by dural artery stimulation. *Pain* 1986; 25:395–401.
27. Davis KD and Dostrovsky JO. Responses of feline trigeminal spinal tract nucleus neurons to stimulation of the middle meningeal artery and sagittal sinus. *J Neurophysiol* 1988; 59:648–666.
28. Strassman A, Mason P, Moskowitz MA, and Maciewicz R. Response of brainstem trigeminal neurons to electrical stimulation of the dura. *Brain Res* 1986; 379:242–250.

25

Extracellular Changes of Aspartate and Glutamate During Generation and During Propagation of Cortical Spreading Depressions in Rats

Dieter Scheller, Ulrike Heister, Karin Dengler, and Frank Tegtmeier

Janssen Research Foundation, 4040 Neuss 21, Germany

Cortical spreading depression (CSD) is suggested to represent an animal correlate of human migraine: a transient increase of local cortical blood flow (LCBF) followed by a long-lasting hypoperfusion could be observed during a migraine attack of humans as well as during CSD in animal experiments (3). CSD can be evoked by glutamate (6) indicating a possible participation of the N-methyl-D-aspartate (NMDA) receptors. Recently, NMDA antagonists have been shown to suppress CSD (4,5), thus supporting an essential role of the NMDA receptor in generation of CSD. NMDA receptor antagonists, therefore, might be of therapeutic interest. However, no *in vivo* studies have been performed to demonstrate a possible contribution of the NMDA receptor in the propagating mechanism of CSD.

The aim of this study was to measure the release of aspartate (asp) and glutamate (glu) during generation and propagation of CSD by means of two microdialysis (MD) probes implanted in sensory and motorcortex: one MD probe served to apply KCl locally as well as to measure the amino acids; the other MD probe was used to detect the changes of asp and glu at a remote site toward which the CSD was propagating. In addition, NMDA antagonists were applied separately to the remote MD probe in order to selectively affect the propagating CSD.

METHODS

Rats were anesthetized with urethane (1.75 g/kg) and fixed within a stereotaxic frame. Two holes [rostral (r) and caudal (c) to the bregma] were drilled into the skull at a distance of 6–10 mm and the dura was incised. Two microelectrodes (ME; rostral ME: MEr; caudal ME: MEc) were inserted, each to a depth of 1,000 μm and at a distance of about 100–500 μm from one of the two MD probes (2 mm length, 0.5 mm outer diameter, from Carnegie Medicine, Stockholm, Sweden), which were implanted separately within both burr holes (rostral probe: MDr; caudal probe: MDc). Four or 10 μl samples were collected at a flow rate of 2 μl/min. Perfusate consisted of artificial cerebrospinal fluid (CSF). Asp, glu, and taurine (tau) were identified by fluorescence detection after derivatization with o-phthaldialdehyde (OPA) and reversed phase high performance liquid chromatography (HPLC).

To induce a single CSD, CSF was switched to high K^+-CSF (NaCl replaced by KCl, K^+ = 128 mmol/l) for 2 min at either the caudal or the rostral MD probe. KCl was perfused repetitively with recovery periods of 45–90 min between each application. 2-APV (0.1 mmol/l in CSF) was added to the perfusate of the remote MD probe and started variable times before the corresponding KCl application.

RESULTS

Figure 1 shows the DC shifts occurring at the site of generation of CSD due to KCl application (Fig. 1a, DC r) and at the site of propagating CSD (Fig. 1a, DC c). The shapes of CSDs at their origin were similar to their appearance at a remote site: the negative deflection varied between 15 and 20 mV and lasted for about 30 sec. Propagation velocity was 3.5 ± 1.04 mm/min.

The inserts (Fig. 1b,c) show the extracellular changes of asp and glu at the site of origin of CSD (Fig. 1b) or at the site of propagation (Fig. 1c): both amino acids increased at the site of KCl application (3) but were rarely detectable at the remote site. Asp and glu reached their maximum more or less concomitantly with DC shift. Baseline was reached again 6.4 ± 1.5 min later. Tau has been monitored additionally as a measure of specific (homeostatic?) events secondary to CSD (5): tau increased at the site of CSD generation (reaching maximum later than DC and returning to baseline within 22.3 ± 4.8 min) but increased only rarely at the site of propagation. Fig. 1a

FIG. 1. DC changes (**a**) and extracellular amino acid alterations (**b,c**) during generation (DC r) and propagation (DC c) of CSD. Two MEs and 2 MD probes were implanted rostrally and caudally to the bregma. At the time indicated (*arrowhead*) a first CSD was induced by perfusing MDr for 2 min with high K^+ CSF: CSD propagated toward both MEs (DC r, DC c). Fifty min later, a second CSD was induced at MDr (*arrowhead*); at the same time, the remote MD probe (DCc) was perfused with 2-APV: propagating CSD could not be detected (*arrow*). Inserts: Amino acid concentrations in perfusate during K^+ application to generate CSD (**b**) and during propagation toward the remote MD probe (**c**).

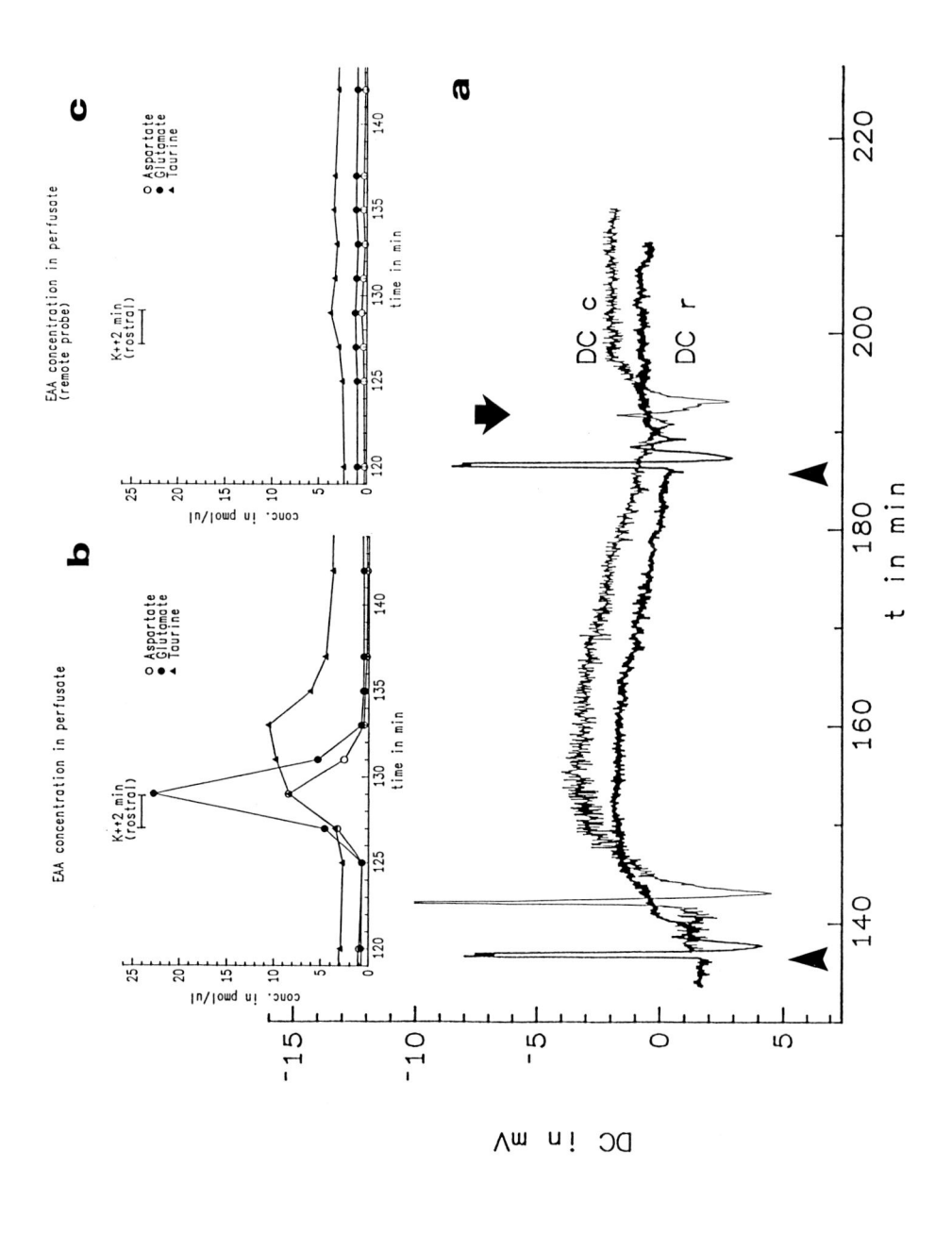

also shows the effect of 2-APV application at the remote MD probe on the propagating CSD (arrow): in 6 of 12 applications, the propagating CSD could be blocked.

DISCUSSION

The MD technique has been used to apply K^+ locally and to measure asp and glu changes at the same time. In parallel, MEs have been used to identify the electrophysiological events accompanying K^+ application. From earlier experiments (5) it has been concluded that local K^+ application evokes a depolarization-mediated release of asp and glu. These transmitters activate NMDA receptors leading to massive electrolyte fluxes and DC shifts identified as CSDs. It has also been shown that application of NMDA induces CSD. K^+-induced and NMDA-induced CSD can be blocked by either ketamine or 2-APV (5).

The CSD, being generated either in motor cortex or sensory cortex, spreads across the hemisphere. As shown here, such propagating CSDs could be blocked by the competitive NMDA-antagonist 2-APV applied in a certain distance from the site of CSD generation. Although 2-APV was efficient in only 50% of applications (possibly due to tissue heterogeneity and nonhomogeneous diffusion of the antagonist in the extracellular space with respect to the location of CSD detecting electrode and/or contribution of non-NMDA receptors or other transmitter-receptor complexes), the results indicate a participation of the NMDA receptor in propagation of CSD. Accordingly, the transmitters mediating the spreading of CSD should be asp and/or glu as the endogenous agonists of the NMDA receptor. However, only tiny changes of both asp and glu were measurable by MD technique at the site of CSD propagation, as opposed to the observation of a dramatic increase at the triggering site. This might be explained methodologically: at the triggering site, K^+ application not only induces neuronal transmitter release but also blocks reuptake of transmitters (1). Only with the aid of this additional effect of K^+ may the synaptic events become detectable. At the remote site, such supporting effect of K^+ is missing. Reuptake of transmitters may still be efficient enough to restrict detectability of the amino acids to only small quantities. Alternatively, endogenous agonists of the NMDA receptor other than asp and glu [e.g., L-homocysteinic acid, quinolinic acid, or N-acetylaspartylglutamate (2)] could have been involved (but were not measured).

The results suggest a participation of the NMDA receptor in propagation of CSD (and, as shown earlier, in generation of CSD) pointing to NMDA antagonists as possible therapeutics to prevent CSD and thus migraine attacks. The role of asp and/or glu or other endogenous agonists on propagation of CSD remains to be established as well as the participation of non-NMDA receptors.

REFERENCES

1. Erecinska M. The neurotransmitter amino acid transport systems: a fresh outlook on an old problem. *Biochem Pharmacol* 1987; 36:3547–3555.
2. Headley PM and Grillner S. Excitatory amino acids and synaptic transmission: the evidence for a physiological function. *TIPS* 1990; 11:205–211.
3. Lauritzen M. Cerebral blood flow in migraine and cortical spreading depression. *Acta Neurol Scand* 1987; 76 [Suppl 111]:9–40.
4. Marrannes R, Willems R, De Prins E, and Wauquier A. Evidence for a role of the N-methyl-D-aspartate (NMDA) receptor in cortical spreading depression in the rat. *Brain Res* 1988; 457:226–240.
5. Scheller D, Heister U, Dengler K, and Peters T. Do the excitatory amino acids aspartate and glutamate generate spreading depressions in vivo? In: Krieglestein J, ed. *Pharmacology of cerebral ischemia*. Stuttgart: Wissenschaftliche Verlagsgesellschaft, 1990: 205–210.
6. Van Harreveld A. Compounds of brain extracts causing spreading depression of cerebral cortical activity and contraction of crustacean muscle. *J Neurochem* 1959; 3:300–315.

26

Noninvasive DC Recordings from the Skull and the Skin During Cortical Spreading Depression: A Model of Detection of Migraine

*Alfred Lehmenkühler, †Frank Richter, ‡Dieter Scheller, and *§Erwin-Josef Speckmann

*Institut für Physiologie, Westfälische-Wilhelms-Universität, W-4400 Münster, †Institut für Physiologie, Friedrich-Schiller-Universität, O-6900 Jena, ‡Janssen Research Foundation, W-4040 Neuss, §Institut für Experimentelle Epilepsieforschung, Westfälische-Wilhelms-Universität, W-4400 Münster, Germany

Evidence is growing that cortical spreading depression (SD), first described by Leão (1), is the underlying event in the aura phase of human migraine (2–4). Therefore, electrophysiological detection of SD in the human brain by measurements of DC potentials and/or magnetic fields (2,5,6) could have great clinical significance for early diagnosis and treatment of migraine attack. The aim of our experiments was to establish an animal model for noninvasive monitoring of SD by DC electroencephalography.

METHODS

The experiments were performed on 12 Wistar rats weighing between 250 and 300 g. The rats were anesthetized with urethane (1,000 mg/kg injected i.p.), paralyzed with suxamethonium chloride (20 mg/kg/hr), and artificially ventilated with oxygen. After hair removal with a depilatory cream, DC potentials were recorded from the skin surface by means of outflow electrodes (Ag-AgCl wire, glass tube, porous ceramic membrane consisting of magnesia; filling solution: 150 mmol/l NaCl, tip diameter: 1.5 mm). A small burr hole (diameter: 0.5 mm) was made near the bregma. Recording electrodes were placed in one row lateral to the sagittal midline so that the first was positioned over the hole and did not contact the brain. The rear electrodes were placed 5 mm apart on the hairless skin. The common reference electrode was positioned on the bone or on the skin of the nose (Fig. 1, B1 and B2). SD was elicited at the trephination hole either by a slight prick with a sharp needle that affected the upper cortical layers, or by replacing 125 mmol/l Na$^+$ by an equimolar amount of K$^+$ in the perfusate (artificial cerebrospinal fluid, perfusion rate: 2 μl/min) of a microdialysis probe for 2 min (Carnegie Medicine, Stockholm, Sweden) lowered into the motorcortex. In

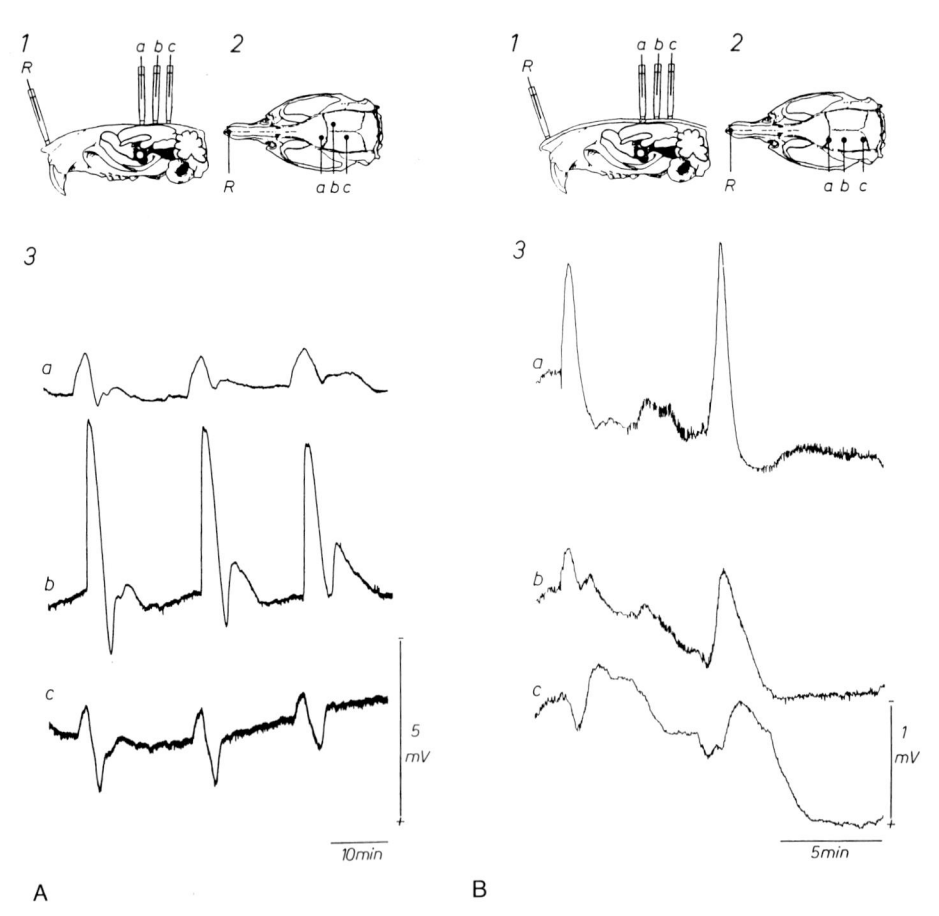

FIG. 1. DC potential shifts recorded at the surface of the skull (**A**) and of the skin (**B**) during cortical spreading depression (SD). Anesthetized and artificially ventilated rat. **A1,A2** and **B1,B2:** Electrodes (a,b,c) and their locations. **A3a,b,c** and **B3a,b,c:** Corresponding simultaneous recordings of SD-related DC potential fluctuations. In A electrode b was filled with 1 M KCl solution to elicit SD. Potassium diffused via the porous membrane in the electrode tip through the bone and resulted in a critical increase of extracellular potassium in upper cortical layers. This increase triggered SD. Electrodes a,c, and R (common reference electrode) were filled with 150 mmol/l NaCl solution and served solely as recording electrodes. In B all electrodes contained 150 mmol/l NaCl solution. The electrode a was positioned over the trephination hole and electrodes b and c recorded from the hairless skin. First SD was elicited by a prick of a needle; the second SD occurred spontaneously. Note different calibrations in A and B. (Panel A from Lehmenkühler and Pöppelmann, ref. 7, with permission.)

some experiments recordings were made from the surface of the intact skull. In these experiments SD waves were produced without any trephination hole by continuous local application of KCl to the skull surface. This was made by replacing the normal filling solution (NaCl, 150 mmol/l) with a solution containing 1,000 mmol/l KCl in the recording outflow electrode overlying the motor cortex. Two additional electrodes filled with isotonic NaCl solution (150 mmol/l) were placed on the skull 2 mm ipsilaterally and contralaterally to the KCl electrode (Fig. 1, A1 and A2).

The signals were recorded using high impedance buffer amplifiers (AD 515L) and stored on digital storage oscilloscope (Nicolet 410V, Nicolet, Madison, WI). The output was made to a laser printer (Hewlett Packard) via a plotter emulating cartridge (Pacific Data Products, Inc., San Diego, CA).

RESULTS

Skull Recordings

Typical negative DC potential shifts as known to occur in the brain during SD started repetitively approximately 1 hr after positioning a KCl electrode on the skull near the bregma (Fig. 1, A3). They were observed only if the KCl electrode was placed above the motor cortex. In this region amplitudes of DC potential shifts accompanying SD reached maximum values and amounted to -4 to -6 mV (Fig. 1A, 3b). Their duration was 5–7 min. Negative DC shifts of lower amplitude were recorded simultaneously from the contralateral site and had lower amplitudes that amounted to -1 to -2 mV (Fig. 1A, 3a,c). The conventional electroencephalogram (EEG) covering the DC recordings was significantly diminished during these transient DC negative shifts.

Skin Recordings

SD was also recorded from the skin surface (Fig. 1, B). SD recorded from the trephination site had DC amplitudes of -1.2 to -1.5 mV (Fig. 1, Ba). They were accompanied by a diminution of the normal EEG and reached their peak about 45 sec after the mechanical stimulus. Recovery to baseline was observed within 130–150 sec. In contrast to the frontal electrode, the rear skin electrodes recorded a smaller negative deflection reaching amplitudes up to -0.9 mV. The negative slope was slowed and recovery was delayed. In some experiments the negative DC shift recorded from the electrode over occipital regions was double-peaked or triple-peaked. SD evoked by switching the perfusate of the microdialysis probe to K^+-rich solution (not shown) were as distinct as those produced by mechanical stimulus, but latencies between application and negative peak of SD were prolonged.

DISCUSSION

In contrast to data in literature achieved by means of DC potential measurements in the brain cortex using microelectrodes, we found SD duration on the skin and on the skull lasting up to 5 times longer. The duration increased with the distance of the point of origin of SD and the point of recording of SD. Therefore, we assume that SD moves within the brain cortex with different speed in different laminae, leading to a large dispersal of the SD wave. This assumption is corroborated by the observation of a triple-peaked DC deviation at distant recording sites. Our data regarding induction of SD solely above motor cortical areas probably could be explained by the relatively small thickness of the bone in this region. Potassium that penetrated this thin bone could therefore accumulate to a critical concentration at the cortical surface that elicited SD. The contralateral electrodes recorded weak negative DC shifts that did not differ in latencies compared with the ipsilateral registered DC shifts. Since the contralateral occurrence of SD-related DC deviation cannot be caused by interhemispheric movement of SD, we assume that SD-related current loops within the skull bones extend to the contralateral site.

As a whole, the study demonstrates that noninvasive DC recording in rats is a useful approach to monitor SD. Comparison with recordings from the brain suggests that skin and skull recordings integratively contain field potentials from a very large brain area. We conclude that the clinical use of DC potential measurements from the skin may resolve the question of whether or not a classical migraine attack is accompanied by SD in human cortex.

REFERENCES

1. Leão AAP. Spreading depression of activity in the cerebral cortex. *J Neurophysiol* 1944; 7:359–390.
2. Welch KMA. Migraine pathogenesis examined with contemporary techniques for analysing brain function. In: Sandler M, Collins GM, eds. *Migraine: A Spectrum of Ideas*, Oxford–New York–Tokyo: Oxford University Press, 1990; 105–113.
3. Olesen J, Skyhøj-Olsen T, Friberg L. Regional cerebral blood flow in migraine. In: Sandler M, Collins GM, eds. *Migraine: a spectrum of ideas*, Oxford–New York–Tokyo: Oxford University Press, 1990; 84–101.
4. Lauritzen M and Olesen J. Regional blood flow during migraine attacks by Xenon-133 inhalation and emission tomography. *Brain* 1984; 107:447–461.
5. Okada YC, Lauritzen M, and Nicholson C. Magnetic field associated with spreading depression: A model for the detection of migraine. *Brain Res* 1988; 442:185–190.
6. Gardener-Medwin AR, Tepley N, Barkley GL, et al. Observation of spreading cortical depression in rabbits. *Proceedings of the 7th International Conference on Biomagnetism, New York* 1989; 127–128.
7. Lehmenkühler A and Pöppelmann Th. Nachweis der corticalen "spreading depression"-reaktion mit hilfe von DC-registrierungen an der schädeloberfläche. In: Wolf P, ed. *Epilepsie 88*, Reinbek: Einhorn-Presse Verlag, 1989; 364–367.

27

Changes in Cerebral Blood Flow Associated with Cortical Spreading Depression in the Cat

Richard Piper, Geoffrey Lambert, John Duckworth, and James Lance

The Institute of Neurological Sciences, The Prince Henry Hospital, Sydney, Australia, 2036

Central to the theory that cortical spreading depression (CSD) may account for the "spreading oligemia" seen during the aura of migraine (1) is the assumption that it results in a prolonged cortical oligemia in the animal model. Unfortunately, apart from the work of Wahl et al. (2), who demonstrated that CSD is followed by prolonged pial dilatation in the cat, animal studies have been confined to the lissencephalic cortex of the rat (3). In this study we have examined the changes in cortical blood flow and cerebrovascular reactivity occurring after CSD in the gyrencephalic cortex of the cat.

METHODS

Thirty two cats weighing 2.3 ± 0.9 kg were anesthetized with α-chloralose (60 mg/kg), intubated, and ventilated to maintain an end-expiratory CO_2 of 4.0–4.5%. Cortical blood flow (CBF_{LD}) was measured through the intact dura and periosteum using a laser Doppler probe (Laserflo BPM403 monitor, Probe-431, TSI, U.S.A.) placed over the suprasylvian gyrus or the posteromedial composite gyrus (visual cortex).

CSD was initiated by cortical pinprick to a depth of 1–2 mm with a 26-gauge needle, 5–22 mm from the recording site. We have previously demonstrated that this stimulus consistently results in a wave of hyperemia, which is associated with electroencephalogram (EEG) flattening and a DC potential shift typical of CSD (4). To avoid any carryover effect, the blood flow changes associated with the first spreading depression in each hemisphere were analyzed. Evidence of subdural hemorrhage at the end of the experiment excluded the animal from the analysis.

Blood Flow Measurements

In animals in whom the delayed effect of CSD or CBF_{LD} was examined, cortical blood flow was recorded for a 2-hr control period in the intact animal, spreading depression was then induced, and CBF_{LD} monitored for another 2 hr. If supplementary anesthesia was required during the recording period, the animal was not included in the data analysis. Only animals demonstrating a normal increase in CBF_{LD} during arterial hypercapnia (>100%) and evidence of active autoregulation as assessed by a gain factor greater than 0.65 (see below) were included in the study.

Assessment of Cerebrovascular Reactivity

Autoregulation of cortical blood flow was assessed by bleeding and subsequently reinfusing the animals to allow calculation of the gain factor ($G_f = 1 - (\Delta CBF_{LD}/CBF_{LD})/(\Delta P/P)$), as described by Norris et al. (5). Cortical vasodilatation after arterial hypercapnia was assessed by passing 8% CO_2, 30% oxygen, and air through the ventilatory circuit for 5 min.

RESULTS

Changes in Cortical Blood Flow

In all animals (n = 32) cortical pinprick resulted in a wave of spreading depression after the initial attempt. In 14 animals the immediate effect of spreading depression on CBF_{LD} was examined. In these animals CSD was associated with a 215 ± 48% (mean ± SE) increase in CBF_{LD}. This period of intense hyperemia lasted for a mean duration of 2.5 ± 0.2 min and in 11 of these animals a period of more prolonged but less intense hyperemia followed (mean duration 5.8 ± 1.1 min).

In 11 animals the more prolonged effect of CSD on cerebral blood flow was examined. After CSD, CBF_{LD} was decreased by 20 ± 4% at 60 min and 28 ± 4% at 120 min compared with initial flow (Table 1). These reductions in CBF_{LD} were statistically significant when compared with CBF_{LD} at the beginning of the 2 hr recording period ($p < 0.01$ at 60 min and $p < 0.01$ at 120 min, paired t-test after Bonferroni correction, n = 11, Table 1). During the 2-hr control period there was no significant change in CBF_{LD} at 60 and 120 min, assessed using a paired t test ($p > 0.05$).

TABLE 1. *Effect of cortical spreading depression on CBF$_{LD}$ and systemic variables*

	Control			CSD		
	0 min	60 min	120 min	0 min	60 min	120 min
CBF$_{LD}$	17.6 ± 2.3	17.1 ± 2.0	18.2 ± 2.2	18.0 ± 2.1	14.3 ± 1.8[a,b]	12.7 ± 1.3[b,c]
% Δ CBF$_{LD}$	—	−2 ± 4	+6 ± 6	—	−20 ± 4	−28 ± 4
MECO$_2$ (%)	2.6 ± 0.1	2.7 ± 0.1	2.8 ± 0.2	2.8 ± 0.1	2.8 ± 0.1	2.8 ± 0.2
BP (mm Hg)	109 ± 5	116 ± 5	118 ± 3	115 ± 6	113 ± 6	113 ± 5

CBF$_{LD}$ is decreased after CSD. Values are expressed as mean ± SE.
[a] $p = 0.001$.
[b] Significant at the $p < 0.01$ level after the Bonferroni procedure.
[c] $p = 0.002$.

Changes in Cerebrovascular Reactivity

The time course of the change in cerebrovascular reactivity to the inhalation of 8% CO$_2$ was followed serially in 12 animals (Fig. 1). The mean increase in cerebral blood flow after the inhalation of CO$_2$ (P$_a$CO$_2$ before = 32 ± 0.9 mm Hg, P$_a$CO$_2$ after = 60 ± 2 mm Hg) was plotted for each successive 200-min interval after the initiation of CSD. These data suggest that cerebrovascular reactivity to the inhalation of CO$_2$ is impaired for as long as 12 hr after the initiation of CSD.

Autoregulation was unaffected when assessed by venesection before and then 30–60 min after CSD (n = 7, G$_f$ pre–CSD 0.80 ± 0.04, G$_f$ post–CSD 0.86 ± 0.03).

DISCUSSION

Crucial to the hypothesis that CSD is responsible for the "spreading oligemia" seen during the aura of migraine (1) is the assumption that it results in prolonged oligemia, not only in the lissencephalic cortex of the rat but also in other experimental animals. This study demonstrates that in the gyrencephalic cortex of the cat, an initial hyperemic phase is followed by prolonged cortical oligemia. In addition, in the cat CSD has effects on cerebrovascular reactivity, characterized by an initial complete abolition of the cortical vasodilatation during arterial hypercapnia, with preservation of autoregulation. These changes in cerebrovascular reactivity are prolonged, as the response to hypercapnia is reduced for up to 10 hr. Wahl et al. (2) have demonstrated dilatation of the pial vessels 15–120 min after CSD in the cat. Our observation that CBF$_{LD}$ at this time is decreased suggests that while the pial vessels dilate the resistance vessels constrict. These animal studies suggest that should CSD occur in the human neocortex it may well result in

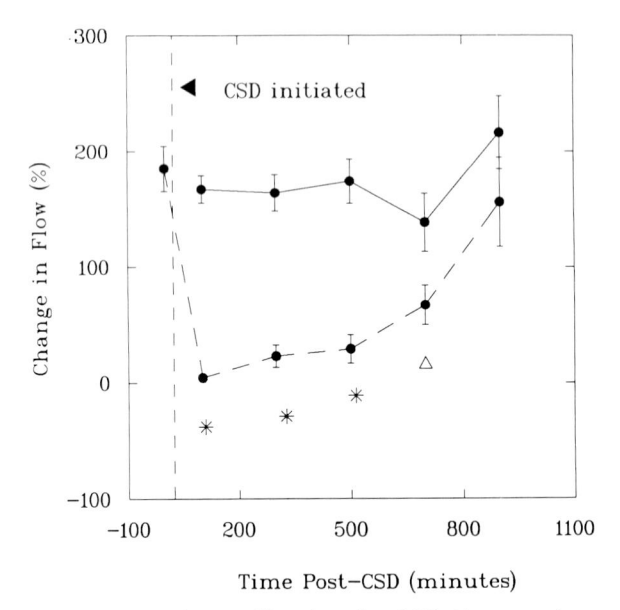

[FIGURE: Plot of Change in Flow (%) vs Time Post-CSD (minutes), showing CSD initiated marker, with two curves comparing responses]

FIG. 1. Reduction in hypercapnic vasodilatation after CSD. Hypercapnia was induced after the inhalation of a mixture of 8% CO_2, 30% oxygen, and air for 5 min. The response before CSD is plotted, followed by the mean response over periods of 200 min after CSD. The mean response in animals in which CSD had not been induced is also plotted over periods of 200 min after the commencement of cortical recordings (* = $p < 0.001$; △ = $p < 0.05$; unpaired t test). Values are expressed as mean ± SE.

significant changes in cerebrovascular hemodynamics of relevance to the migrainous aura.

ACKNOWLEDGMENTS

This work was supported by the National Health and Medical Research Council of Australia, the Basser Trust, the J. A. Perini Family Trust, and Warren and Cheryl Anderson.

REFERENCES

1. Olesen J, Larsen B, and Lauritzen M. Focal hyperaemia followed by spreading oligemia and impaired activation of rCBF in classic migraine. *Ann Neurol* 1981; 9:344–352.
2. Wahl M, Lauritzen M, and Schilling L. Changes in cerebrovascular reactivity after cortical spreading depression in cats and rats. *Brain Res* 1987; 411(1):72–80.
3. Lauritzen M. Long-lasting reduction of cortical blood flow of the rat brain after spreading

depression with preserved autoregulation and impaired CO_2 response. *J Cereb Blood Flow Metab* 1984; 4:546–554.
4. Piper RD, Lambert GA, and Duckworth JW. Cortical blood flow changes during spreading depression in the cat. *Am J Physiol* (*Heart Circ Physiol*) 1991; (in press).
5. Norris CP, Barnes GE, Smith EE, and Granger HJ. Autoregulation of superior mesenteric flow in fasted and fed dogs. *Am J Physiol* 1979; 237(Heart Circ Physiol 6):H174–H177.

28

Effects of Spreading Depression on Physiological Activation of the Cerebral Cortex in the Cat

Richard Piper

The Institute of Neurological Sciences, The Prince Henry Hospital, Sydney, Australia, 2036

Coupling of cerebral blood flow and metabolism was first suggested by Roy and Sherrington in 1890 (1). Fulton in 1928 (2) provided the first evidence to support this hypothesis when he reported a patient with an occipital arteriovenous malformation that was associated with a bruit that increased during reading and visual stimuli. Modern studies using ^{133}Xe clearance and positron emission tomography have since established that metabolism and blood flow in the brain are normally tightly coupled. Roland and Skinhøj (3) using ^{133}Xe clearance have shown that visual stimuli result in widespread changes in cortical blood flow, which are most marked in the primary visual cortex. During the cortical hypoperfusion seen during the migrainous aura, Olesen et al. (4) and others have observed that the changes in cortical blood flow after functional activation are impaired. There is evidence in experimental animals to suggest that cortical spreading depression (CSD) could account for the cortical oligemia seen during the migrainous aura, but its importance in accounting for altered physiological activation of blood flow is uncertain.

With present techniques it is difficult to demonstrate the time course of blood flow changes after activation of discrete areas of cerebral cortex. Laser Doppler is a method that allows localized cortical blood flow to be monitored continuously. This study undertakes to demonstrate that, using this method with computerized averaging, it is possible to study the blood flow changes in the occipital cortex after retinal flash stimulation. The effect of CSD on this response is also examined.

METHODS

Fourteen male cats of mean weight 1.9 ± 0.4 kg were anesthetized with α-chloralose (60 mg/kg) administered intraperitoneally. Depth of anesthesia was checked regularly throughout the experiments and small supplementary doses were given to maintain a stable level of anesthesia. Animals were paralyzed with intravenous vecuronium bromide 0.3 mg/kg to minimize cortical movement artifact caused by ventilation. Before the use of muscle relaxants, the depth of anesthesia was checked to ensure absence of flexion to painful limb stimuli and absence of startle to retinal flash stimulus. The animals were intubated and ventilated to maintain an end-expiratory CO_2 of 4.5–5.0%. Arterial and venous catheters were inserted to monitor blood pressure and administer drugs. Cerebral blood flow (CBF_{LD}) was monitored with a laser doppler perfusion monitor (TSI Laserflo, BPM403, U.S.A.) and pencil probe (P-431). A small occipital craniotomy was performed and the laser Doppler probe placed perpendicular to the cortical surface in gentle contact with the dura. The pupils were dilated with topical homatropine hydrobromide 2%. The ipsilateral eye was covered and a xenon flash positioned 5 cm from the contralateral eye.

CSD was initiated by cortical pinprick to a depth of 1–2 mm with a 26-gauge needle, 5–22 mm from the recording site. We have previously demonstrated that this stimulus consistently results in a wave of hyperemia that is associated with electroencephalogram (EEG) flattening and a DC potential shift typical of CSD (5). To avoid any carryover effect, the blood flow changes associated with the first spreading depression in each hemisphere were analyzed. Evidence of subdural hemorrhage at the end of the experiment excluded the animal from the analysis.

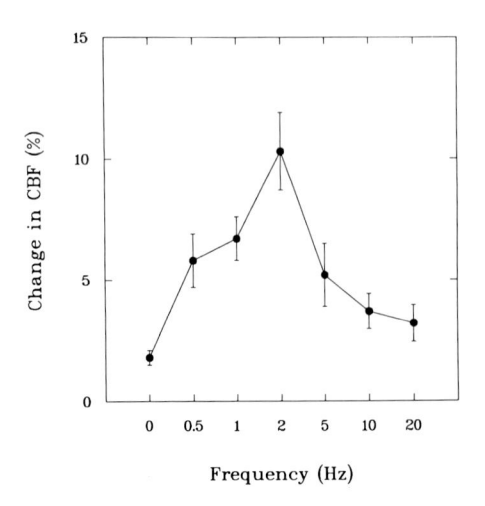

FIG. 1. Cerebral vascular response to activation. Retinal flash stimuli resulted in a frequency-dependent increase in blood flow in the contralateral occipital cortex. Trains of stimuli were 10 sec in duration. Values are expressed as mean ± SE. The maximum response was at 2 Hz. 0 Hz represents the response with the eye covered.

Data were collected on computer after A/D conversion using a fixed data collection cycle of between 30 and 120 sec. The first 25% of the collection cycle was used to accumulate control data; this was immediately followed by a train of retinal flash stimuli. Online averaging was performed over 20–40 such cycles. Cortical vasomotor activity, which results in spontaneous fluctuation in baseline flow at a frequency of 5–10 Hz, made assessment of changes in occipital blood flow difficult because of the large number of data collection cycles required for averaging. In some animals recordings had to be deferred until stable baseline recordings could be achieved. An index of cortical resistance (RES_{Ld}) was obtained by dividing the blood pressure by CBF_{LD}. Changes in CBF_{LD} and RES_{LD} are expressed as a percentage of the initial control period. All values are expressed as mean ± SE unless otherwise stated.

RESULTS

Strobe stimulation of the retina resulted in a frequency-dependent increase in cerebral blood flow in the contralateral occipital cortex (Fig. 1). The response was maximal at 2 Hz (10.3 ± 1.6%) with a latency of 6.8 ± 0.2 sec.

In a group of eight animals the effect of CSD on the changes in CBF_{LD} and RES_{LD} after retinal flash stimulation (2 Hz for 10 sec) was studied. After CSD in the ipsilateral cortex, the change in CBF_{LD} was decreased from 11.4 ± 4.0% to 3.3 ± 1.4% (n = 8, p = 0.03, paired t test) and RES_{LD} from −10.6 ± 3.3% to −4.7 ± 1.9% (p = 0.013, Table 1). Cortical activation after retinal flash stimulation was diminished for up to 80 min with the response being decreased by −77 ± 4.5% at 0–40 min, post-CSD, −49 ± 9.5% at 40–80 min and returning to control values at 80–120 min post-CSD (17 ± 7.4%).

DISCUSSION

Blood flow changes in the occipital cortex after retinal flash stimulation can be detected using laser Doppler velocimetry and computerized averaging. The blood flow changes seen in the cat (10%) are small compared with

TABLE 1. *Effect of CSD on activation of occipital CBF_{LD}*

	Before CSD	After CSD	n	p
BP (mm Hg)	109 ± 10.1	108 ± 8.8	8	0.738
Mean exp CO_2 (%)	2.8 ± 0.18	2.8 ± 0.19	8	0.74
CBF_{LD} (% change)	11.5 ± 4.04	3.35 ± 1.4	8	0.037[a]
RES_{LD} (% change)	10.6 ± 3.3	4.7 ± 1.9	8	0.013[a]

[a] Paired *t* test significant at $p < 0.05$.

those demonstrated using other methods in the awake human (30–40%). It is likely that this is the result of the anesthetic agent used in this study. Blood flow changes were frequency-dependent, being maximal at 2 Hz. After CSD, the visually evoked changes in occipital blood flow were significantly decreased. This result was not due to increased signal variability causing decreased efficiency of the averaging routine, as we have previously observed that cortical vasomotor activity is decreased after CSD (5). There are striking similarities between the blood flow changes seen after CSD and those observed during migraine with aura. In migraine with aura Olesen et al. (4) have demonstrated that cortical blood flow does not increase as expected after cortical activation, consistent with the observations reported here during CSD. Our data thus support the concept of CSD being associated with the migrainous aura and suggest that active vasoconstriction suppresses the usual vasodilator response to metabolic demand.

ACKNOWLEDGMENTS

This work was supported by the National Health and Medical Research Council of Australia, the Basser Trust, the J. A. Perini Family Trust, and Warren and Cheryl Anderson.

REFERENCES

1. Roy CS and Sherrington CS. On regulation of the blood supply to the brain. *J Physiol* 1890; 11:85–108.
2. Fulton JF. Observations made upon vascularity of the human occipital lobe during visual activity. *Brain* 1928; 51:310–320.
3. Roland PE and Skinhøj E. Focal activation of the cerebral cortex during visual discrimination in man. *Brain Res* 1981; 222:166–171.
4. Olesen J, Larsen B, and Lauritzen M. Focal hyperaemia followed by spreading oligemia and impaired activation of rCBF in classic migraine. *Ann Neurol* 1981; 9:344–352.
5. Piper RD, Lambert GA, and Duckworth JD. Cortical blood flow changes during spreading depression in the cat. *Am J Physiol (Heart Circ Physiol)* 1991; (in press).

29

Hypercapnic but Not Neurogenic Cortical Vasodilatation is Blocked by Spreading Depression in Rat

*Peter J. Goadsby, †Jacques Seylaz, and †Sima Mraovitch

*The National Hospital for Neurology and Neurosurgery, Maida Vale, London, England, and †Laboratoire de Physiologie et Physiopathologie Cerebrovasculaire, INSERM U. 182, CNRS U.A. 641, Universite VII, Paris, France

The cortical spreading depression of Leao (SD) was first reported to occur in the exposed rabbit cortex as a negative shift in DC potential that was measured and thus defined electrically. This shift corresponds ionically to a redistribution of K, Na, Cl, Ca, and H ions that has been carefully characterized by micropipette studies (1). Several features of SD have been used to characterize it. These include a rate of propagation of 2–6 mm/min, limitation to one hemisphere, and a refractory period for further SD of up to 3 min. SD has been observed in a number of species including rat and cat, and distinct changes in cerebral blood flow have been described. Initially flow may increase after SD has been initiated and the increase has been reported to be up to 200% and postulated to be related to the pre-SD level of blood flow (2). This is followed by a prolonged moderate reduction in cerebral blood flow that is associated with a marked blunting of cerebrovascular responses to hypercapnia with normal autoregulation (2).

Recently we have shown that the reduction in cerebral blood flow seen after SD may involve not only the cortex but may also include subcortical structures and even the brain stem (3). In this study we have monitored SD as reflected by changes in cerebral cortical perfusion measured by laser doppler flowmetry (CBF_{LDF}) in order to look at the possible basis for the paralysis of the hypercapnic vasodilator response. A comparison to the well described central neurogenic vasodilator response elicited from the centromedian parafasicular thalamus has also been considered (4).

METHODS

Male Wistar rats weighing 300–350 g were anesthetized initially with halothane (0.5–3.0% in 25% O_2/75% N_2) and maintained with α-chloralose (40 mg/kg sc followed by 10 mg/kg iv supplemental). The femoral vessels were cannulated with thin-walled polyethylene tubing and the trachea was cannulated. The animals were paralyzed with *d*-tubocurarine (initially 0.5 mg/kg iv followed by 0.2 mg/kg/hr) and ventilated. Periodically during the experiment the PaO_2, P_aCO_2, and the pH of the arterial blood were measured with a blood gas analyzer (Corning 178). Blood pressure was continuously monitored by connecting the arterial catheter to a Statham pressure transducer and displaying the arterial pressure, mean arterial pressure, and heart rate on a polygraph (Gould).

Stimulation of the CMPf

A parietal burr hole was placed to permit a 100-μm diameter electrode bare only at the tip to be inserted into the CMPf. The anode was connected by a clip to the dorsal neck muscles and square wave pulses (250 μsec duration, 150 μA, 200/sec) were delivered for 10 sec.

Cerebral Cortical Perfusion with LDF (CBF_{LDF})

The use of the laser doppler in the study of cerebral cortical blood flow has been described in detail elsewhere (5). Briefly, a frontal burr hole was placed with care to avoid damage to the underlying cortex. The dura was left intact for these studies. CBF_{LDF} was measured with a BPM 403a (TSI Instruments, St Paul, Minn.) laser Doppler flowmeter and a probe mounted in a stereotaxic holder. The flow signal from the monitor was recorded on the polygraph and changes in CBF_{LDF} determined directly from the tracing.

Experiment Design

The CBF_{LDF} response to acute hypercapnia was checked by introducing CO_2 into the respiratory circuit and a brisk rise in flow observed. After a short recovery period the electrode was lowered into the CMPf and the ensuing flow changes of SD observed. The animal was again challenged with a hypercapnic mixture of gases and immediately or some minutes later, after restoration of normocapnia, the CMPf stimulated and flow responses observed. The responses to both hypercapnia and CMPf stimulation were followed for up to 4 hr.

Statistics

Data are expressed as mean ± SEM. CBF_{LDF} data have been expressed as the percentage change from the preceding control period before any statistical analysis. Experiments were evaluated using a single way ANOVA with Dunnett's test. Significance was assessed at the $p < 0.05$ level.

RESULTS

Hemodynamic and arterial blood gas data for the animals included in the analysis were within the normal range for the anesthetized rat (Table 1).

Effect of Hypercapnia on CBF_{LDF}

Increasing the proportion of CO_2 in the inspired gas mixture increased the $Paco_2$ to 57 ± 2 mm Hg, which resulted in an overall increase in CBF_{LDF} of 225 ± 51%. This response was time-locked and highly reproducible (Fig. 1). The latency of onset was 60–90 sec and the time to peak 120–150 sec, with a total duration of 4 min.

SD and CBF_{LDF}

After insertion of the stimulating electrode into the CMPf at a latency consistent with a rate of propagation of 3–5 mm/min a wave of SD passed under the laser doppler probe. This consisted initially of a marked brisk increase in flow of 566 ± 124% and was followed by a diminution in flow of 19 ± 4% (Fig. 1).

CBF_{LDF} Responses After SD

After a SD, increasing the $Paco_2$ (Table 1) produced little if any response in the CBF_{LDF} (Fig. 1). The mean change over the cohort studied was a 10

TABLE 1. *Physiologic data[a]*

	pH	pCO_2	pO_2	Blood pressure (mm Hg)	Heart rate (/min)
Control	7.48 ± 0.02	35 ± 1	164 ± 13	125 ± 5	505 ± 35
Hypercapnia	7.33 ± 0.02	57 ± 2	127 ± 17	126 ± 6	442 ± 32
SD[b]	7.32 ± 0.02	59 ± 2	139 ± 14	120 ± 7	447 ± 37

[a]Physiologic data for the rats (n = 6, weight 334 ± 23g) included in the anaylsis.
[b]SD, data for hypercapnic response after induction of spreading depression.

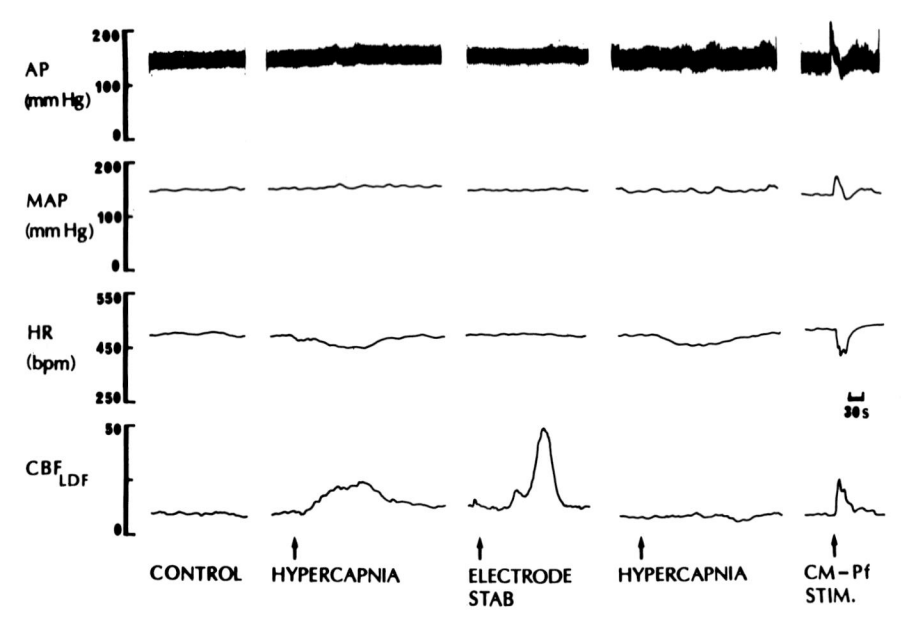

FIG. 1. Chart recordings from a typical experiment with the blood pressure (BP, top trace pulsatile and second mean), heart rate (HR, beats/min) and cerebral cortical perfusion (CBF$_{LDF}$) data. The control period is shown after preparatory surgery. A response to hypercapnia is shown in the second panel with the change in inspiratory CO$_2$ marked. Small pressor and bradycardic responses are seen with a marked increase in CBF$_{LDF}$. The introduction of the electrode into the cortex is followed by a very large increase in CBF$_{LDF}$ with minimal systemic changes. In panel 4 the hypercapnic vasodilator response is blocked whereas in panel 5 the CMPf is stimulated shortly after normocapnia is restored and the flow response is clearly intact. A 30 sec time bar is shown.

± 8% increase. In contrast a strong (120 ± 7%) vasodilator response was seen with CMPf stimulation (Fig. 1). After SD the cardiovascular responses seen with hypercapnia were unaffected (Fig. 1).

DISCUSSION

The experiments presented demonstrate that there is a fundamental difference between hypercapnic vasodilatation and vasodilatation that is neurogenically mediated, at least certainly for that mediated from the CMPf, in that the two may be completely dissociated. By checking cortical vascular reactivity both before and after electrode implantation and induction of SD, these experiments confirm recent observations of SD induction (see Piper, this volume) and that after SD hypercapnic vasodilatation is blocked (2). The neurogenic response mediated from the CMPf is clearly intact even when there is virtually no change with hypercapnia.

The increase in CBF_{LDF} and subsequent reduction in flow observed in these experiments is typical of the changes in cerebral blood flow that characterize SD. Flow may initially increase in SD and this has been considered to be a function of the control flow level. The coupling of the characteristic immediate hyperemia followed by a longer lasting oligemia with a blunted hypercapnic response and normal autoregulation is typical of SD (2). Interestingly, it has recently been shown that some alteration in contralateral flow can be seen with iodoantipyrine autoradiography (Duckrow, personal communication), a phenomenon that may imply that a subcortical or even a brain stem mechanism may play a role in SD. Uniquely in this study stimulation of a central structure that does not alter cerebral glucose utilization (4), the CMPf increases cerebral blood flow when hypercapnia has no effect. The marked vasodilatation that remains is, therefore, not related to any change in either pH or pCO_2 since these no longer have an effect. Furthermore, it can be deduced that the smooth muscle mechanisms for relaxation are primarily unaffected by SD.

The cerebrovascular physiology associated with SD is of particular interest in the clinical setting of migraine. Lashley some years ago plotted the progress of his visual scotoma across his visual field and calculated that it was moving at a rate consistent with a wave of SD. A number of authors have confirmed that there is a reduction in cerebral blood flow at the onset of migraine and that this reduction moves across the cortex at a rate of 3–5 mm/min (6). It has also been observed in some migraineurs that this oligemia is preceded by a focal hyperemia and that after the passage of the oligemia the cerebrovascular response to hypercapnia is blunted while autoregulation is intact (6). All these observations in man are clearly consistent with a wave of SD at the onset of headache. The data presented in this study suggest that neural mechanisms involved in cerebrovascular control and vascular pain, such as those in the brain stem and trigeminovascular system (7), could still influence cerebral blood flow during headache. Furthermore, the cerebral smooth muscle is plainly functional, a fact that may have immense importance in considering the action and design of future antimigraine drugs.

In summary, these data have demonstrated the characteristics of the cerebral cortical blood flow during SD, with a hyperemia that propagates at a rate of 3–5 mm/min followed by a long-lasting cortical oligemia. Hypercapnic vasodilatation is blocked after SD while neurogenic vasodilatation arising from electrical stimulation of the CMPf is intact and powerful. This study demonstrates a fundamental difference in the mechanism of both these responses and provides the exciting prospect of a simple reproducible model to dissociate neurogenic and nonneurogenic cerebrovascular mechanisms. The data also have important implications in the understanding and future management of migraine.

REFERENCES

1. Kraig RP and Nicholson C. Extracellular ionic variations during spreading depression. *Neuroscience* 1978;3:1045–1059.
2. Lauritzen M. Long-lasting reduction of cortical blood flow of the rat brain after spreading depression with preserved autoregulation and impaired CO_2 response. *J Cereb Blood Flow Metab* 1984;4:546–554.
3. Mraovitch S, Calando Y, and Seylaz J. Long-lasting cerebral blood flow and metabolic changes within the limbic and brainstem regions following cortical spreading depression in rat. *J Cereb Blood Flow Metab* 1989;9:S508.
4. Mraovitch S and Seylaz J. Metabolism-independent cerebral vasodilation elicited by electrical stimulation of the centromedian-parafasicular complex in the rat. *Neurosci Lett* 1987;83:269–274.
5. Goadsby PJ. Characteristics of facial nerve elicited cerebral vasodilatation determined with laser Doppler flowmetry. *Am J Physiol* 1991; (in press).
6. Lauritzen M, Olsen TS, Lassen NA, and Paulson OB. Regulation of regional cerebral blood flow during and between migraine attacks. *Ann Neurol* 1983;14:569–572.
7. Goadsby PJ and Lance JW. Brainstem effects on intra- and extracerebral circulations. Relation to migraine and cluster headache. In: Olesen J, Edvinsson L, eds. *Basic mechanisms of headache*. Amsterdam: Elsevier Science Publishers, 1988:413–427.

30

Magnetoencephalographic Signals During and Between Migraine Attacks: Possible Relationship to Spreading Cortical Depression

*Gregory L. Barkley, *†Norman Tepley, *†John E. Moran, *Sandra Nagel-Leiby, and *K. M. A. Welch

*Neuromagnetism Laboratory, Department of Neurology, Henry Ford Hospital, Detroit, Michigan 48202, and †Physics Department, Oakland University, Rochester, Michigan 48309

METHODS

Patients were classified according to criteria of the International Headache Society (1) and consent was obtained. Seventeen migraine patients (4 men, 13 women) from 18 to 43 years old were studied. Eleven women and three men had migraine with aura (MA) and two women and one man had migraine without aura (MO). Three MA patients were studied both during attacks and interictally, four during attacks only, and six interictally only (including one during a failed trigger attempt). One MO patient was studied both during an attack and interictally and two were studied interictally only. Eight volunteers aged 25–46 years old (five men, three women) with rare episodic tension-type headaches, three patients aged 38–61 years old with chronic tension-type headaches, and one woman aged 43 years with headaches due to an Arnold-Chiari malformation were studied as controls.

Subjects were studied in a magnetically shielded room for 30–60 min using a seven-channel DC-coupled Squid Neuromagnetometer (BTI Model 607) consisting of hexagonal array and central second-order gradiometers (18 mm diameter pick-up coils, 21.5 mm axial spacing) within a dewar vessel. The dewar was placed close to but not touching the scalp. Magnetic signals from distant sources were measured continuously with three orthogonal reference magnetometers and reference gradiometer located within the dewar about 300 mm above the seven gradiometer channels. Patients were recumbant and the probe was positioned over the temporoparietooccipital (TPO) junction of the hemisphere felt to be responsible for the migrainous aura in MA patients or on the side of the headache (MO and other headache patients). Where possible, migraine patients were studied (11 cases) under DC-coupled conditions (bandpass 0–50 Hz). When patient or environmental magnetic noise was high (11 cases), data were collected AC-coupled (bandpass 0.1–50 Hz). A sampling rate of 130 Hz/channel was used in all cases. Extensive precautions were taken to recognize and when possible to prevent artifacts. A series of head movements, blinks, swallowing, and so on were performed at the beginning of each study except for patients rushed to the laboratory with migrainous aura, where these maneuvers were performed at the end of the recording. An observer also signaled any perceptible inadvertent movements by event marker pulses during each study. All data contaminated by artifact were excluded from analysis. Only 17 of 56 migraine patients and 12 of 15 nonmigraine patients had studies sufficiently free of artifact to be analyzed.

RESULTS

Two magnetic signals lasting many minutes have been seen during migraine attacks and once after a failed attempt to trigger an attack. These signals consist of: (a) DC field shifts and (b) suppression of ongoing neuromagnetic activity. DC field shifts are large amplitude 2–10 picotesla field changes lasting 10–30 min. Figure 1 shows an example of such a shift recorded over the right TPO junction in a 29-year-old woman. The recording began 20 min after the onset of a left homonymous visual aura. The aura persisted for the initial 6 min of the study before being succeeded by a throbbing right-sided headache. The study was interrupted for administration of medicine (as shown). DC shifts were seen in two of three DC-coupled studies during attacks in MA patients and in the only MO patient studied during an attack. The second ictal signal seen during migraine is suppression of amplitude of spontaneous activity. This attenuation lasts from 2 to 10 min and can be seen both in AC-coupled and DC-coupled studies. The suppression can be seen more easily when spontaneous activity is displayed as consecutive 2-sec averages or the standard deviation of these averages as shown in Fig. 2 taken from a 26-year-old male MA patient after a failed attempt to trigger an attack by vigorous exercise. In this study the greatest attenuation is seen in the 2,300–2,400 sec interval, which is shown by further analysis by a mimetic technique we have developed called Dynamic Period Analysis (DPA) to represent a reduction in neuromagnetic activity in a widespread fashion at all frequency bands. In Fig. 3 the spectrum of magnetic activity occurring during the interval of suppression is compared to the interval from 100 to 200 sec when the patient was known to be awake and also differs from

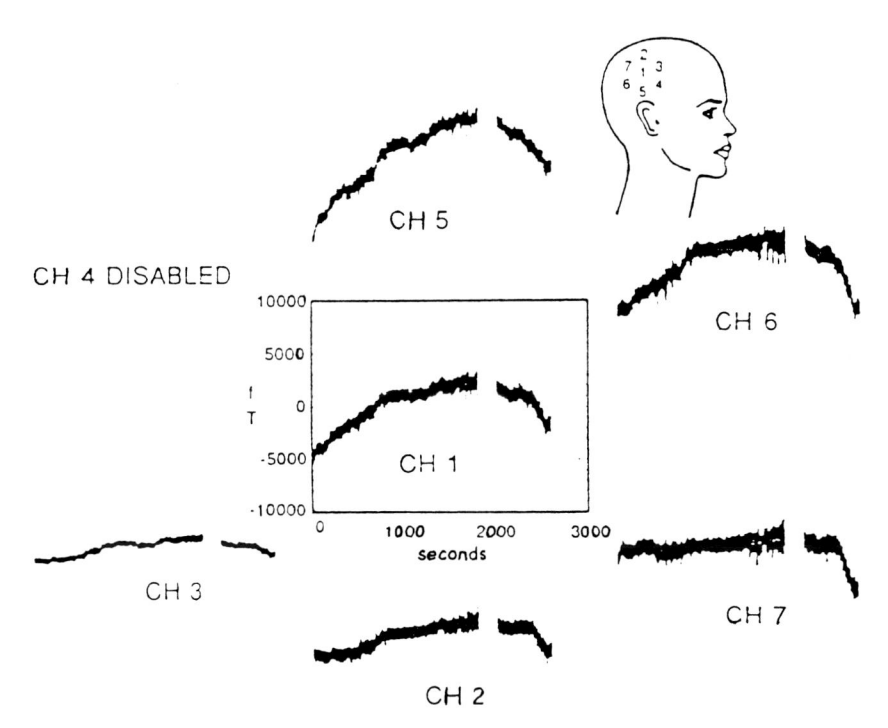

FIG. 1. DC shift during migraine with aura.

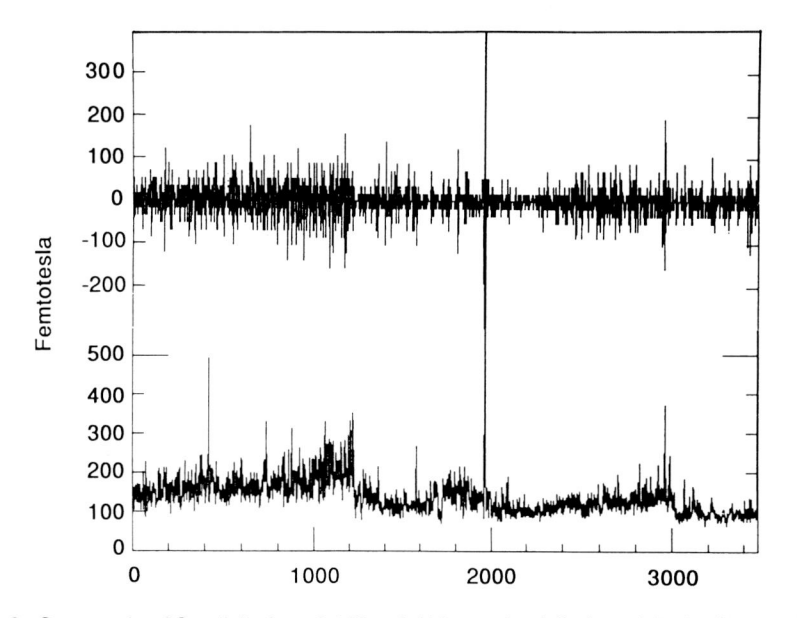

FIG. 2. Suppression AC activity from 2,300 to 2,400 sec after failed precipitation by exercise. **Top:** 2-sec average data. **Bottom:** standard deviation of 2-sec average data.

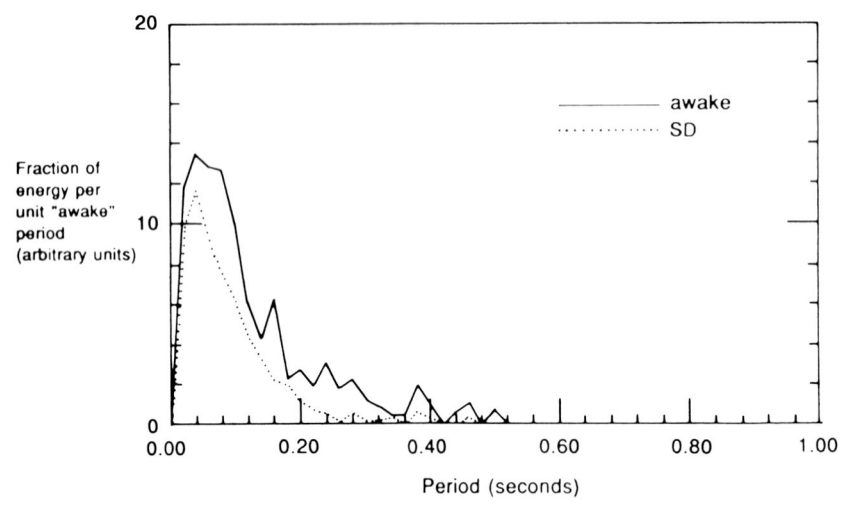

FIG. 3. Reduced amplitudes at all frequencies during suppressed period compared to baseline (from Fig. 2).

spectra obtained during sleep (not shown). Suppression of this type was seen in five of eight MA patients during attacks (and after a failed trigger attempt) as well as in the only MO patient seen during an attack.

The third signal we found consists of large amplitude waves (LAW) lasting 5–10 sec ranging 800 femtotesla to 13 picotesla (Fig. 4). These waves vary in appearance in each channel but are typically biphasic. Several LAWs are frequently seen during a typical study, with each LAW varying in morphology from the others. LAWs have been seen both during attacks and interictally. In MA patients, LAWs were seen in four of eight attacks and in 4 of 10 interictal studies, including the failed trigger attempt. In MO patients, LAWs were not seen in the only attack studied but were present in one of three interictal studies.

The three signals just described are summarized in Table 1. None of these signals was seen in control patients with nonmigraine headaches.

In the 19th century, Gowers speculated on the origins of migraine and felt that its genesis lay in a primary disturbance of brain function (2). In 1941, Lashley calculated that the advancing positive phenomena of his migrainous visual aura could be explained by a propagating cortical dysfunction in his occipital lobe spreading at a rate of 3 mm/min (3). Three years later Leao described a slowly propagating cortical process, detectable only by electrocorticography (ECoG), now called spreading cortical depression (SCD), characterized by suppression of neuronal activity (4) and a DC potential shift that expands annularly at a rate of 2–4 mm/mm (5), which he postulated might play a role in migraine. The similarity between Lashley's scotoma and

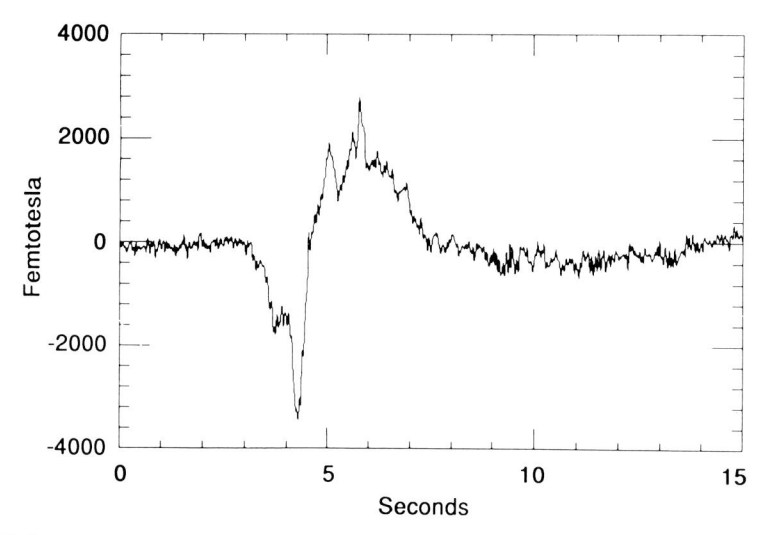

FIG. 4. LAWs from patient in Fig. 2 that occurred just before suppressed interval.

SCD of Leao was first noted by Milner in 1958 (6). Olesen et al. in 1981 showed spreading oligemia is produced during migrainous aura in a pattern suggestive of the spread of SCD (7). Skyhoj-Olsen et al. reexamined these data and concluded that cerebral blood flow actually reached ischemic levels during the attacks (8).

Magnetoencephalography (MEG) represents a major technical advancement in the study of neurophysiology. This is particularly true for measurement of slowly changing phenomenon such as SCD, which previously could be detected only by invasive techniques such as ECoG. MEG can be used to make noninvasive DC recordings. In addition, MEG measures primary currents arising intracellularly in neurons and is inherently more sensitive to local changes such as the type generated by SCD than is electroencephalography (EEG), which not only averages potential changes over a larger vol-

TABLE 1. *MEG signals in migraine*

	LAW	DC shift	Suppression
Migraine with aura (18 studies)			
Ictal	4/8 (50%)	2/3 (67%)	5/8 (63%)
Interictal	4/10 (40%)	0/6 (0%)	1/10 (10%)[a]
Migraine without aura (4 studies)			
Ictal	0/1 (0%)	1/1 (100%)	1/1 (100%)
Interictal	1/3 (33%)	0/1 (0%)	0/3 (0%)
Control (12 studies)	0/12 (0%)	0/6 (0%)	0/12 (0%)

[a] Failed precipitation.

ume of tissue than MEG but also unlike MEG requires a reference electrode, a possible source of artifact.

We have seen three signals in our MEG studies of migraine, none of which has been seen in controls with other headache types. Two of the three signals we have recorded in migraine patients are typical of SCD. The suppression of spontaneous activity and DC field shifts lasting many minutes are similar to the suppression of DC field shifts seen in our rabbit model of SCD (9). The third signal is a novel wave form of high amplitude and varying morphology that typically lasts 5–10 sec (10). This signal, which we call LAWs, has not been seen in our SCD experiments in the rabbit. LAWs have been seen both during and between migraine attacks in contrast to DC shifts and suppression, which have been seen only during migraine attacks with one exception. That lone exception was after a failed precipitation of migraine in a MA patient with exercise induced migraine.

We are uncertain of what LAWs represent. We initially thought that LAWs were a manifestation of SCD as it propagated across a sulcus, the ideal orientation of pyramidal neurons felt responsible for the generation of fields detectable by MEG. We now think that this is not sufficient to explain the presence of LAWs in interictal studies. We postulate that LAWs represent the abortive onset of SCD that fails to exceed the threshold necessary to sustain propagation. Geometric constraints again would suggest that these signals arise in sulci. This explanation is consistent with our hypothesis that migraine represents a state of central neuronal hyperexcitability (11). Conceivably, LAWs occasionally might be seen in nonmigrainous relatives of migraine patients analogous to the findings of certain EEG patterns in relatives of individuals with primary generalized epilepsies. We are in the midst of an extended project involving many migraine and tension-type headache patients measuring brain activity by MEG and simultaneous EEG. Patients are being studied both ictally and interictally. Interpretations are being made in a blinded fashion. We hope that this project will further delineate the nature and occurrence of the intriguing signals we have identified with this initial work.

REFERENCES

1. Headache Classification Committee of the International Headache Society. Classification and diagnostic criteria for headache disorders, cranial neuralgias, and facial pain. *Cephalalgia* 1988; 8:10–92.
2. Gowers WR. *The border-land of epilepsy*. London: Churchill, 1907. Reprinted by Old Hickory Bookshop, Brinklow, Maryland.
3. Lashley KS. Patterns of cerebral integration indicated by the scotomatas of migraine. *Arch Neurol Psychiatry* 1941; 46:331–339.
4. Leao AAP. Spreading depression of activity in the cerebral cortex. *J Neurophysiol* 1944; 8:379–390.
5. Leao AAP. Further observation on the spreading depression of activity in the cerebral cortex. *J Neurophysiol* 1947; 10:409–419.

30

Magnetoencephalographic Signals During and Between Migraine Attacks: Possible Relationship to Spreading Cortical Depression

*Gregory L. Barkley, *†Norman Tepley, *†John E. Moran, *Sandra Nagel-Leiby, and *K. M. A. Welch

*Neuromagnetism Laboratory, Department of Neurology, Henry Ford Hospital, Detroit, Michigan 48202, and †Physics Department, Oakland University, Rochester, Michigan 48309

METHODS

Patients were classified according to criteria of the International Headache Society (1) and consent was obtained. Seventeen migraine patients (4 men, 13 women) from 18 to 43 years old were studied. Eleven women and three men had migraine with aura (MA) and two women and one man had migraine without aura (MO). Three MA patients were studied both during attacks and interictally, four during attacks only, and six interictally only (including one during a failed trigger attempt). One MO patient was studied both during an attack and interictally and two were studied interictally only. Eight volunteers aged 25–46 years old (five men, three women) with rare episodic tension-type headaches, three patients aged 38–61 years old with chronic tension-type headaches, and one woman aged 43 years with headaches due to an Arnold-Chiari malformation were studied as controls.

Subjects were studied in a magnetically shielded room for 30–60 min using a seven-channel DC-coupled Squid Neuromagnetometer (BTI Model 607) consisting of hexagonal array and central second-order gradiometers (18 mm diameter pick-up coils, 21.5 mm axial spacing) within a dewar vessel. The dewar was placed close to but not touching the scalp. Magnetic signals from distant sources were measured continuously with three orthogonal reference magnetometers and reference gradiometer located within the dewar about 300 mm above the seven gradiometer channels. Patients were recumbant and the probe was positioned over the temporoparietooccipital (TPO) junction of the hemisphere felt to be responsible for the migrainous aura in MA patients or on the side of the headache (MO and other headache patients). Where possible, migraine patients were studied (11 cases) under DC-coupled conditions (bandpass 0–50 Hz). When patient or environmental magnetic noise was high (11 cases), data were collected AC-coupled (bandpass 0.1–50 Hz). A sampling rate of 130 Hz/channel was used in all cases. Extensive precautions were taken to recognize and when possible to prevent artifacts. A series of head movements, blinks, swallowing, and so on were performed at the beginning of each study except for patients rushed to the laboratory with migrainous aura, where these maneuvers were performed at the end of the recording. An observer also signaled any perceptible inadvertent movements by event marker pulses during each study. All data contaminated by artifact were excluded from analysis. Only 17 of 56 migraine patients and 12 of 15 nonmigraine patients had studies sufficiently free of artifact to be analyzed.

RESULTS

Two magnetic signals lasting many minutes have been seen during migraine attacks and once after a failed attempt to trigger an attack. These signals consist of: (a) DC field shifts and (b) suppression of ongoing neuromagnetic activity. DC field shifts are large amplitude 2–10 picotesla field changes lasting 10–30 min. Figure 1 shows an example of such a shift recorded over the right TPO junction in a 29-year-old woman. The recording began 20 min after the onset of a left homonymous visual aura. The aura persisted for the initial 6 min of the study before being succeeded by a throbbing right-sided headache. The study was interrupted for administration of medicine (as shown). DC shifts were seen in two of three DC-coupled studies during attacks in MA patients and in the only MO patient studied during an attack. The second ictal signal seen during migraine is suppression of amplitude of spontaneous activity. This attenuation lasts from 2 to 10 min and can be seen both in AC-coupled and DC-coupled studies. The suppression can be seen more easily when spontaneous activity is displayed as consecutive 2-sec averages or the standard deviation of these averages as shown in Fig. 2 taken from a 26-year-old male MA patient after a failed attempt to trigger an attack by vigorous exercise. In this study the greatest attenuation is seen in the 2,300–2,400 sec interval, which is shown by further analysis by a mimetic technique we have developed called Dynamic Period Analysis (DPA) to represent a reduction in neuromagnetic activity in a widespread fashion at all frequency bands. In Fig. 3 the spectrum of magnetic activity occurring during the interval of suppression is compared to the interval from 100 to 200 sec when the patient was known to be awake and also differs from

6. Milner PM. Note on a possible correspondence between scotomas of migraine and spreading depression of Leao. *Electroencephal Clin Neurophysiol* 1958; 10:705.
7. Olesen J, Larsen B, and Lauritizen M. Focal hyperemia followed by spreading oligemia and impaired activation of rCBF in classic migraine. *Ann Neurol* 1981; 9:344–352.
8. Skyhøj-Olsen TS, Friberg L, and Lassen NA. Ischemia may be the primary cause of the neurologic deficits in classic migraine. *Arch Neurol* 1987; 44:156–161.
9. Gardner-Medwin AR, Tepley N, Barkley GL, Moran JE, Nagel-Leiby S, Simkins RT, and Welch KMA. Magnetic fields associated with spreading depression in anaesthetised rabbits. *Brain Res* 1991; 540:153–158.
10. Barkley GL, Tepley N, Nagel-Leiby S, Moran JE, Simkins RT, and Welch KMA. Magnetoencephalographic studies of migraine. *Headache* 1990; 30:428–434.
11. Welch KMA, D'Andrea G, Tepley N, Barkley G, and Ramadan NM. The concept of migraine as a state of central neuronal hyperexcitability. *Neurol Clin* 1990; 8:817–828.

31

Mechanisms of Migraine with Aura: Discussion Summary

John Stirling Meyer and Michael A. Moskowitz

The problem of Compton scatter utilizing the intraarterial injection method was found to be considerable, although clearly less than with inhalation or intravenous (iv) injection of ^{133}Xe. Simulation experiments reported in the discussion confirm that scattered radiation makes it impossible to evaluate exactly how low the flow is in the hypoperfused area of migraine patients.

The discussion thereafter focuses on spreading depression as a possible mechanism of migraine aura. It was asked whether activation by visual stimulation of cerebral blood flow (CBF) is inhibited in migraine with aura as it is in animal models of spreading depression. There was agreement that such functional activation is abolished in the low flow areas of migraine patients. It has not been possible to prove that ischemia produces spreading depression (SD) but N-methyl-D-aspartate (NMDA) receptors are definitely involved. The speed of SD is relatively constant at 3–4 mm/min but depends on the degree and severity of the stimulus and other experimental conditions. There is no hyperperfusion for up to 4 hr after SD but it has not been evaluated beyond this time interval. There is an increased production of lactate during SD as also occurs in the aura of migraine where cerebrospinal fluid (CSF) lactate has been shown to be increased. SD moves at different rates in different layers of the cortex. During SD no permeability change of the blood-brain barrier has been demonstrated after trypan blue and albumin injections. It was concluded that SD is an interesting model in experimental animals of possible relevance to the migraine aura, but although some similarities exist there is no confirmatory evidence that the two phenomena are the same or that SD occurs in humans.

The correlation of migraine with stroke as a complication was discussed. In general, it was agreed that whereas aura may, and sometimes does, progress to stroke, once stroke has occurred the characteristic migraine phenomena cease. Transient ischemic attacks may be confused with migraine but are identifiably different and may be separated by careful history and neurological evaluation.

Sumatriptan crosses the blood-brain barrier only poorly in part because of its hydrophilic properties. These results were obtained from three experimental paradigms. The first used isotopically labeled sumatriptan injected intravenously and demonstrated that only a small fraction of the drug was able to pass into the brain. The second demonstrated that intravenously administered sumatriptan did not inhibit the release of brain sterotonin, as measured by *in vivo* dialysis, but was able to block serotonin (5-HT) release when injected intracerebrally. The third demonstrated that sumatriptan given intravenously did not constrict pial arterioles but did so when applied topically. One unresolved question was whether sumatriptan's effects are restricted to the dura mater or whether they might also involve the pial vasculature. Another concerned whether or not the receptors involved in inhibition of neurogenic inflammation were 5-HT_1–like or $5\text{-HT}_1\text{-D}$. The point was made that $5\text{-HT}_1\text{-D}$ receptors are scarce in rats; the 1B-receptor dominates in that species. Hence, the blockade of neurogenic inflammation in the rat was likely to be 1-B whereas in the guinea pig it is $5\text{-HT}_1\text{-D}$. It is difficult to distinguish between the B and the D receptors, but $5\text{-HT}_1\text{-A}$ and $5\text{-HT}_1\text{-C}$ were unlikely to mediate the antiinflammatory response based on the pharmacological profile presented. It is still premature to say $5\text{-HT}_1\text{-D}$ since there may be more than one subtype. It is better to use the term $5\text{-HT}_1\text{-D}$–like. In a model involving arteriovenous shunts it was unclear whether there is a specific $5\text{-HT}_1\text{-D}$ response.

The development of drug strategies for interrupting individual processes leading to neurogenic inflammation might be important for migraine treatment. For example, calcium-dependent release of neurotransmitters might be blocked by calcium antagonists. Prostaglandin-like agents or nonsteroid-like inflammatory drugs are important as well.

The neurogenic inflammatory response serves to increase blood flow and clear offending toxin or toxins from the tissue at risk and therefore is a protective mechanism that should limit the phenomena of headache. The downside of course is that neurogenic inflammation might be associated with agents that affect the primary afferent fibers with prolongation of headache. Additional studies are needed to clarify this point.

PART VI

Interictal Studies of Migraine Without Aura

32

Regional Cerebral Blood Flow Patterns in Migraine Without Aura: An Interictal SPECT Study

*Lars Friberg, *Bjørn Sperling, †Jes Olesen, †Helle Iversen, *Ida Nicolic, ‡Peer Tfelt-Hansen, and *Niels A. Lassen

*Department of Clinical Physiology and Nuclear Medicine, Bispebjerg Hospital, DK-2400 Copenhagen NV, †Department of Neurology, Gentofte Hospital, DK-2900 Hellerup, and ‡Department of Neurology, Bispebjerg Hospital, DK-2400 Copenhagen NV, Denmark

There are conflicting reports on cerebral blood flow (CBF) during migraine attacks without aura. In the course of some investigations it has not been possible to show any abnormal changes in either regional or global CBF (1–3). Others have found CBF values consistent with global hyperemia during attacks, but without signs of redistribution of focal CBF (4,5). The two types of migraine, now classified as migraine *with aura* and migraine *without aura*, were previously commonly termed "vascular headaches" because of the similarity between the symptomatology of the two types of attacks—except for the *aura*.

This study on interictal regional CBF (rCBF) in patients, with migraine attacks without aura, was carried out in order to explore whether focal abnormalities could be detected in the rCBF patterns. This preliminary report focuses on regional side-to-side asymmetries.

PATIENTS AND CONTROL MATERIAL

According to a prospective, consecutive protocol we examined rCBF in 40 patients who fulfilled the International Headache Society criteria for having solely or predominantly migraine attacks without aura (6). They were all examined when they were completely free from symptoms, including other types of headache than migraine. After examination eight patients were excluded either because they reported having had a migraine attack less than 5 days before examination or because of a technically unsatisfactory examination, including rCBF measurements on a slice level different from OM + 50 mm. Included in this report are 32 patients. Twenty two patients were studied with the ^{133}Xe inhalation technique (18 women, 4 men, mean age 39 years, range 14–58 years). Ten patients were examined with the intravenous ^{99m}Tc-HMPAO (hexamethyl-propylene-amine-oxime) technique (nine women, one man, mean age 42 years, range 25–55 years). Thirty healthy non-migraineurs served as a control material: 10 were examined with the ^{133}Xe inhalation technique (four women, six men, mean age 24 years, range 20–29 years) and 20 with the intravenous (iv) ^{99m}Tc-HMPAO technique (9 women, 11 men, mean age 24 years, range 20–29 years).

METHODS AND DATA ANALYSIS

The examination methods and way of data analysis are explained in detail elsewhere (see Friberg et al.) Briefly, a single photon emission computed tomography (SPECT) rCBF examination was performed using either inhaled ^{133}Xe or iv injected ^{99m}Tc-HMPAO as a blood flow tracer. Quantitated rCBF values (ml/100 g/min) were obtained from the ^{133}Xe inhalation studies and a semiquantitated rCBF distribution was obtained from the ^{99m}Tc-HMPAO examinations. All ^{99m}Tc-HMPAO pictures were normalized and linearized according to the method described by Lassen et al. (7).

Data were analyzed for asymmetries between mirrored regions in the hemispheres in two ways: (a) an independent visual evaluation by four experienced observers, each scoring from 1 (normal) through 4 points (clear asymmetry) and (b) a quantitative analysis by means of a computer, calculating side-to-side asymmetry indices between a set of symmetric, predefined regions of interest (ROIs) corresponded approximately to the supply territories of the large intracranial arteries at the slice level OM + 50 mm. Regional *asymmetry* in the patient's rCBF distribution was defined as an asymmetry index value below or above 2.5 times the standard deviation from the mean value of the same region in the relevant control group. The referral index values for the control groups are given in Tables 1 and 2.

TABLE 1. *Control material: ^{133}Xe inhalation, OM + 50 mm, n = 10*

Region	Right–left asymmetry in %		
	−2.5 SD	Mean	+2.5 SD
Hemisphere	−3.5	0.7	4.9
ACA	−3.3	3.5	10.3
MCA	−4.2	0.9	6.0
MCA 1	−6.5	−1.2	4.1
MCA 2	−4.5	2.8	10.1
PCA	−9.5	−2.2	5.1
Migraine ROI	−6.2	1.0	8.2

TABLE 2. Control material: ^{99m}Tc-HMPAO iv injection, OM + 50 mm, n = 20

Region	Right–left asymmetry in %		
	−2.5 SD	Mean	+2.5 SD
Hemisphere	−3.0	0.7	4.4
ACA	−13.1	−2.4	8.3
MCA	−4.0	1.2	6.4
MCA 1	−5.0	1.9	8.8
MCA 2	−6.3	−0.1	6.1
PCA	−8.5	0.9	10.3
Migraine ROI	−7.2	1.0	9.2

RESULTS

Visual Evaluation

Six migraine patients without aura (19%) were scored as having asymmetrical rCBF patterns (total score between 9 and 16). Twenty six (81%) patients were scored as normal (total score between 4 and 8). All 30 rCBF patterns from the control group were evaluated as being normal. However, when comparing the individual assessments there was lack of consensus of asymmetry among the observers in all patients without aura (not all observers scored either 3 or 4). Full interobserver consensus of normality was found in 43 of 62 patients and controls (all observers scoring 1 or 2). Thus, there was absence of agreement among observers in 19 of 62 (31%) of the evaluated pictures.

Quantitative Evaluation

Asymmetry had to be present between only one set of ROIs to cause the picture to be considered asymmetrical. Asymmetry was found in 3 of 10 (30%) of the patients examined with ^{99m}Tc-HMPAO. Among the patients examined with ^{133}Xe inhalation no less than 18 of 22 (82%) were calculated to be asymmetrical. The high overall rate of asymmetries in the ^{133}Xe studies was influenced by a high incidence of asymmetries between the anterior cerebral artery (ACA) ROIs, in whom 15 of 22 (68%) had asymmetry. However, in none of the ^{99m}Tc-HMPAO studied patients did we find significant asymmetries between the ACA ROIs. As explained previously (in this volume), for technical reasons we left out the ACA ROIs in the analysis. Excluding the ACA ROIs the results showed that 12 of 22 (55%) had asymmetries in one or more ROIs. When more than one hypoperfused ROI was found, they were all located in the same hemisphere. The distribution of number of ROIs with asymmetry was: 1 ROI = 7 patients, 2 ROIs = 10, 33 ROIs = 1, 4 ROIs = 0, and 5 ROIs = 1 patient. The large middle cerebral artery (MCA) ROI was affected less frequently than MCA1, MCA2, PCA, and "migraine ROI." In 4 of 12 the asymmetry in smaller ROIs affected mean CBF in the whole hemisphere, causing mean hemisphere asymmetry.

DISCUSSION

It is interesting that the proportion of patients having migraine *without aura* with asymmetrical rCBF patterns does not differ grossly from the number of asymmetrical patterns seen among patients having migraine *with aura* (see Friberg et al.). It is well established that migraine attacks *without aura* are not associated with focal decrease of brain tissue perfusion as seen in patients *with aura*. However, the clinical characteristics, both concerning pain and accompanying symptoms, are exactly the same in the two types of migraine attacks. Furthermore, pharmaceutical compounds as ergotamine and a new effective antimigraine drug, sumatriptan, exerts a comparable beneficial effect on both types of attacks (8,9). Finally, migraine patients often report both types of attacks, although the majority of attacks are of one type. It therefore seems that the pain in both types of migraine are the same. The present findings indicate that there may also be a common vascular factor involved.

REFERENCES

1. Olesen J, Tfelt-Hansen P, Henriksen L, and Larsen B. The common migraine attack may not be initiated by cerebral ischemia. *Lancet* 1981;2:438–440.
2. Lauritzen M and Olesen J. Regional cerebral blood flow during migraine attacks by Xenon-133 inhalation and emission tomography. *Brain* 1984;107:447–461.
3. Friberg L, Olesen J, and Iversen HK. Regional cerebral blood flow during attacks and when free of symptoms in a large group of migraine patients. *Cephalalgia* 1989;9 [Suppl 10]:29–30.
4. Sakai F and Meyer JS. Regional cerebral hemodynamics during migraine and cluster headache measured by the Xe-133 inhalation method. *Headache* 1978;18:122–132.
5. Juge O and Gauthier G. Mésures de debit sanguin cérebral régional (DSCR) par inhalation de Xenon 133; application cliniques. *Bulletin der Schweizerishn Akadamie der Medizinischen Wissenschaften* 1980;36:101–115.
6. Headache Classification Committee of the International Headache Society. Classification and diagnostic criteria for headache disorders, cranial neuralgias and facial pain. *Cephalalgia* 1988;8[Suppl 7]:1–96.
7. Lassen NA, Andersen AR, Friberg L, and Paulson OB. The retention of [99mTc]-d,l-HM-PAO in the human brain after intracarotid bolus injection: a kinetic analysis. *J Cereb Blood Flow Metab* 1988;8:S13–S22.
8. Doenicke A, Brand J, and Perrin VL. Possible benefit of GR 43175, a novel 5-HT$_1$-like receptor agonist, for the treatment of severe migraine. *Lancet* 1988;i:1309–1311.
9. Tfelt-Hansen P, Brand J, Dano P, Doenicke A, Findley LJ, Iversen HK, Melchart D, and Sahlender HM. Early clinical experience with subcutaneous GR43175 in acute migraine: an overview. *Cephalalgia* 1989;9 [Suppl 9]:73–77.

33

^{99m}Tc-d,l-HMPAO SPECT in Migraine Without Aura

P. Wessely, E. Suess, G. Koch, and I. Podreka

Department of Headache, Neurological Clinic, University of Vienna, Vienna, Austria

In the evolution of theories concerning the pathogenesis of migraine, complementary approaches have been developed. Initially, the vascular theory assumed cerebral vasoconstriction followed by vasodilatation to be responsible for headache in classic migraine (1). Later, spreading oligemia (2) was assumed to be a corresponding hemodynamic phenomenon to spreading cortical depression (3). Advances in the development of regional cerebral blood flow (rCBF) imaging techniques today have encouraged clinical studies to resume a modified vascular theory of migraine. It is widely accepted that rCBF alterations play an important role in different stages of the time course of an attack. In this study, the ^{99m}Tc-d,l-hexamethyl-propylene-amine-oxime (d,l-HMPAO) single photon emission computed tomography (SPECT) technique was used to investigate whether persistent alterations in regional cerebral perfusion can be shown in migraineurs in the symptom-free interval.

MATERIAL AND METHODS

Ten female patients (mean age, 39.5 ± 13.8) with headache classified as *migraine without aura* (according to ref. 4) were investigated in the symptom-free interval using ^{99m}Tc-d,l-HMPAO-SPECT. After clinical investigation, electroencephalogram (EEG) recordings and computed tomography CT investigations were performed in all patients. Except slight cortical atrophy in two cases, CT was normal in all instances. EEG was normal in seven patients, whereas three patients showed diffuse or predominantly lateralized abnormalities (one left, one right). Although the course of migraine attacks frequently implies alternating sites of pain, most patients were able to specify a predominant localization. Five patients described diffuse or bilateral pain, three predominantly right-sided, and two predominantly left-sided.

Since the first onset of migraine, the mean time was 9.42 years (2 month to 35 years). In seven patients, attacks occurred once or several times a week; in three patients once a month or less. SPECT was performed within 2–7 days after the last attack in four cases; in six cases the symptom-free interval exceeded 2 or more weeks. Only one patient was drug-free for several weeks at the time of investigation. The others were under therapy with calcium antagonists (n = 5), ergotamine derivates (n = 4), or other analgesic drugs (n = 8). Three patients took oral contraceptives. For control, a group of 51 healthy volunteers (mean age, 26.3 ± 4.6; 32 women, 19 men) were investigated after informed consent was given, following the procedure described below. SPECT was performed with a dual-head rotating scintillation camera (SIEMENS Dual Rota ZLC 37) under resting state conditions. The patients were placed in a supine position with eyes closed in a room with dim light and white background noise. Parallel hole HIRES collimators (FWHM 12 mm) were used. Sodium perchlorate (500 mg) was given before tracer administration. Eighteen to 25 mCi (666–925MBq) of ^{99m}Tc-d,l-HMPAO was injected intravenously immediately after formulation of the kit, 10 min before starting data acquisition. Sixty (2 × 30) projections were achieved within 30 min (60 sec/angle) with a linear sampling distance of 3.125 mm. Preconstructional filtering of angle views, using a weighted filter of variable shape and size (5) and correction for tissue absorption, was performed (6). For final evaluation, seven single slices (3.125 mm thick) were summed consecutively to obtain a set of 21.9-mm thick transverse sections covering the whole brain. For statistical data evaluation, 16 regions of interest (ROIs) per hemisphere were drawn in four representative cross-sections. The ROIs circumscribe visually discriminable anatomical structures in high-resolution SPECT images (SF1, SF2, SF3: superior frontal gyrus; MF: mesofrontal gyrus; IF: inferior frontal gyrus; C1, C2: central regions; SP, IP: superior and inferior parietal regions; SO, IO: superior and inferior occipital regions; ST, IT: superior and inferior temporal regions; BG: anterior basal ganglia; TH: thalamus; HI: hippocampus). Finally, a regional index [RI = mean cts per voxel (ROI)/ mean cts per voxel (all ROIs)] was calculated, indicating relative hyperperfused or hypoperfused areas.

RESULTS

The comparison of regional indices between patients and normal controls revealed areas with relative hyperperfusion or relative hypoperfusion when mean RIs ± 2 × SD of controls were taken as normal range limits. Both relative hyperperfusion and hypoperfusion were found equally frequent in 23 regions (7.19% of all ROIs or 2.3 ROIs per patient). Significant hemispheric differences (paired t test, n = 10) were found only in one superior frontal region (SF1: t = 2.27, $p < 0.05$), inferior frontal (IF: t = 3.74, $p <$

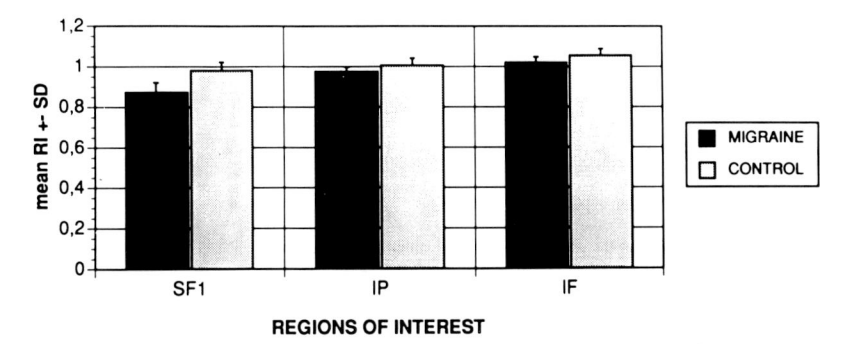

FIG. 1. Hemispheric asymmetries in migraine without aura (paired t test, n = 10).

0.005), and inferior parietal (IP: t = 3.78, $p < 0.005$). The left-sided indices were consistently lower than those on the contralateral side (Fig. 1).

Statistical comparison of RIs between the patient group and normal controls (ANOVA $p < 0.05$) revealed abnormal perfusion in five left-sided and eight right-sided regions. Left-sided, a significant hypoperfusion was observed in one superior frontal region (SF2) and mesofrontal (MF). A significant hyperperfusion was found superior frontal (SF3), superior temporal (ST), and in the hippocampus (HI). Likewise, hypoperfusion occurred in two central regions (C1, C2), superior parietal (SP), and mesofrontal (MF) on the right side. A significant hyperperfusion was observed superior occipital (SO), frontal (SF3), and in the hippocampus (HI). Thus, a distinct pattern of regional hypoperfusion in the frontal and central regions combined with regional hyperperfusion in the distribution area of the posterior artery (occipitotemporal region and hippocampus) can be described in migraine without aura in the symptom-free interval (Fig. 2).

Considering the relatively small caseload and the classification problems due to frequently alternating symptoms, statistical results must be interpreted carefully. However, when the predominant side of headache is taken as classification criterion, ANOVA ($p < 0.05$) allows an approximate estimation of how individual clinical features contribute to the result.

Patients with predominantly left-sided pain (n = 2) showed significant regional alterations only in the left central region and in the right hippocampus. Patients with predominantly right-sided symptoms (n = 3) showed abnormalities in five right-sided (C1, C2, MF, SO, HI) and three left-sided (SF2, MF, SO) regions. Those patients with predominantly diffuse headache (n = 5) contributed to four left-sided and to six right-sided regions with abnormal perfusion. While no abnormalities in the left central and superior occipital regions of both sides were found in the latter group, it is conspicuous that all clinical subgroups contribute to the hippocampal hyperperfusion. According to the observation that a significant lateralization is seen only in

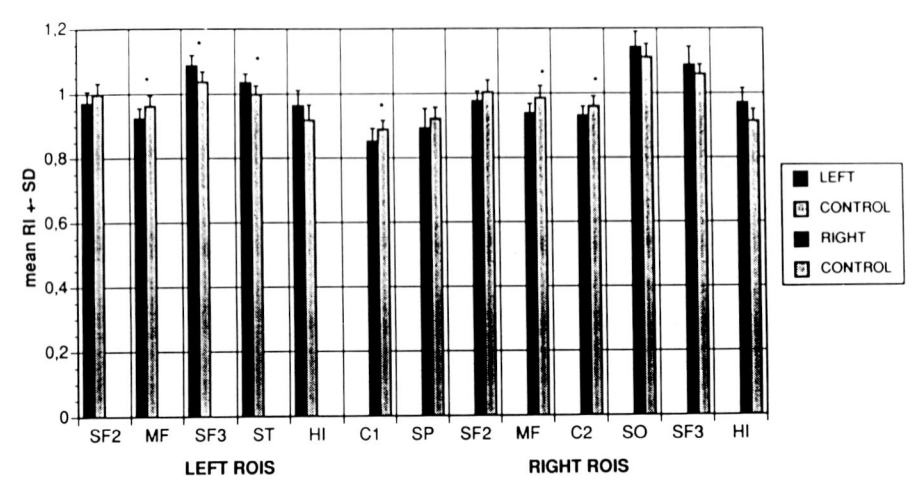

FIG. 2. Comparison (ANOVA $p < 0.05$. (*) $p < 0.01$) of RIs between patients (n = 10) and controls (n = 51).

three regions, the predominant side of headache does not correlate with the number of corresponding abnormally perfused regions. On the contrary, the coincidence of bilateral regional hyperperfusion or hypoperfusion is evident in this type of migraine. Likewise, since EEG recordings were normal in 70% of the patients, neither individual clinical symptoms occurring during the attack nor SPECT findings correlate in the headache-free interval.

DISCUSSION

In this study, three observations characterize a typical pattern of rCBF alterations in migraineurs without aura in the headache-free interval. First, a significant frontal hypoperfusion combined with a hyperperfusion in the posterior region could be shown. Second, compared with the observations made in patients with *migraine with aura*, the number of abnormally perfused regions is relatively high (n = 13), whereas the extent of significant hemispheric asymmetries is comparatively low (n = 3). Finally, all patients investigated in this study contribute to a bilateral hyperperfusion in a subcortical region: the hippocampus.

Similarities between rCBF patterns in different types of headache, as described recently (7), do not necessarily contradict our result, but may reflect common pathogenic factors. Persistent rCBF alterations in the headache-free interval, as observed in this study, may, however, support the assumption of predisposing autonomic dysfunction in migraineurs.

REFERENCES

1. Juge O. Regional cerebral blood flow in the different clinical types of migraine. *Headache* 1988; 28:537-549.
2. Olesen J, Larsen B, and Lauritzen M. Focal hyperemia followed by spreading oligemia and impaired activation of rCBF in classic migraine. *Ann Neurol* 1981; 9: 344-352.
3. Leao AAP. Spreading depression of activity in the cerebral cortex. *J Neurophysiol* 1944; 7:359-390.
4. Headache Classification Committee of the International Headache Society: Classification and diagnostic criteria for headache disorders, cranial neuralgias and facial pain. *Cephalgia* 1988; 8 [Suppl 7]: 1-96.
5. Todd-Prokopek A and Di Paola R. The use of computers for image processing in nuclear medicine. *IEEE Trans Nucl Sci* 1982; 21:1299-1309.
6. Bellini S, Piacentini M, Cafforio C, et al. Compensation of tissue absorption in emission tomography. *IEEE Trans Acous Speech and Sign Proc ASSP* 1979; 27:213-218.
7. Kobari M, Meyer JS, Ichijo M, et al. Cortical and subcortical hyperperfusion during migraine and cluster headache measured by Xe CT-CBF. *Neuroradiology* 1990; 32:4-11.

Migraine and Other Headaches:
The Vascular Mechanisms,
edited by Jes Olesen.
Raven Press, Ltd., New York © 1991.

34

Brain Imaging with ^{99m}Tc-HMPAO and SPECT in Migraine Without Aura: An Interictal Study

*Hans-Peter Schlake, †Ingolf G. Böttger, *Karl-Heinz Grotemeyer, *Ingo W. Husstedt, and †Otmar Schober

*Departments of *Neurology and †Nuclear Medicine, Westfälische Wilhelms-Universität, D-4400 Münster, Germany*

Regional alterations of cerebral perfusion have been demonstrated to occur in migraine with aura even during the interictal state (1–3). However, in patients suffering from migraine without aura, regional cerebral blood flow (rCBF) studies by means of ^{133}Xe inhalation technique gave contradictory results (2,3).

Based on our previous findings with single photon emission computed tomography (SPECT) and Iodoamphetamine (^{123}I-IMP) in interictal classic migraine (1), we investigated headache-free patients suffering from migraine without aura by means of SPECT and the flow tracer ^{99m}Tc-HMPAO (hexamethyl-propylene-amine-oxime).

In contrast to radiopharmaceuticals used in conventional brain scintigraphy, this lipophilic compound crosses the intact blood-brain barrier; it shows a high first-pass extraction into the brain proportionally to blood flow with a maximum of cerebral uptake after 1–2 min and a nearly constant maintenance of the regional distribution over several hours (4,5). It also could be demonstrated that ^{99m}Tc-HMPAO as compared to ^{133}Xe might be superior concerning the spatial resolution of rCBF (5).

MATERIAL AND METHODS

Twenty-two patients (4 men/16 women, aged 16–53 years) suffering from migraine without aura were investigated during the interictal phase. At the time of investigation all patients were headache-free and had not taken any medication for at least 2 weeks.

SPECT investigation of rCBF was performed under standardized environmental conditions (quiet room, dimmed light, eyes open). Fifteen min after intravenous (iv) administration of 400–600 MBq ^{99m}Tc-HMPAO, 64 single images were obtained within a 360° circle using a rotating gamma camera (General Electric 400 ACT). Imaging time per projection was 30 sec and 40 min per examination. Tomographic slices of 12.5 mm width were reconstructed in sagittal, coronal, and horizontal projections by filtered backprojection employing a Butterworth filter with a cut-off frequency of 0.2 cycles/pixel. Interpretation was performed qualitatively and semiquantitatively by a specialist in nuclear medicine in a quasi-blinded way, as he only knew the diagnosis "migraine," but did not get any information on individual migraine subtype or pain localization.

By visual inspection, SPECT findings were divided into four categories:

1. symmetrical perfusion
2. inhomogeneous regional perfusion (bilateral)
3. slight hypoperfusion (regional side difference 2–4 of 16 steps on the color scale, representing a regional hypoperfusion of 14–28%)
4. marked hypoperfusion (regional side difference >4 of 16 steps on the color scale, representing a regional hypoperfusion of >28%)

According to ^{99m}Tc-HMPAO SPECT findings in healthy volunteers reported in the literature (4), a regional difference of cerebral tracer uptake exceeding two steps (approximately 14%) was considered to be significant.

RESULTS

Clinical neurological investigation gave normal findings in all patients. There was no evidence of morphologic alterations in either computed tomography (CT; n = 13) or magnetic resonance imaging (MRI; n = 8) of the brain, except two patients with a few vascular white matter lesions in the MRI. Electroencephalographic patterns (n = 22) were normal in 15 patients, whereas 7 patients revealed pathological alterations (focal changes: n = 2; unspecific dysrhythmic paroxysms: n = 3; dysrhythmic paroxysms with spike-/sharp-waves: n = 2).

Table 1 summarizes ^{99m}Tc-HMPAO SPECT findings in all patients and their relation to pain localization during attacks.

Cerebral tracer uptake was normal in 9 of 22 patients suffering from migraine without aura. A bilaterally inhomogeneous or decreased perfusion was found in four patients. Eight patients showed a slight decrease of rCBF, of whom six showed a corresponding hypoperfusion of the contralateral cerebellar hemisphere ["cerebellar diaschisis" (6)]. In one female patient regional tracer uptake was markedly reduced.

In all nine patients demonstrating a unilateral hypoperfusion, the areas of decreased tracer uptake were localized in the left hemisphere. In six of these

TABLE 1. ^{99m}TC-HMPAO SPECT findings in patients suffering from migraine without aura

Results of ^{99m}Tc-HMPAO SPECT	N (n = 22)	Positive relation of cerebral hypoperfusion to pain localization
Normal perfusion	9	—
Bilaterally inhomogeneous or reduced perfusion	4	—
Slight hypoperfusion[a]	8	6
Marked hypoperfusion[b]	1	0
Cerebellar diaschisis	3	3

[a] Side difference of rCBF amounting to 2–4 steps on the color scale (approx. 14–28%).
[b] Side difference of rCBF amounting to >4 steps on the color scale (approx. >28%).

patients headache during migraine attacks also was localized on the left side (Fig. 1). ^{99m}Tc-HMPAO SPECT showed a marked hypoperfusion (→) in the left-sided temporobasal region (horizontal projections).

DISCUSSION

In contrast to our findings in interictal migraine with aura, rCBF was normal or only unspecifically altered in 13 of 22 patients suffering from migraine without aura. However, nine patients revealed a decrease of regional tracer uptake. In all these cases the observed areas of regional hypoperfusion were localized in the left hemisphere—mostly within the temporal lobe—and corresponded to the side of headache during migraine attacks in six of them. Except one case, the observed side differences were only slight, but clearly

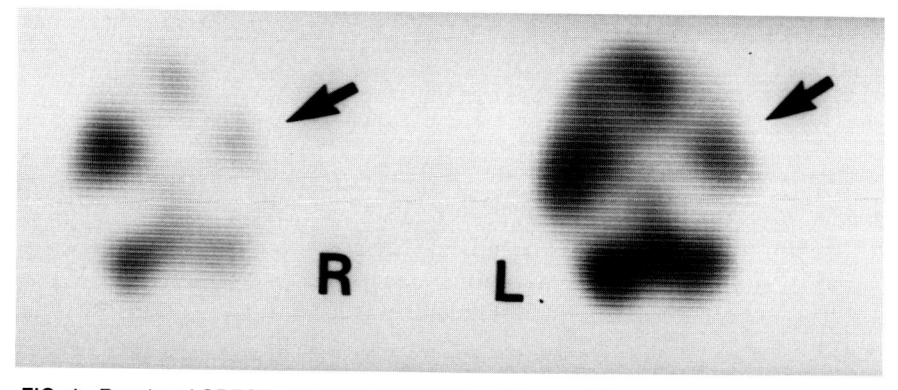

FIG. 1. Results of SPECT with ^{99m}Tc-HMPAO in a 51-year-old woman suffering from typical migraine without aura for about 40 years. Pain localization during attacks was half-sided, but alternated from attack to attack without any side preference. CT of the brain and electroencephalography were normal.

exceeded the values reported for healthy persons, ranging between 0.42 ± 2.45% SD (4).

The question of whether or not the observed preference of rCBF alterations in the left hemisphere is of any significance in the pathogenesis of migraine or represents only an accidental phenomenon requires further investigations in a greater number of patients.

REFERENCES

1. Schlake H-P, Böttger IG, Grotemeyer K-H, and Husstedt IW. Brain imaging with ^{123}I-IMP-SPECT in migraine between attacks. *Headache* 1989;29:344–349.
2. Lagréze HL, Dettmers C, and Hartmann A. Abnormalities of interictal perfusion in classic but not common migraine. *Stroke* 1988;19:1108–1111.
3. Levine SR, Welch KMA, Ewing JR, and Robertson W. Cerebral blood flow asymmetries in headache-free migraineurs. *Stroke* 1987;18:1164–1165.
4. Podreka E, Suess E, Goldenberg G, et al. Initial experience with Technetium-99m brain SPECT. *J Nucl Med* 1987;28:1657–1666.
5. Nakano S, Kinoshita K, Jinnouchi S, Hoshi H, and Watanabe K. Comparative study of regional cerebral blood flow images by SPECT using Xenon-133, Iodine-123 IMP, and Technetium-99m HM-PAO. *J Nucl Med* 1989;30:157–164.
6. Baron JC, Bousser MF, and Comar D. "Crossed cerebellar diaschisis" in human supratentorial brain infarction. *Trans Am Neurol Ass* 1980; 105:459–461.

35

Age-Related Changes in Cerebral Blood Flow in Patients with Migraine

Wendy M. Robertson, K. M. A. Welch, Steven R. Levine, and Lonni R. Schultz

Center for Stroke Research, Department of Neurology, Henry Ford Hospital, Detroit, Michigan 48202

Migraine is predominantly a disease of the young. Since an age-related decline in cerebral blood flow is found in the normal population, we considered the possibility that such changes differ in the aging migraine sufferer. We studied regional cerebral blood flow (rCBF) in a large population of migraine patients (with and without aura) and compared results with those of normal subjects.

PATIENTS AND METHODS

We studied 92 patients with a clinical diagnosis of recurrent migraine (Table 1). The duration of migraine history was 14.6 ± 12.8 years with a mean frequency of 4.5 ± 5.1 attacks per month. All were symptom-free at least 48 hours before the study and had a normal neurological examination. Controls had no history or examination findings to suggest neurological deficit. rCBF was measured by the ^{133}Xe inhalation technique (1) using 16 scintillation detectors placed in a symmetrical hemispheric array of eight probe pairs over each hemisphere. The initial slope index (ISI) was the measure of blood flow used in this study (2).

TABLE 1. *Patient population*

	N	Mean age (yrs)	Age range (yrs)	% Female
Migraine without aura	43	42.4	19–61	90.7
Migraine with aura	49	38.3	19–85	68.6
Control	49	50.4	22–80	55.1

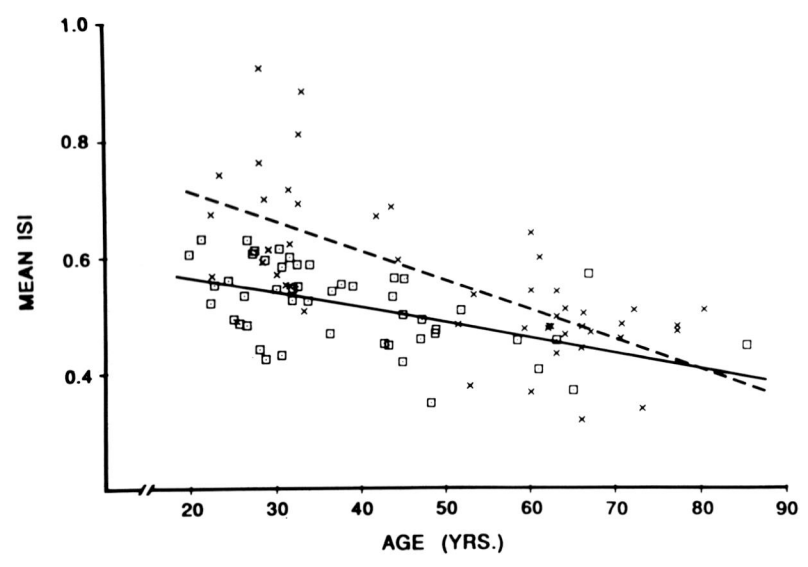

FIG. 1. Regression lines of mean ISI vs. age for migraine with aura patients (□——□) and controls (X----X).

RESULTS

The rate of decline of ISI with age was lower in the migraine population (-0.26 per year) than controls (-0.52 per year, $p < 0.005$). The migraine with aura group (Fig. 1) had a significantly lower rate of decline compared to controls (-0.26, $p < 0.02$). The rate of decline of CBF with age in the migraine without aura group (-0.31, Fig. 2) was lower than controls but did not reach statistical significance ($p < 0.14$).

The mean ISI did not differ between groups as a whole (migraine 52.3 ± 0.7 vs. controls 55.9 ± 1.9). However, the mean ISI was significantly lower in migraine with aura patients under 48 years of age and in migraine without aura patients between 32 and 48 years of age (Table 2).

The percentage of patients with at least one regional probe of major asymmetry, defined as >7% difference in ISI ratio =

$$\frac{|ISI_R - ISI_L|}{(ISI_R + ISI_L)/2} 100$$

was higher (69%) than controls (36%) under 32 years of age (Table 3). This was statistically significant for posterior probe pair asymmetries. With increased age (>48 years), this relationship differed as the percentage of con-

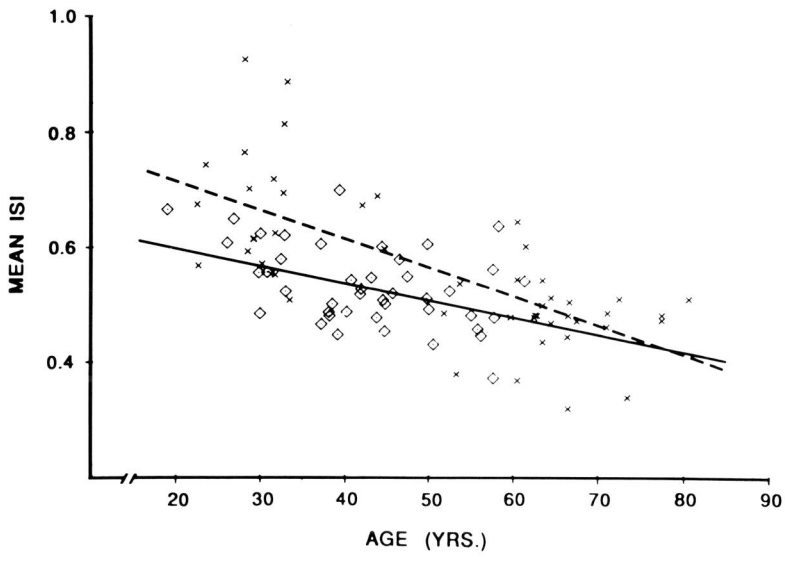

FIG. 2. Regression lines of mean ISI vs. age for migraine without aura patients (◊——◊) and controls (X-----X).

trol subjects with at least one probe of asymmetry increased (75%). There was no significant change in the percentage of migraine patients with asymmetries with advancing age.

DISCUSSION

Interictal differences in rCBF asymmetry have previously been demonstrated in the migraine population (3). This study reveals that asymmetries

TABLE 2. *Mean ISI of migraineurs and controls in three age groups*

		Age				
		<32 yrs		32–48 yrs		>48 yrs
	N	Mean ISI ± SEM	N	Mean ISI ± SEM	N	Mean ISI ± SEM
Migraine without aura	7	59.1 ± 2.4	23	53.0 ± 1.3[a]	13	50.1 ± 2.0
Migraine with aura	22	54.6 ± 1.4[b]	20	50.4 ± 1.4[b]	7	45.9 ± 2.5
All migraine	29	55.7 ± 1.2[b]	43	51.8 ± 1.0[a]	20	48.6 ± 1.6
Controls	14	65.8 ± 2.8	7	69.4 ± 4.8	28	47.7 ± 1.3

[a] $p < 0.01$ *t* test compared to controls of the same age group.
[b] $p < 0.005$ *t* test compared to controls of the same age group.

TABLE 3. Number of patients with one regional probe of major asymmetry (> 7% difference in ISI ratio)

Age	(yrs)	Patients with asymmetric PP/N	%	Patients with asymmetric posterior PP/N	%	Patients with asymmetric anterior PP/N	%
All migraine	< 32	20/29	69	9/29	31[a]	15/29	52
Without aura	< 32	5/7	71	3/7	43[a]	4/7	57
With aura	< 32	15/22	68	6/22	27	11/22	50
Controls	< 32	5/14	36	0/14	0	5/14	36
All migraine	> 48	12/20	60	5/20	25	9/20	45
Without aura	> 48	7/13	54	3/13	23	5/13	38
With aura	> 48	5/7	71	2/7	29	4/7	57
Controls	> 48	21/28	75[b]	8/28	29[b]	17/28	61

PP = Probe pair, N = Group number.
[a] $p < 0.03$ compared to controls by Fisher's exact text.
[b] Chi-square test for trend indicates significant increase in the number of controls with at least one asymmetric probe pair with increasing age ($p < 0.03$).

are found in the young migraine brain, but that asymmetries develop in the aging normal population, so that differences between migraineurs and controls are not apparent in the older age groups.

The age-related decline of blood flow is slower in migraine patients. However, the mean ISI is starting at a lower level in the young migraine groups. In the rat model, it has been demonstrated that the initial hyperperfusion accompanying the depolarization of spreading depression is inversely related to the preexisting blood flow levels (4). The lower preexisting blood flow found in the migraine population in this study could render the migraine brain more susceptible to the changes accompanying spreading depression and the subsequent migraine attack.

Differences from controls were found in both migraine groups, but were more pronounced in migraine with aura. These results suggest that migraine with and without aura represents a continuum of differences in the migraine brain with different clinical manifestations.

REFERENCES

1. Obrist WD, Thompson HK, King CH, and Wang HS. Determination of regional cerebral blood flow by inhalation of ^{133}Xenon. *Circ Res* 1967; 20:124–135.
2. Risberg J, Ali Z, Wilson EM, Wills EL, and Halsey JH. Regional cerebral blood flow estimated by ^{133}Xe inhalation: Preliminary evaluation of an initial slope index in patients with unstable flow compartments. *Stroke* 1975; 6:142–148.
3. Levine SR, Welch KMA, Ewing JR, and Robertson WM. Asymmetric cerebral blood flow patterns in migraine. *Cephalalgia* 1987; 7:245–248.
4. Lauritzen M. Regional cerebral blood flow during cortical spreading depression in rat brain: increased reactive hyperperfusion in low-flow states. *Acta Neurol Scand* 1987; 75:1–8.

36

Interictal Studies of Migraine Without Aura: Discussion Summary

Jes Olesen

The studies presented in this section describe areas of increased and/or decreased blood flow outside of attacks in patients suffering from migraine without aura. The changes are minor and the abnormal areas differ from one study to the other. Furthermore, the abnormalities do not correspond to patients' symptomatology even in cases in which the headache is always or almost always on the same side. It is unclear whether the changes are a stable trait or if they vary over time. The changes cannot be disclosed by simple visual inspection according to two studies, whereas one study found a few minor changes by visual analysis. The latter study suffers from a lack of control material, which is absolutely necessary. Furthermore, visual analysis of these subtle changes is completely unreliable according to one of the presentations, in which three experienced scientists blindly evaluated blood flow maps and scored the abnormalities by visual inspection. The agreement rate was miserable. Thus, the strict statistical approach seems to be the more valid, but here the risk would be to overinterpret data, and it is not always clear if mass significance due to multiple comparisons can account for some of the results.

Perhaps the most important result of this section is that blood flow asymmetries are definitely less pronounced in migraine without aura than in migraine with aura, in keeping with the marked differences in results obtained during actual attacks.

PART VII
Attacks of Migraine Without Aura

37

^{99m}Tc-HMPAO Studies in Migraine Without Aura

T. J. Steiner and Paul T. G. Davies

The Princess Margaret Migraine Clinic, Charing Cross Hospital, London W6 8RF, England

There is no one ideal method for regional cerebral blood flow (rCBF) assessment in acute migraine attacks. Xenon-133 (^{133}Xe) is valuable in allowing serial examinations during the same migraine attack (1) but the images suffer from poor spatial resolution and are distorted by Compton scatter (2; see Davies and Steiner). The CBF marker ^{99m}Tc-hexamethyl-propylene-amine-oxime (HMPAO) offers good spatial resolution (9 mm at full width half maximum, using the Novo 810 SPET scanner). It is fixed intracellularly with a decay half-life of about 11 hr, making it considerably difficult to perform repeated studies during one acute attack. Timing of studies in spontaneous attacks is dictated by when patients present, plus the time required (10 min) to make up the tracer. In migraine without aura, time from onset at presentation may be considerably later than in migraine with aura because of the greater uncertainty of onset. This factor applies equally to all imaging techniques.

METHODS

Patients (Table 1)

Patients were selected in two ways from those attending The Princess Margaret Migraine Clinic: they were either first seen when reporting spontaneously for acute headache treatment or they were kept under follow-up in the routine clinic and encouraged to return, untreated, during a further attack. Migraine has been diagnosed largely according to Vahlquist's (3) criteria, but more recently by International Headache Society criteria (4). Pa-

TABLE 1. Characteristics of the patients studied

Headache type	N (M:F)	Age range (yrs)	Symptoms at time of injection		
			Aura	Headache	Asymptomatic
Migraine without aura	27 (4:23)	(18–63)	—	15	24
Migraine with aura	20 (6:14)	(25–65)	6	19	10
Tension-type	22 (5:17)	(18–68)	—	21	2
Cluster	10 (10:0)	(36–62)	—	5	10

tients with abnormal neurological signs were excluded from the diagnosis of migraine and from this series. All migraine attacks were spontaneous: we have made no studies of induced attacks. Most were untreated before tracer injection. Patients with other types of headache were studied for comparison.

Preparation of ^{99m}Tc-HMPAO

HMPAO (Ceretec, Amersham) was mixed with freshly eluted technetium and 7–10 MBq/kg injected intravenously, within 30 min. Injections were given under standardized conditions of ambient light and noise levels.

Scanning of Cranial Tracer Distribution

Patients were scanned within 30 min of tracer injection, using the Novo 810 high-resolution single-slice acquisition SPET scanner (Table 2). Images were obtained in eight 12.5-mm transverse slices, parallel to the orbitomeatal line, at intervals of 1 cm, each being acquired over 5 min (total scan time: 35–45 min). Images were displayed by computer on a color monitor where regional coloration represented flow as a percentage of the maximum rCBF seen in that slice, according to a calibrated color scale depicted by the computer alongside the image. Quantification was thus relative per slice. Pola-

TABLE 2. Novo 810 parameters for acquisition of data

Energy window	110–170 keV
Number of slices	1–12 (8)
Time per slice	Limited only by computer memory (300 sec)
Slice thickness	1–25 mm (12.5)
Space between slices	5–15 mm (10)
Number of detectors	12
Pixel size	1.5 mm × 1.5 mm
Field of view	21 cm

() = Routine setting.

roid photographs were taken for easy reference. Image analysis was visual and was performed by two independent reporters, one blinded to the patient's clinical details. No "abnormality" was regarded as significant unless there was agreement between both.

RESULTS

In all 27 migraine patients without aura, whether symptomatic at the time of tracer injection or not, CBF images were no different from our series of scans from the 22 chronic tension-type headache patients. That is, in all cases rCBF appeared symmetrical and otherwise normal. In two patients with chronic tension-type headache, there was marked uptake of tracer in both temporal muscles, an appearance not seen in other muscle groups or in other headache syndromes. In one of these, the headache persisted and he was restudied a year later, with care to ensure that muscles of mastication were inactive; the same changes were seen (see tension-type headache case history).

CASE HISTORIES

Migraine Without Aura

A healthy 35-year-old woman had suffered from menstrual migraine for several years. Attacks occurred exclusively within 48 hr of menstruation and consisted of unilateral headache, nausea, vomiting, and photophobia. She presented about 5 hr into her typical, untreated attack with frontal headache on the right side. There were no abnormal neurological signs on examination. The normal rCBF image is shown in Fig. 1.

Chronic Tension-Type Headache

A 29-year-old man presented with a 2-month history of constant headache that had started suddenly one morning for no apparent reason. The headache was dull, bilateral, and mainly occipital but would spread around the sides of the head to both temples; it could be eased by conscious relaxation and was aggravated by activity. There was no previous history of headache or other illness, nor relevant family history. He was taking no regular medication and denied alcohol abuse. Examination showed a tense nervous individual, neurologically otherwise normal. A single photon emission computed tomography (SPECT) scan carried out when headache was mild

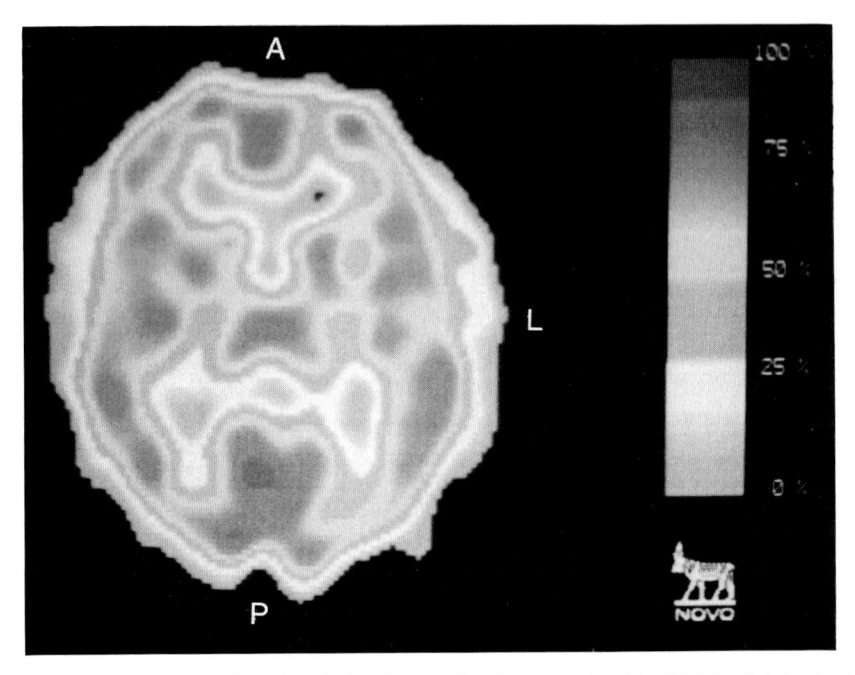

FIG. 1. Representative Novo 810 SPET image showing normal ^{99m}Tc-HMPAO distribution in a case of acute migraine without aura. The slice cuts the occipital and frontal lobes at the level of the thalami in a transverse plane 30 mm above the orbitomeatal line. Regional tracer distribution is expressed as a percentage of maximum according to the color scale alongside. A, anterior; P, posterior; L, left side.

showed marked uptake of tracer outside the skull in areas corresponding to the temporal muscles (Fig. 2). Treatment was commenced with amitriptyline, 25 mg each night, with improvement, but his headache continued. Another SPECT scan performed nearly a year later showed the same abnormalities.

DISCUSSION

High-resolution CBF images have been obtained with HMPAO and SPECT, but assessment of these has some limitations (see Davies and Steiner). Absolute quantification is currently not possible with this technique, rCBF in each slice being expressed as a percentage of the maximum tracer uptake in any region of the plane of the scan. Side-to-side asymmetries or other focal derangements of rCBF may be visualized, depending to some extent on the experience of the reporter, but generalized changes may be undetectable. In addition, hyperemia may be underestimated because of the

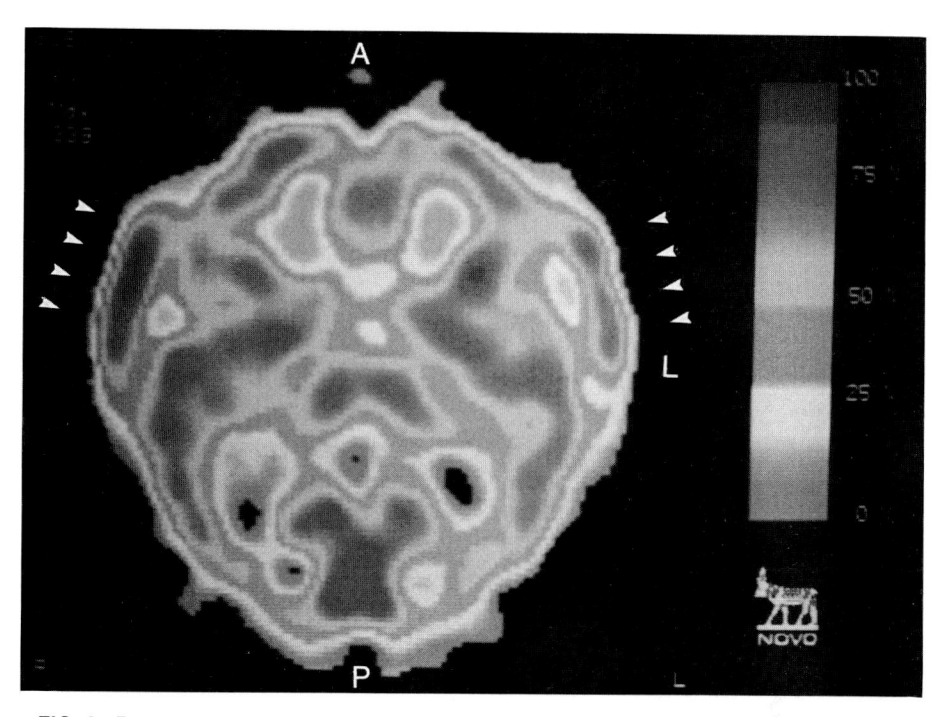

FIG. 2. Representative Novo 810 SPET image showing ^{99m}Tc-HMPAO distribution in a case of chronic tension-type headache. The slice cuts the occipital and frontal lobes at the level of the thalami in a transverse plane 30 mm above the orbitomeatal line. Regional tracer distribution is expressed as a percentage of maximum according to the color scale alongside. There is marked tracer uptake in the both temporal muscles (*arrows*). A, anterior; P, posterior; L, left side.

uptake characteristics of HMPAO. Consequently, a normal series of images does not exclude a range of abnormality especially encompassing flow increases. Nevertheless, our normal findings are not in discord with ^{133}Xe studies that show no changes in rCBF in migraine without aura.

Unlike ^{133}Xe, HMPAO has the resolution to demonstrate extracranial changes. For the moment these should be considered of uncertain significance since the uptake characteristics of HMPAO into muscle, for example, have not been well studied. In two cases of acute migraine without aura studied with HMPAO, Podreka (5) considered, probably erroneously, that foci of extracranial uptake similar to our images in two tension-type headache patients represented temporal artery tracer. We have no doubt from the disposition of the areas in our images that they represent the temporal muscles, and may indicate abnormalities in temporal muscle blood flow or metabolism. At least this is a question for further investigation, especially if similar appearances occur occasionally in migraine without aura.

REFERENCES

1. Olesen J. Migraine and regional cerebral blood flow. Trends *Neurosci* 1985; 7:318–321.
2. Olesen TS. Migraine with and without aura: The same disease due to cerebral vasospasm of different intensity. A hypothesis based on CBF studies during migraine. *Headache* 1990; 30:269–272.
3. Vahlquist B. Migraine in children. *Int Arch Allergy* 1955; 7:348–355.
4. Headache Classification Committee of the International Headache Society. *Cephalalgia* 1988; 8 [Suppl 7]: 1–96.
5. Podreka I. HMPAO in clinical practice. *Nuc Med Commun* 1987; 8:559–572.

38

CT-CBF and ^{133}Xe CBF Studies in Migraine Without Aura

John Stirling Meyer, Jun Kawamura, and Yasuo Terayama

Cerebral Blood Flow Laboratory, Department of Veterans Affairs Medical Center and Department of Neurology, Baylor College of Medicine, Houston, Texas 77030

Some progress has been made in the past five decades concerning the pathogenesis and treatment of migraine (1,2). The introduction of ^{133}Xe inhalation methods for measuring cerebral blood flow (CBF) made possible several studies that reported cerebral hyperperfusion during migraine headaches (3–5), which supported Wolff's vascular theory (6). On the other hand, Olesen et al. (7,8) concluded that spreading cortical depression, described by Leao in lissencephalic animal models (9), may be a phenomenon accounting for migraine headaches, based on observations of spreading oligemia moving forward from occipital regions of the brain. These two theories do not necessarily contradict each other but could be part of an evolving cascade during the migraine attack, as proposed in the unifying hypothesis of Welch (10).

This chapter, which includes data that have not been published before, was designed to elucidate cerebral hemodynamic changes during both the headache and headache-free intervals of migraineurs without aura using both the [133]Xenon inhalation and stable xenon-enhanced computed tomography (Xe CT-CBF) methods.

PATIENTS AND METHODS

[133]Xe Inhalation Study

Regional cerebral blood flow (rCBF) was measured in two dimensions by a modification of the ^{133}Xe inhalation method described by Obrist et al. (11).

Serial measurements of noninvasive rCBF were made in 68 patients suffering from migraine without aura (35 ± 14 years old; 16 men, 52 women) and compared with age-matched normal volunteers (n = 32; 35 ± 12 years old, 17 men, 15 women). Attempts were made to obtain rCBF measurements during either the headache, postheadache (2–48 hr after headache had subsided), and headache-free intervals.

Cerebral autoregulation was tested by decreasing cerebral perfusion pressure during orthostatic hypotension induced by tilting the patient 30° head-up by the use of a tilt table in six patients without migraine during either the headache, postheadache, or headache-free intervals. Quantitative analysis of impairment of cerebral autoregulation was made by means of the Autoregulation Index (AI) (12).

Cerebral vasomotor responsiveness to either 5% CO_2 in air or during hypocapnia induced by hyperventilation, expressed as $\Delta\%Fg$ (Δgray matter blood flow) per Δmm Hg $PECO_2$ (Δend-tidal CO_2 tension), was measured during the headache (n = 6), postheadache (n = 12), or headache-free (n = 16) intervals. Testing the effect of 100% oxygen inhalation on rCBF was measured in 11 patients with migraine without aura (during headache; n = 4, headache-free; n = 7) and compared with those measured in normal volunteers.

Normal CO_2 and O_2 responsiveness was tested in normal volunteers by hypercapnia (5% CO_2 inhalation) in 21 patients (53 ± 17 years), hypocapnia (voluntary hyperventilation) in 17 patients (45 ± 15 years), and hyperoxia (100% O_2 inhalation) in 10 patients (57 ± 10 years) for purposes of comparison.

Xe CT-CBF Study

Eighteen patients with migraine without aura (40 ± 13 years; 5 men, 13 women) participated in the Xe CT-CBF studies for measuring LCBF in three dimensions. The patients were told to discontinue all medications, particularly those used for migraine prophylaxis, for at least 48 hr before their scheduled appointment. For purposes of data analysis, patients were divided into two groups according to whether or not headaches were present during the local CBF (LCBF) measurements. LCBF values were compared between groups of patients during headache (nine patients, 43 ± 16 years; four men and five women) and without headache (nine patients, 37 ± 9 years; one man and eight women). Furthermore, asymmetries of LCBF changes with respect to the reported side of headache were analyzed.

Details of the stable Xe CT-CBF method have been reported previously (13,14) and in our chapter in Part I of this volume.

RESULTS

Serial Measurements of rCBF Using [133]Xe Inhalation Methods

During the headache interval, mean Fg values in a group of 23 patients with migraine without aura (29 ± 12 years old; 5 men, 18 women) were significantly higher than those during the headache-free interval (headache absent for 5 days or longer) of 29 migraineurs (39 ± 13 years old; 5 men, 24 women; $p < 0.01$). In 16 patients (31 ± 12 years old; 6 men, 10 women) with severe migraine studied 2–24 hr after the headache subsided, mean Fg values remained significantly increased ($p < 0.01$) during the immediate postheadache interval compared with patients who had remained headache-free for 6 days or longer and compared with normal volunteers (83.5 ± 8.9) (Fig. 1).

Dysautoregulation was found to be present in three patients during either the headache phase or the period up to 36 hr after the subsidence of headache (AI = 2.0 ± 1.6), but dysautoregulation was no longer present after the second day in three patients.

As shown in Fig. 2, CO_2 responsiveness in patients during headache (n = 6) was significantly impaired throughout both hemispheres compared with similar testing among age-matched normal volunteers ($p < 0.01$). To the contrary, during the headache-free interval among migraineurs (n = 16), there was excessive cerebrovascular CO_2 responsiveness with significantly greater increases in CO_2-induced vasodilator CBF increases on the side where the headache usually occurred compared with the nonheadache side ($p < 0.05$).

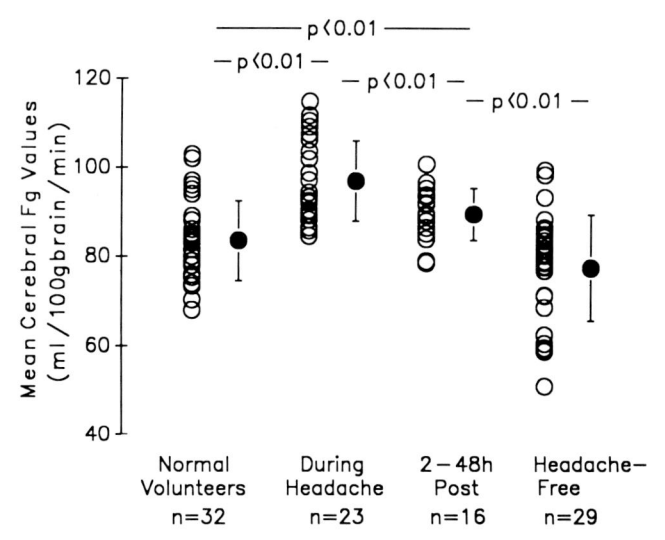

FIG. 1. Mean cerebral Fg values in patients suffering from migraine without aura compared with normal volunteers. During headache, the mean Fg values in a group of 23 patients was significantly higher (96.9 ± 9.1 ml/100 g brain/min) than that of the headache-free interval (headache absent for 5 days or longer) in a group of 29 migraineurs (77.4 ± 11.9 ml/100 g brain/min; $p < 0.01$). In 16 patients with severe migraine studied 2–24 hr after the headache subsided, the mean Fg values remained significantly increased (89.4 ± 5.9 ml/100 g brain/min) compared with patients who were headache-free for 6 days or longer and with normal volunteers ($p < 0.01$).

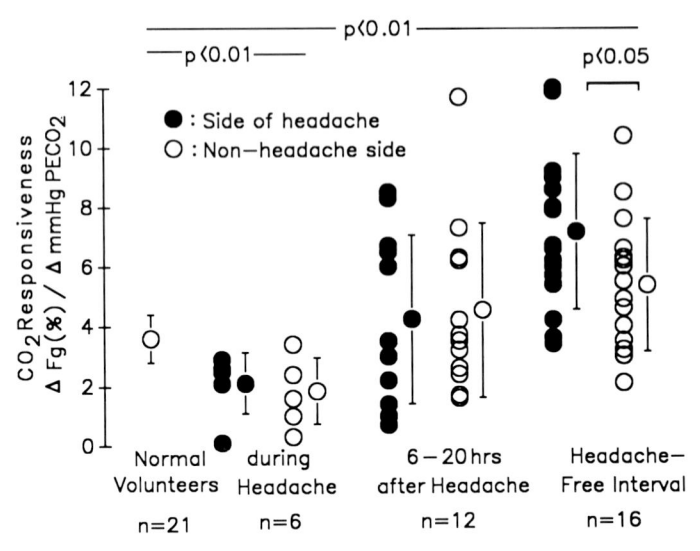

FIG. 2. Mean hemispheric vasodilator responsiveness to 5% CO_2 in patients with migraine without aura comparing the side of the most recent headache with nonheadache side. CO_2 responsiveness in six patients during headache was impaired throughout both hemispheres (mean value: 1.93 ± 1.03 $\triangle Fg(\%)/\triangle$ mm Hg $PECO_2$; $p < 0.01$) compared with normal volunteers. During the headache-free intervals (n = 16), CO_2 responsiveness was excessive (6.23 ± 2.21) with greater increases in CO_2 responsiveness on the side of the headache (7.16 ± 2.53) compared with the noninvolved side (5.37 ± 2.14; $p < 0.01$).

Testing effects of 100% oxygen inhalation on rCBF (15) measured in 11 patients with migraine without aura showed similar cerebral vasoconstrictive responsiveness to 100% oxygen inhalation (during headache; 10.2 ± 3.7%, headache-free; 12.3 ± 7.5%) as was measured in normal volunteers (n = 10; 6.0 ± 5.6%).

Three-Dimensional Analysis of LCBF Using Xenon-Enhanced CT-CBF Methods

Figure 3 illustrates the noncontrasted CT image of the brain and corresponding LCBF map of a 47-year-old man with migraine without aura. The patient had a moderate bilateral headache at the time of the LCBF measurements. LCBF values are increased in cerebral cortex, thalamus, and basal ganglia of both hemispheres.

Mean LCBF values for nine representative brain regions were compared during headaches and headache-free intervals (Fig. 4). LCBF values for cortical and subcortical gray matter are markedly increased during intervals of the headaches compared to headache-free intervals.

CT-CBF AND ^{133}Xe STUDIES 231

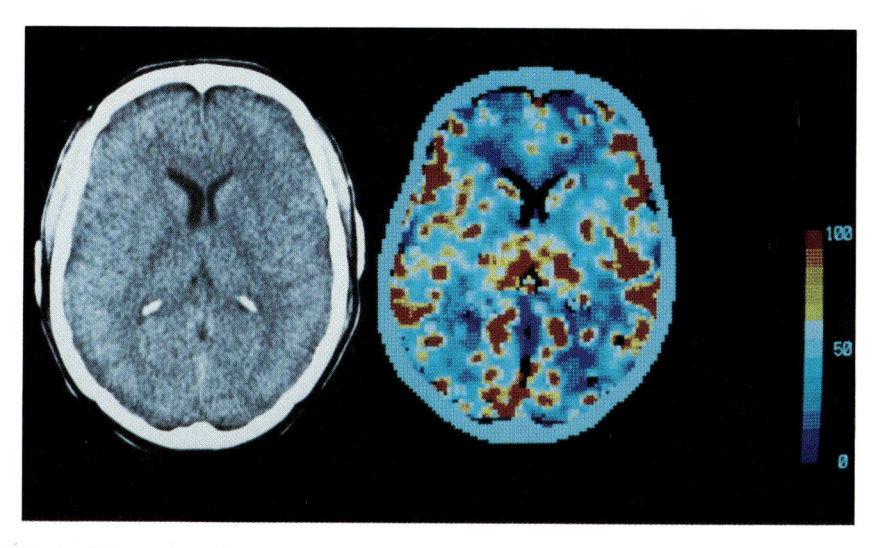

FIG. 3. Plain cranial CT (left) and corresponding LCBF image (right) of a 47-year-old man diagnosed as migraine without aura. The patient complained of a moderate bilateral headache and nausea during the LCBF measurement. LCBF values are increased in cerebral cortex, thalamus, and basal ganglia of both hemispheres.

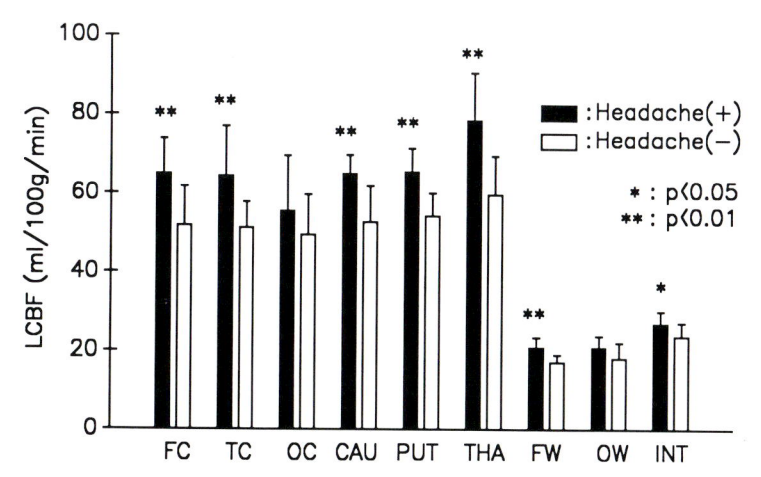

FIG. 4. Mean LCBF values of nine representative cerebral regions of nine migraineurs without headache compared among the headache-free interval and the headache phase. Each LCBF value is given as the average value for both hemispheres. During headaches, LCBF are increased especially in frontotemporal cortex, thalamus, and basal ganglia. FC, frontal cortex, TC, temporal cortex, OC, occipital cortex, CAU, caudate nucleus, PUT, putamen, THA, thalamus, FW, frontal white matter, OW, occipital white matter, INT, internal capsule.

TABLE 1. LCBF in migraine patients with and without headache

	Without headache	With headache	Percentage change
Frontal cortex	51.8 ± 10.0	65.0 ± 8.8	+25.5[a]
Temporal cortex	51.2 ± 6.6	64.4 ± 12.6	+25.8[a]
Occipital cortex	49.4 ± 10.3	55.5 ± 14.1	+12.3
Caudate nucleus	52.7 ± 9.2	65.0 ± 4.8	+23.3[a]
Putamen	54.3 ± 5.8	65.5 ± 5.9	+20.9[a]
Thalamus	59.7 ± 9.8	78.5 ± 12.1	+31.5[a]
Frontal white matter	17.2 ± 1.9	20.9 ± 2.6	+21.5[a]
Occipital white matter	18.2 ± 4.0	20.9 ± 3.0	+14.8
Internal capsule	23.8 ± 3.4	28.0 ± 3.2	+17.6[b]
n	9	9	

LCBF = Local cerebral blood flow (ml/100 g brain/min).
[a]
[b]

Table 1 summarizes mean LCBF values for the nine representative cerebral regions among migraine patients with (n = 9) and without (n = 9) headaches at the time of LCBF measurements. When headache-free, LCBF values of all regions are comparable to those of age-matched normal volunteers reported previously (14). In the group of patients reporting severe headache during the LCBF measurements, LCBF values are significantly increased not only in cerebral cortex but also in thalamus and basal ganglia as well as white matter, except for the occipital lobes. The thalamus shows the greatest mean LCBF increases of +31.5% from normal resting values of 54.3 ± 5.8 ml/100 g brain/min to 78.5 ± 12.1 ml/100 g brain/min during headaches ($p < 0.01$). Other regions of gray matter showing hyperperfusion are as follows: temporal cortex (+25.8%), frontal cortex (+25.5%), caudate nucleus (+23.3%), and putamen (+20.9%). Although less remarkably so, LCBF values for white matter are also increased during headaches. There were no significant differences in the level of Paco$_2$ while headache-free and during headaches. No electroencephalogram (EEG) abnormalities were observed throughout all the LCBF measurements made among migraineurs with and without headaches.

Figure 5 compares the nine brain regions between the right and left hemispheres of patients (n = 5) who complained of bilateral migraine headaches during LCBF measurements. All showed hyperperfusion of both hemispheres not only in the cerebral hemisphere ipsilateral to the headache but also in the contralateral hemisphere (with no statistically significant differences being noted between the two sides). There are no statistically significant differences in the degree of LCBF increases for any of the nine regions between right and left hemispheres.

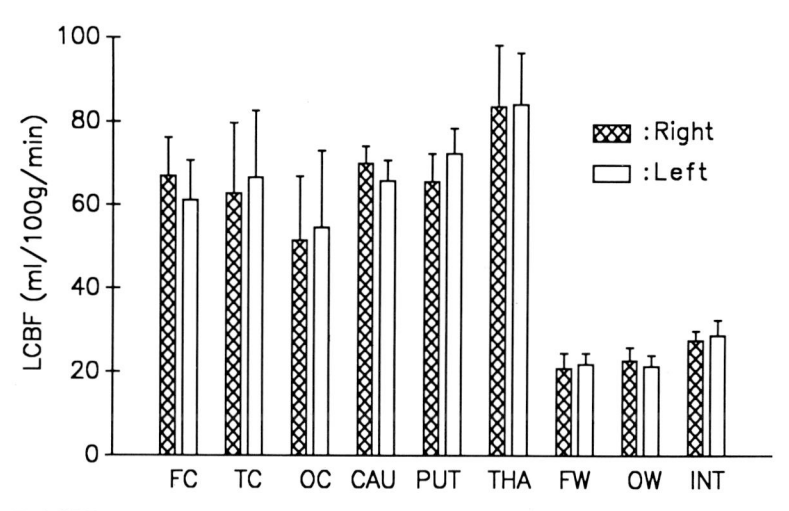

[Figure showing bar chart with LCBF values on y-axis (ml/100g/min) from 0 to 100, and brain regions on x-axis: FC, TC, OC, CAU, PUT, THA, FW, OW, INT. Right and Left hemispheres shown.]

FIG. 5. LCBF values for nine brain regions measured in five patients with migraine without aura during bilateral headaches. LCBF values for the nine regions are compared between the right and left hemispheres. There are no statistically significant differences in the LCBF increases for all regions between right and left hemispheres. Abbreviations are the same as in Fig. 4.

DISCUSSION

Cerebrovascular reactivity in patients with migraine without aura during the headache-free interval is characterized by excessive and asymmetric cerebral vasodilator responses to hypercapnia with greater responses on the side of the predominant head pain, despite the fact that cerebral vasodilator responses to hypercapnia are lost or impaired during headache intervals.

While cerebral lactic acidosis, secondary to cerebral ischemia, has been logically invoked in migraine with aura as a contributory cause for impaired cerebral vasomotor responsiveness to end-tidal CO_2 changes during the prodrome or headache phase of migraine (3,16), excessive CO_2 responsiveness during headache-free intervals cannot be attributed to this mechanism in migraine without aura. Increased cerebral vasomotor CO_2 responsiveness during headache-free intervals, in patients with migraine without aura, is best attributed to abnormalities of neurotransmitter receptor sites, including alpha- and beta-adrenergic types. This hypothesis for abnormal cerebrovascular hemodynamic changes in migraineurs is consonant with reports in the literature citing excessive vasomotor responsivity elsewhere in the body (17,18), as well as with abnormalities of innervation and pharmacological responses of receptor sites in the iris of the eye (19) indicating increased norepinephrine release (16). These data from numerous sources are adduced to indicate disorders of the autonomic nervous system and vascular receptor sites among migraineurs. The fact that CO_2 responsiveness is exaggerated to a greater degree on the side of the head pain, as observed in the present study, implies that cerebrovascular receptor sites become abnormally activated and may be disordered more in one cephalic region than another.

The present study of patients with migraine without aura utilizing three-dimensional analyses of cerebral perfusion by Xe CT-CBF method revealed that LCBF increases during headaches did not correlate with the preponderant side of the headache, that is, cerebral hyperperfusion was bilateral and relatively symmetrical during unilateral headaches. This suggests that the head pain cannot be caused solely by distention of the pain-sensitive intracerebral vessels. As originally proposed by Wolff and his coworkers, it appears probable that extracranial vessels play a major role in the occurrence and laterality of the head pain of migraine (4,6). Since subcortical structures were involved in the hyperperfusion, spreading cortical depression, which involves only the cortex and not subcortical structures, cannot be invoked to explain the headaches and changes in cerebrovascular hemodynamics.

In conclusion, the present study confirms previously reported observations of cerebral hyperperfusion during attacks of migraine without aura. Furthermore, these observations provide evidence suggesting sympathetic hypofunction with denervation hypersensitivity in migraineurs with aura. Derangements of sympathetic innervation of the cranial arteries are believed to account for the instability of CBF observed in migraineurs when headache-free and this contributes to hemodynamic changes during the aura and headache interval. Present results do not support spreading cortical depression as the cause of migraine without aura.

REFERENCES

1. Meyer JS, Hata T, and Imai A. Evidence supporting a vascular pathogenesis of migraine and cluster headache. In: Blau JN, ed. *Migraine: clinical, therapeutic, conceptual and research aspects.* London: Chapman and Hall, 1987;265–302.
2. Lance JW. The pathophysiology of migraine. In: Dalessio DJ, ed. *Wolff's headache and other head pain, 5th ed.* New York: Oxford University Press, 1987;58–86.
3. Skinhøj E. Hemodynamic studies within the brain during migraine. *Arch Neurol* 1973;29:95–98.
4. Sakai F and Meyer JS. Regional cerebral hemodynamics during migraine and cluster headaches measured by the ^{133}Xe inhalation method. *Headache* 1978;18:122–132.
5. Meyer JS, Zetusky W, Jonsdottir M, and Mortel K. Cephalic hyperemia during migraine headaches: A prospective study. *Headache* 1986;26:388–397.
6. Schumacher GA and Wolff HG. Experimental studies on headache. A. Contrast of histamine headache with the headache of migraine and that associated with hypertension. B. Contrast of vascular mechanisms in preheadache and in headache phenomena of migraine. *Arch Neurol Psychiatry* 1941;45:199–214.
7. Olesen J, Larsen B, and Lauritzen M. Focal hyperemia followed by spreading oligemia and impaired activation of rCBF in classic migraine. *Ann Neurol* 1981;9:344–352.
8. Lauritzen M, Skinhøj E, Olesen T, Lassen NA, and Paulson OB. Changes in regional

cerebral blood flow during the course of classic migraine attacks. *Ann Neurol* 1983;13:633–641.
9. Leao AAP. Spreading depression of activity in the cerebral cortex. *J Neurophysiol* 1944;7:359–390.
10. Welch KMA. Migraine: a biobehavioral disorder. *Arch Neurol* 1987;44:323–327.
11. Obrist WD, Thompson HK, Wang HS, and Wilkinson WE. Regional cerebral blood flow estimated by ^{133}Xe inhalation. *Stroke* 1975;6:245–256.
12. Meyer JS, Shimazu K, Fukuuchi Y, Ohuchi T, Okamoto S, Koto A, and Ericsson AD. Impaired cerebrovascular control and dysautoregulation after stroke. *Stroke* 1973;4:169–186.
13. Meyer JS, Shinohara T, Imai A, Kobari M, Sakai F, Hata T, Oravez WT, Timpe GM, Deville T, and Solomon E. Imaging local cerebral blood flow by xenon-enhanced computed tomography-Technical optimization procedures. *Neuroradiology* 1988;30:283–292.
14. Imai A, Meyer JS, Kobari M, Ichijo M, Shinohara T, and Oravez WT. LCBF values decline while Lλ values increase during normal human aging measured by stable xenon-enhanced computed tomography. *Neuroradiology* 1988;30:463–472.
15. Deshmukh VD and Meyer JS. *Noninvasive measurement of regional cerebral blood flow in man*. New York: Spectrum Publication, 1978.
16. O'Brien MD. Cerebral cortex perfusion rates in migraine. *Lancet* 1967;1:1036.
17. Appenzeller O, Davidson K, and Marshall J. Reflex vasomotor abnormalities in the hands of migrainous subjects. *J Neurol Neurosurg Psychiat* 1963;26:447–450.
18. Price RP and Tursky B. Vascular reactivity of migraineurs and nonmigraineurs: A comparison of responses to self control procedures. *Headache* 1976;16:210–217.
19. Fanciullacci M. Iris adrenergic impairment in idiopathic headache. *Headache* 1979;19:8–13.

39

Xenon-133 SPECT Studies in Migraine Without Aura

*Jes Olesen and †Lars Friberg

*Department of Neurology, Gentofte Hospital, University of Copenhagen, DK-2900 Hellerup, Denmark, and †Department of Clinical Physiology and Nuclear Medicine, Bispebjerg Hospital, DK-2400 Copenhagen NV, Denmark

Migraine attacks without aura often begin insidiously, like a tension headache, then gradually worsen and become lateralized, throbbing, intense, and associated with nausea, vomiting, photophobia, and phonophobia. Before the advent of the operational diagnostic criteria of the International Headache Society (1), there was no clear guidance as to whether an episode with headache was a tension headache or a common migraine. Several previous studies have not documented the attacks well enough to ascertain that they really studied migraine. In the past, migraine without aura was often regarded as a milder form of migraine with aura, and it was anticipated that the initial hypoperfusion observed in migraine with aura could also be found in migraine without aura, although less severe and asymptomatic. This hypothesis was difficult to explore because of the necessary time lag from recognition of symptoms until the patient could be studied.

REVIEW OF PUBLISHED STUDIES

Olesen et al. (2) overcame the above-mentioned difficulties by studying attacks induced by red wine or food stuffs. From a large series, 12 patients were selected who by history reliably could induce attacks within 1 hr and who were willing to participate in a study during induced attacks. These patients fulfilled the usual criteria for common migraine and also the more operational criteria suggested by Olesen et al. (3). These latter criteria were close to the subsequent diagnostic criteria of the International Headache Society (1). Characteristics of patients and of the studied attacks are given in Table 1. Regional cerebral blood flow (rCBF) was measured in the resting state, after ingestion of the provoking substance, and measurements were

TABLE 1. *Characteristics of patients and attacks in rCBF study of migraine without aura.*

	Patients (n = 6)	Studied attacks (n = 8)
Mean age (range)	37 (31–51 yrs)	
Sex	M 1, F 5	
Provokation	Red wine 5	
	Chocolate 1	
Interval headache	Never 3	
	Monthly 2	
	Weekly 1	
Severe or moderate pain	—	8
Pulsating pain	2	3
Unilateral pain	3	4
Nausea	6	6
Photophobia or phonophobia	6	8
Effect of ergotamine	5	6

Modified from Olesen et al., ref. 2, with permission.

then repeated until either a migraine attack developed or four measurements had been taken without development of an attack. The provocation was successful in six patients and two patients were studied twice. Three studies were taken with ^{133}Xe inhalation and stationary detectors, four with ^{133}Xe inhalation and single photon emission computed tomography (SPECT), and one was studied with the ^{133}Xe intracarotid injection method. The most important findings are shown in Table 2. Mean rCBF was almost constant during the development of migraine attacks (95% confidence limits for mean alteration of rCBF from rest to onset of migraine -4.4 to $+9.4\%$, and from rest to fully developed attack -2.0 to $+10.2\%$). The regional distribution of cerebral blood flow in each patient was also studied. No focal hypoperfused areas were observed in any patient or during any measurement. It was concluded that an early asymptomatic period of focal hypoperfusion is not likely to accompany the attack of migraine without aura. Unfortunately, no later studies have focused at this early phase of migraine without aura.

Lauritzen and Olesen (4) studied 12 patients during attacks without aura. Patients were again characterized in operational terms similar to the present criteria of the International Headache Society. The usual symptoms of the patients as well as the actually recorded symptoms in association with the rCBF study were given and the studied attacks were typical of migraine without aura. Patients were between 18 and 65 years old and suffered from four or fewer attacks each month. Patients with frequent attacks were excluded because in such patients migraine attacks often mix with chronic daily headache, making attacks difficult to define. For the same reasons, patients having interval headache more than once a week were excluded, as were patients who had taken drugs acting on the circulatory system and patients studied more than 24 hr after onset of the attack. rCBF was measured one to five times at 20– to 45-min intervals before treatment, then after

TABLE 2. Hemodynamic variables during development of common migraine attacks

	Resting state	Onset of migraine	Migraine	Percentage change from resting state			
				To onset		To full attack	
				Mean	Range	Mean	Range
Mean arterial blood pressure (mm Hg) (n = 8)	95.5	93.0	93.5	−1.3%	+7.5 to −11.1%	−1.1%	+11.1 to −21.6%
Arterial PCO_2[a] (mm Hg) (n = 5)	36.3	36.1	37.1	−2.0%	+5.9 to −10.8%	+1.3%	+19.9 to −7.3%
Mean cerebral blood flow (ml/100 g/min) (n = 8)	70.1	72.5	73.5	+2.5% NS[b]	+12.5 to −11.6%	+4.1% NS[b]	+20 to −4.7%

[a] Calculated from end-expiratory CO_2% in two patients and from warmed hand vein blood in two patients.
[b] Wilcoxon's test for paired data.
Modified from Olesen et al., ref. 2, with permission.

TABLE 3. *Tomographic rCBF in migraine*

rCBF in common migraine absolute levels in regions of interest

Case no.	CBF no.[a]	Hemisphere CBF (ml/100 g/min) L	R	Total cortex L	R	Basal ganglia L	R	Blood pressure (mm Hg)	PaCO$_2$ (mm Hg)
1	a	78	76	75	72	91	88	115/80	38.9
	b	76	75	75	76	96	86	—	44.6
	c	60	60	61	61	—	—	110/80	35.8
2	a	87	88	80	79	98	94	190/90	45.0
	b	84	92	84	97	—	—	160/90	43.9
	c	64	64	62	63	73	71	150/70	40.3
3	a	51	54	51	51	58	58	120/90	33.1
	b	49	48	49	49	55	53	125/90	—
	c	61	59	61	60	74	73	115/90	40.3
4	a	75	72	74	71	80	77	160/100	36.0
	b	65	65	62	63	81	75	—	41.8
	c	59	56	57	54	63	61	135/95	34.6
5	a	51	49	49	45	61	49	140/80	33.1
	b	57	54	56	51	68	67	—	37.4
	c	—	—	—	—	—	—	—	—
6	a	59	58	56	56	71	66	110/80	37.8
	b	46	44	44	41	56	55	—	40.3
	c	64	64	61	62	77	70	—	34.6
7	a	61	61	58	63	81	73	160/100	—
	b	58	56	58	55	61	57	115/80	31.0
	c	—	—	—	—	—	—	—	—
8	a	49	46	48	48	58	52	140/80	28.8
	b	62	63	62	64	65	62	140/100	39.6
	c	—	—	—	—	—	—	—	—
9	a	55	55	53	53	66	65	100/60	28.8
	b	59	59	58	59	65	64	—	31.7
	c	73	74	71	72	87	81	95/60	36.0
10	a	77	76	78	70	91	87	120/90	45.0
	b	68	64	69	67	—	—	—	—
	c	66	66	67	65	—	—	—	36.7
11	a	76	75	75	74	85	82	—	42.5
	b	76	68	76	68	83	83	—	42.4
	c	65	62	63	60	77	79	110/80	39.6
12	a	69	66	68	62	84	79	130/80	27.4
	b	61	59	63	60	78	65	130/80	29.5
	c	55	52	54	50	60	55	130/90	31.7

[a] The lower case letters refer to rCBF studies before (a) and after (b) treatment with ergotamine and metoclopramide, and in a headache-free period (c).
From Lauritzen and Olesen, ref. 4, with permission.

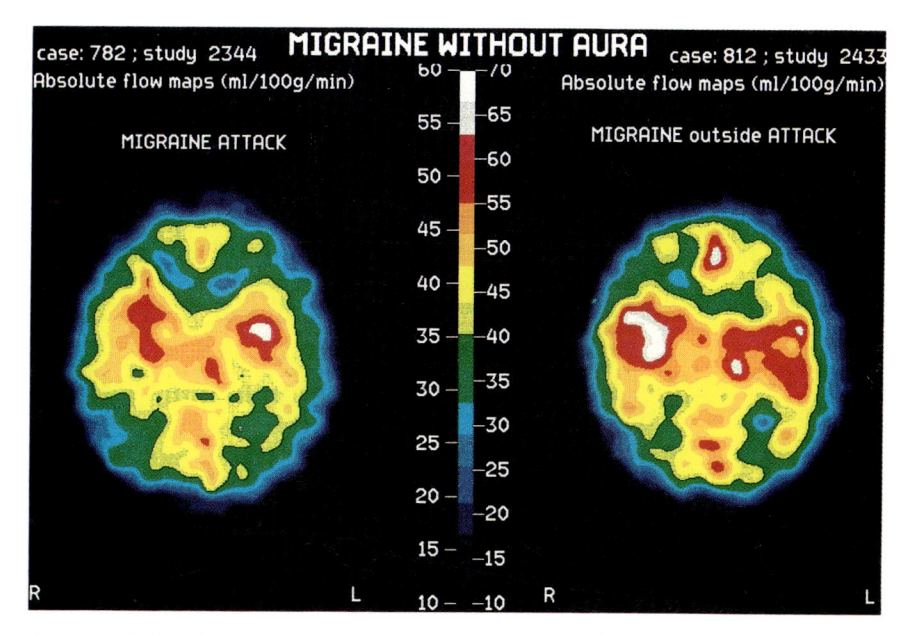

FIG. 1. ^{133}Xe SPECT study of rCBF during an attack of migraine without aura (*left*) and when the patient had been free from migraine for a week (*right*). rCBF in mm/100 g/min is translated into color on the scale to the right. Frontal region is up, right is to the right (the patient is viewed from above). Note that there is no difference in absolute blood flow level between the two situations. Note also that there is perfect symmetry between each region in the two hemispheres on both occasions. This was a uniform finding in our migraine patients without aura.

0.25 mg ergotamine and 10 mg metoclopramid intramuscularly, and again when symptom-free. Finally, a measurement was taken after patients had been free from migraine for at least a week. rCBF was measured with ^{133}Xe inhalation using a rapidly rotating SPECT with 64 sodium iodide crystals. The resolution in the plane with this equipment was 1.7 cm (full width, half maximum count rate). The air curve from the right upper lung was used for calculations of rCBF by a deconvolution procedure. Three slices were recorded, but mean flows in this report are from the second slice (5 cm above the orbitomeatal line). The first measurements were taken at a mean of 7 hr after onset of the attack (range 3–20 hr). Mean hemispheric blood flow and cortical blood flow were normal and symmetrical (Table 3). There were no hypoperfused or hyperperfused regions either ipsilaterally or contralaterally to the side of pain. A typical example is shown in Fig. 1. Blood flow in the basal ganglia, notably in their posterior parts, was calculated to elucidate pain-related activation of this region. No attack-related side-to-side asymmetry was seen. No alterations were noted comparing hemisphere or cortical blood flow during attacks to posttreatment or to the study performed 7 days after the last migraine attack.

A large new series of studies from our group has confirmed the above findings. Some of these data have been presented as an abstract (5). Fourteen patients were studied during an attack as well as outside of an attack. In the group as a whole there was no difference between hemispheric rCBF during and outside of attack, and there were no side-to-side asymmetries comparing headache side to nonheadache side (visual evaluation). Looking at each individual and comparing with our normal interval, rCBF values were normal in 13 patients during attack. In none of these was any definite difference detectable between measurements during attack and outside of attack. In one patient rCBF was globally increased during an attack compared to outside of an attack.

Our three series of studies are thus in perfect agreement. No focal or global rCBF abnormalities have been discovered in migraine without aura either at the onset of the attack, during the fully developed attack, or after treatment, and no significant difference exists between focal or global rCBF during the attack as compared to studies when the patient has been free from attack for 7 days. These results are in agreement with some studies using other methods (6–9), but contrast with other reports (10–13). In these latter reports the patient material was not characterized in detail. One study used discontinuation of medicine 48 hr before a scheduled study to induce migraine attacks. This is not a fully acceptable method because it could induce a mild abstinence that perhaps could be responsible for the increased blood flow. Conversely, when patients were studied outside of attack they were on drugs, which may have depressed blood flow below normal. Methodological differences could also contribute to explain the discrepancy between our findings and those of other groups. This appears unlikely, however, since Schroeder et al. (14) demonstrated a good agreement between ^{133}Xe inhalation SPECT and ^{133}Xe inhalation with external stationary detectors both at rest and during the diamox test. We know too little about the patients in the other studies to evaluate if clinical differences could also play a role. The group comparison approach employed by other authors is not as strong as the longitudinal study of each individual patient in our three series. On the other hand, the large sample size studied by Meyer et al. (11) and Juge (12) should compensate for this.

CONCLUSION

Conflicting rCBF data have been presented in migraine without aura. On the one hand, in carefully described patients studied during attacks that clearly fulfill present-day operational criteria for an attack of migraine without aura, using a sophisticated brain dedicated SPECT equipment, rCBF as well as global flow has been normal at the onset of attack as well as during the fully developed attack. This result has been obtained in four independent series of studies from our group. It is supported by four independent groups using inhalation of ^{133}Xe and stationary detectors, ^{99m}Tc-HMPAO SPECT, and, in one case only, using positron emission tomography (PET). On the other hand, three studies from the Houston group and one from Geneva, three using ^{133}Xe inhalation and stationary detectors and one stable xenon and CT, have demonstrated global hyperperfusion during attacks. With stable xenon this was spotty and in one study it was focal in some patients, whereas it was global in the majority of studied patients. Scarcity of clinical case description, low spatial resolution, the use of induced attacks (stable xenon study), and the use of a group comparison design are factors that weaken the last mentioned studies. On balance, it seems that normal rCBF is most likely to be the true finding during migraine attacks without aura. Caution must, however, still be exercised and the possibility of hyperperfusion should be further explored using PET and other methods. Studies of the regulation of rCBF during attacks of migraine without aura are much needed.

REFERENCES

1. Ad hoc committee on the classification of headache. Classification of Headache. *JAMA* 1962; 179:717–718.
2. Olesen J, Tfelt-Hansen P, Henriksen L, and Larsen B. The common migraine attack may not be initiated by cerebral ischemia. *Lancet* 1981; 2: 438–4402.
3. Olesen J, Krabbe AÆ, and Tfelt-Hansen P. Methodological aspects of prophylactic drug trials in migraine. *Cephalalgia* 1981; 1:127–141.
4. Lauritzen M and Olesen J. Regional cerebral blood flow during migraine attacks by Xenon-133 inhalation and emission tomography. *Brain* 1984; 107:447–461.
5. Friberg F, Olesen J, and Iversen H. Regional cerebral blood flow in a large group of migraine patients. *Cephalalgia* 1989; 9 [Suppl 10]:29–31.
6. Davies PTG, Steiner TJ, Costa DC, Jones BE, Jewkes RF, and Rose FC. Caution in extrapolating from regional cerebral blood flow studies of migraine to hypotheses of pathogenesis. In: Rose FC, ed. *New advances in headache research*. London: Smith-Gordon 1989; 169–174.
7. Gullichsen G and Enevoldsen E. Prolonged changes in rCBF following attacks of migraine accompagnee. *Acta Neurol Scand* 1984; 69 [Suppl 98]:270–271.
8. Lagrèze HL, Dettmers C, and Hartmann A. Abnormalities of interictal cerebral perfusion in classic but not common migraine. *Stroke* 1988; 19:1108–1111.
9. Herold S, Gibbs JM, Jones AKP, Brooks DJ, Frackowiak RSJ, and Legg NJ. Oxygen metabolism in migraine. *J Cereb Blood Flow Metab* 1985; 5 [Suppl 1]:445–446.
10. Sakai F and Meyer JS. Regional cerebral hemodynamics during migraine and cluster headache measured by the 133-Xe inhalation method. *Headache* 1978; 18:122–132.
11. Meyer JS, Zetusky W, Jonsdottir M, and Mortel K. Cephalic hyperemia during migraine headaches. A prospective study. *Headache* 1986; 26:388–397.
12. Juge O. Regional cerebral blood flow in the different clinical types of migraine. *Headache* 1988; 28:537–549.
13. Kobari M, Meyer JS, Ichijo M, and Kawamura J. Cortical and subcortical hyperperfusion during migraine and cluster headache measured by Xe CT-CBF. *Neuroradiology* 1990; 32:4–11.
14. Schroeder T, Vorstrup S, Lassen NA, and Engell HC. Non invasive Xenon-133 measurements of cerebral blood flow using stationary detectors compared with dynamic emission tomography. *J Cereb Blood Flow Metab* 1986; 6:739–746.

40

^{99m}Tc-HMPAO SPECT in Migraine Attacks Without Aura and Effect of Sumatriptan on Regional Cerebral Blood Flow

*Michel D. Ferrari, *Joost Haan, †J. A. Koos Blokland, *Pieter Minnee, ‡Koos H. Zwinderman, and §Pramod R. Saxena

*Departments of *Neurology, †Radiology, Division of Nuclear Medicine, and ‡Medical Statistics, University Hospital, 2300 RC Leiden, and §Department of Pharmacology, Erasmus University, Rotterdam, and the Dutch Migraine Research Group (MDF & PRS), The Netherlands*

The selective 5-hydroxytryptamine$_1$-like receptor agonist sumatriptan is a highly effective novel drug in the acute treatment of migraine attacks (1). Because of its selective pharmacological profile (2), studying the mechanism of action of sumatriptan in migraine may help to elucidate the pathophysiology of migraine. In animals, sumatriptan constricts arteriovenous shunts in the carotid arterial bed (2,3), without clearly affecting the blood flow to the brain (3). Not much is known of the mechanism of action of sumatriptan in humans.

Technetium-99m hexamethyl-propylene-amine-oxime (HMPAO) single photon emission computed tomography (^{99m}Tc-HMPAO SPECT) renders reproducible high resolution static imaging of regional cerebral blood flow (rCBF) (4). The radionuclide rapidly reaches a high intracerebral concentration after intravenous (iv) injection, and its distribution represents the rCBF of the first circulation through the brain. This results in a kind of "frozen" image of rCBF, which remains measurable during several hours. Thus, the tracer can be injected during a migraine attack, but the actual data acquisition can be done after drug-induced resolution of the attack. In addition, a repeated injection of the tracer thereafter will register the rCBF after treatment.

We performed three SPECT scans in each of 13 migraine patients without aura (MO): one outside an attack, one during a migraine attack before treatment, and one after treatment with sumatriptan. Results were determined semiquantitatively and intraindividually compared.

PATIENTS AND METHODS

Ten female and three male drug-free MO patients (mean age 44 years) were studied as part of a clinical trial (1). They came to the hospital as soon as possible (mean 9 hr, 3–24 hr) after the onset of a severe migraine attack with unilateral headache. Here, 20 mCi ^{99m}Tc-HMPAO was injected intravenously. Sumatriptan was given subcutaneously 10–23 min later. The first SPECT registration (Toshiba GCA 90 B) was done 120–255 min after the first injection of the tracer. All patients were (virtually) free of headache at that time. Shortly thereafter, all patients received a second injection with the radionuclide, and 3–45 min later the second registration was done. A third SPECT was performed several weeks later, when they were attack-free for at least 5 days.

Frontal, parietal, occipital, temporal, white matter, and cerebellar regions of interest (ROIs) were chosen. The count density values were averaged for each ROI (= relative counts, RC), related to dose of radionuclide administered (radioactivity of total dose—radioactivity remaining in the injection-device), and to loss of radioactivity over time. The relative perfusion was calculated as follows: [$\alpha \times RC/(1 + \alpha - RC); \alpha = 1.5$].

To calculate the relative perfusion after medication, RCs were first corrected for the still remaining activity from the first examination [RC = RC after medication $-$ RC before medication $\times$ exp. ($-0.693 \times t/T_{1/2}$)] (t = time between the two data acquisitions; $T_{1/2}$ = half-life of the isotope).

An asymmetry index was calculated as follows:

$$\frac{\text{rCBF at the headache-side} - \text{rCBF at the nonheadache side}}{(\text{rCBF right} + \text{rCBF left})/2}$$

We also used conventional cortical/cerebellar ratios: the rCBF of each cortical and white matter ROI was correlated with the rCBF of the contralateral, ipsilateral, and total cerebellum.

Statistics were done with the Wilcoxon Matched Pairs Signed-Ranks test and the Mann Whithney U-Wilcoxon Rank Sum W test.

RESULTS

Asymmetry index (Table 1): There were no significant asymmetries in rCBF between the headache and nonheadache side, both outside and during an attack, before and after sumatriptan.

Cortical/cerebellar ratio (Table 2): No significant overall increase or decrease of rCBF during the attack compared to attack-free or after sumatrip-

TABLE 1. *Asymmetry index (average %) per brain region, outside an attack, during an attack before treatment, and after sumatriptan*

	Outisde	During	Sumatriptan
Frontal	1.4	−1.1	2.1
Parietal	−0.4	−0.7	0.2
Temporal	0.1	2.0	2.9
Occipital	−0.1	0.2	1.0
White matter	−1.6	−0.8	−1.2

tan (as compared to pretreatment) was found. However, when the patients were analyzed individually, two patterns of rCBF changes were observed during attacks (Fig. 1): four patients showed an increase of rCBF whereas the other patients showed a decrease. After sumatriptan, however, the rCBF changed into opposite direction in 11 patients. This effect was significant for the parietal and temporal regions ($p = 0.005$) but not for the other regions.

DISCUSSION

We investigated a clinically homogeneous group of patients with unilateral headache. We could not confirm earlier observations suggesting an overall global 25–31% increase of the rCBF during MO attacks (5). In contrast, both an increase and decrease of the rCBF were found, suggesting two patterns of ictal rCBF changes. In addition, there were no differences in rCBF between the headache and nonheadache side.

More relevant, however, is the finding that during migraine attacks, sumatriptan seems to correct the rCBF, irrespective of the change due to the attack. This normalizing effect seemed restricted to the territory of the middle cerebral artery. Comparing these data with results in placebo-treated patients will tell whether this normalizing effect is really due to the drug, or merely is a result of resolution of the attack.

TABLE 2. *rCBF ratio (average %) per brain region, outside an attack, during an attack before treatment, and after sumatriptan*

	Headache side			Nonheadache side		
	Outside	During	Sumatriptan	Outside	During	Sumatriptan
Frontal	87	84	85	86	87	81
Parietal	83	82	83	83	84	81
Temporal	87	85	87	87	85	83
Occipital	91	88	90	91	90	87
White matter	74	75	76	75	77	75

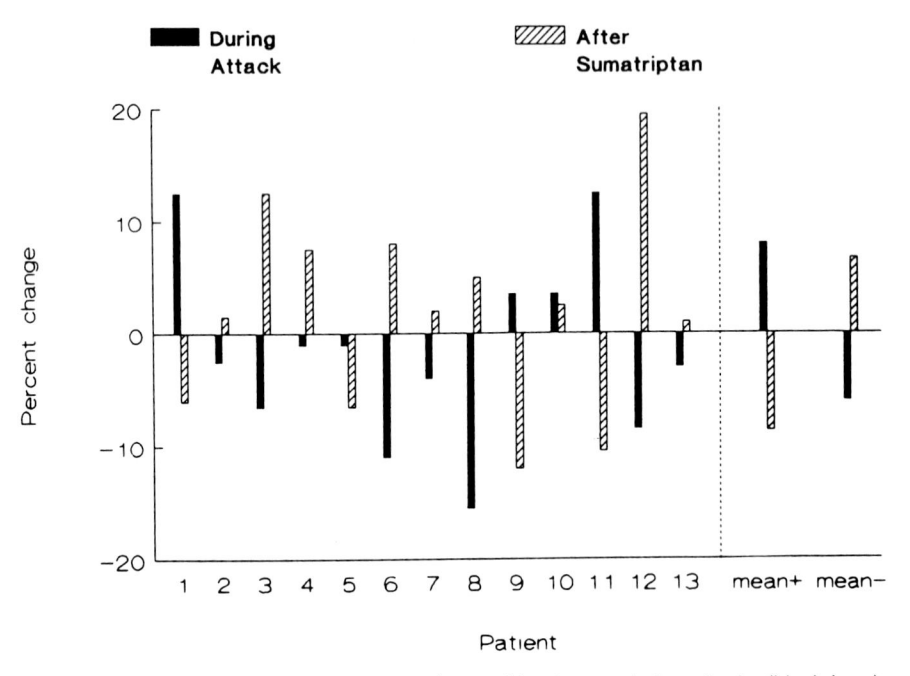

FIG. 1. rCBF ratio changes in migraine patients without aura, during attacks (black bars), and after treatment with sumatriptan (hatched bars). Numbers 1–13 indicate individual patients, mean − indicates the group means of those patients who had a decrease of the rCBF during attacks, and mean + indicates the group means of the patients who had an increase of the rCBF.

REFERENCES

1. The Subcutaneous Sumatriptan International Study Group (Ferrari MD et al). Effective treatment of acute migraine attacks with subcutaneous sumatriptan. A randomised placebo-controlled clinical trial (submitted).
2. Saxena PR and Ferrari MD. 5-Hydroxytryptamine$_1$-like receptor agonists and migraine: Possible impact on the pathophysiology of migraine. *Trends Pharmacol Sci* 1989; 10;5:200–204.
3. Humphrey PPA, Feniuk W, Perren MJ, Connor HE, and Oxford AW. The pharmacology of the novel 5-HT$_1$-like receptor agonist, GR43175. *Cephalalgia* 1989;9[Suppl 9]:23–33.
4. Andersen AR, Friberg HH, Schmidt JR, and Hasselbach SG. Quantitative measurements of cerebral blood flow using SPECT and [^{99m}Tc]-d,l-HM-PAO compared to Xenon-133. *J Cereb Blood Flow Metab* 1988;8:S69–S81.
5. Kobari M, Stirling Meyer J, Ichijo M, Imai A, and Oravez WT. Hyperperfusion of cerebral cortex, thalamus and basal ganglia during spontaneously occurring migraine attacks. *Headache* 1989;29:282–289.

41
Attacks of Migraine Without Aura: Discussion Summary

Jes Olesen and John Stirling Meyer

In migraine without aura virtually all investigators agree that there are no focal abnormalities of regional cerebral blood flow (rCBF). Neither early low flow areas, such as seen in migraine with aura, nor focal areas of increased blood flow in the later phases of attacks have been a consistent finding. In a few cases focal abnormalities in migraine without aura may possibly be explained by the fact that some patients, who predominantly have attacks without aura, also occasionally have attacks with aura.

Regarding global flow no consensus was reached, however. Most studies using ^{133}Xe inhalation with stationary detectors report bilateral and symmetrical increases by 30–40% of CBF (hyperemia) during attacks of migraine without aura. Using inhalation of stable xenon and computed tomography (CT), these bilateral changes have been described as multifocal. During the discussion it was pointed out that the method cannot in fact measure cerebral blood flow with reasonable accuracy in small areas of the brain. Thus, it is probably most fair to describe the changes as bilateral and diffuse. There were no definite clues regarding the possible mechanism of such a hyperemia. It may be caused by activation of the brain by the pain of the headache itself, but it does not appear to cause the headache since there is no correlation of hyperemia with the side of the head pain. Also, hyperemia persists for 8–24 hr after the headache subsides. This finding is similar to the lack of correlation between hyperperfusion and headache in migraine with aura. It was also pointed out that vasodilatation in the brain induced by injection of diamox or breathing of mixtures containing 5% CO_2, which cause similar CBF increases, are not associated with headache.

Contrasting with these findings of global hyperperfusion were the reports using ^{133}Xe inhalation and single photon emission computed tomography (SPECT). The patients were studied longitudinally, and no significant changes in global blood flow were observed when comparing measurements during an attack to values in the same patients after symptoms had been successfully treated a few hours after onset, or, to measurements taken when patients had been migraine-free for a week. To attribute these differing findings to methodologic difficulties is not easy in light of published studies that document that rCBF values measured with the two different techniques correlate well. Ergotamine was used in the SPECT studies to treat attacks and the patients were generally studied rather early, that is, within the first 6 hr. These differences from some of the studies demonstrating hyperemia may perhaps explain the discrepancies.

Studies using rapidly fixed tracers such as technetium hexamethyl-propylene-amine-oxime (HMPAO) cannot provide absolute blood flow values and are therefore unable to detect global blood flow changes. It seems as if the cerebellar blood flow is unchanged during migraine attacks without aura. Therefore, cerebellar blood flow could perhaps be used as a scaling factor to evaluate if hemispheric global flow is increased. The discussion revealed, however, that the documentation of normal cerebellar blood flow is not strong enough to trust such calculations. Technetium HMPAO occasionally is taken up in the temporalis muscle in headache patients. This has been observed in both forms of migraine and in tension-type headache, although rarely, and it remains an unexplained phenomenon.

The regulation of rCBF during migraine attacks without aura has been studied by only one group. Their findings in a small number of patients were interesting in indicating that autoregulation as well as the reactivity to changes in arterial carbon dioxide tension are impaired. Much more should be done to elucidate how the cerebral circulation responds to altered physiological variables during attacks of migraine without aura.

PART VIII

Transcranial Doppler Studies in Migraine

42

Principles of Transcranial Doppler Measurements

Rune Aaslid

Department of Neurosurgery, University of Berne, Inselspital, CH-3010 Berne, Switzerland

The application of the Doppler principle to measure blood flow velocity was first described in 1960 by Satomura and Kaneko (1), working in Osaka. It is interesting to note that Kaneko actually suggested what we now call transcranial Doppler (or simply TCD) (2), but that Satomura thought this was impossible and developed the instrument for investigating the extracranial circulation only. The barrier presented by the skull was, in fact, not that formidable, and the TCD methodology was developed 22 years later, in 1982 (3). It was first applied to the detection of vasospasm (4). Later, the application of the TCD technique to record cerebral blood flow velocity changes after brain activation (5,6) and blood pressure changes (7) demonstrated the possibilities of dynamic measurements of the cerebral circulation. However, it is necessary to verify how such velocity changes are related to changes in flow volume (8). This chapter discusses this problem.

Frequently, pulsatility or "resistance" indices are calculated from the Doppler waveform (9,10), and some authors use these to detect changes in cerebrovascular resistance. Obviously, for many applications, including migraine studies, an easy-to-use and noninvasive method to detect changes in cerebrovascular tone would be of great interest. The problem is, however, that the approaches and indices suggested so far have so many inherent possibilities of errors that a serious investigator would not trust their use. A new and more theoretical valid approach to this problem is under development, and will be discussed below.

THE DOPPLER PRINCIPLE

Basically, the Doppler principle measures velocity, V, by the frequency of shift f of ultrasound with frequency f_0 when it is reflected by the moving blood according to the equation $f = 2 \cdot f_0 \cdot V/c$ (c is the velocity of sound in blood). This Doppler shift is what we hear in the earphones of the Doppler instrument and what we see on the spectrum analyzer. A velocity of 1 m/sec will give a shift of about 2.5 KHz at an f_0 of 2 MHz and 5 KHz if the Doppler ultrasound frequency is 4 MHz. Since different instruments usually use different ultrasonic frequencies, it is best to express readings from such an instrument in velocity units: that is, in cm/sec or m/sec (11) and not in the frequency units KHz or Hz. Normally an angle exists between the ultrasonic beam and the blood flow direction. This must be taken into account when interpreting an observed Doppler shift, and the correction factor is proportional to the cosine of ■. It is good practice in Doppler measurements to try to minimize the angle of insonation. For example, ±30° of variation in angle gives an error of maximum 13.5%, whereas ±60° will increase the error to 50%. The velocity component measured by the Doppler principle is always lower than or equal to the real flow velocities. Unfortunately, angle correction is not usually possible in TCD applications because the arteries are short, curving, and difficult to map accurately. It should always be stated if velocity readings are given as angle corrected and how the angle is determined.

The Doppler shifts are detected from a spatial region which in ultrasound terminology is called the sample volume. The lateral borders of this are given by the focusing of the ultrasonic beam. In TCD application, the focus usually has a lateral diameter of about 3–4 mm, which is about the same as the arteries measured from. In the axial direction, the sample volume is defined by a technique called range-gating. This averages the received signal over a certain time interval after transmission of a burst. Only signals received within this interval, corresponding to an interval in depth, are used to derive the Doppler shift. It is common in TCD applications to use rather long and somewhat undefined sample volumes (approx. 5–12 mm) to achieve an improvement of the signal-to-noise ratios.

It has long been felt that multichannel TCD might be useful in monitoring. The problem with using two conventional TCD units and two probes (usually one on each hemisphere) is the mutual interference between them. The frequencies of the instruments have to be locked in phase, and the PRFs must be identical to avoid acoustic interference. This problem is readily solved if the two channels are integrated into one instrument, with completely synchronous bursts of transmission. Figure 1 shows a simultaneous recording of arterial and venous (straight sinus) flow velocities during a step decrease in arterial blood pressure (ABP) made with such a prototype instrument.

VELOCITY PROFILES AND DOPPLER SPECTRA

For the flowing blood in a basal cerebral artery, the situation is rather complex with regard to the velocity profile and its influence on the received

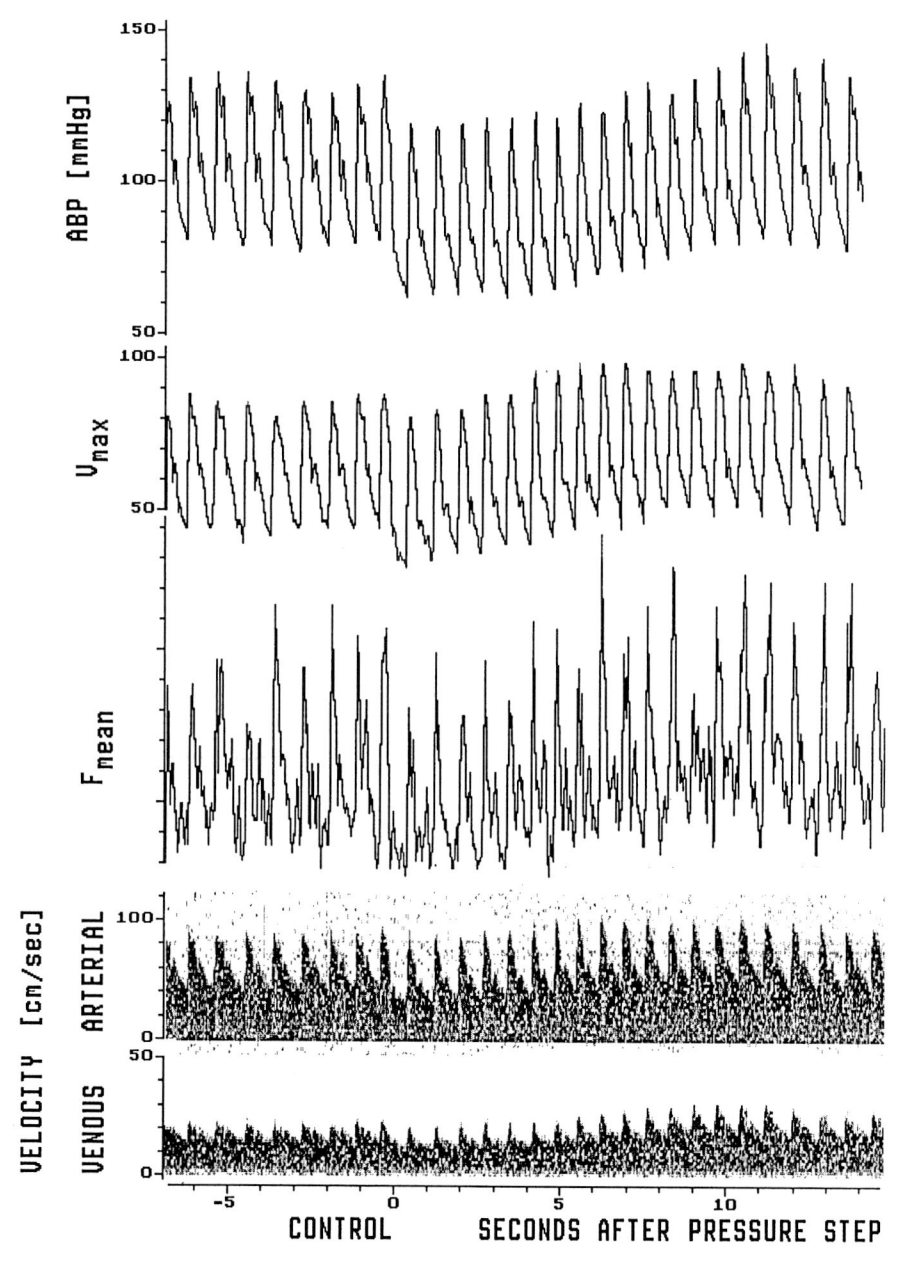

FIG. 1. Simultaneous recordings of arterial and venous Doppler spectra during acute step decreases in arterial blood pressure (ABP). Outline velocity (V_{max}) and relative volume flow (F_{mean}) in the middle tracings are calculated from the arterial spectral recording.

Doppler signal. The entire cross-section of the artery, branches, and maybe proximal or distal curving segments will be within the sample volume. Each moving part of the blood within the sample volume contributes to a mixture of Doppler shifts consisting of many frequencies. By a technique called spectral analysis, we can determine the signal power of each velocity component; this can be coded in color or grayscale on a computer display as shown in Fig. 1. Clearly, such a spectral signal is rather complex and information-heavy, and it is necessary to extract more simple information out of it.

Most of the TCD instrument designs and most authors have chosen the envelope or spectral outline velocity, V_{max}, as a parameter. By definition, this corresponds to the maximum Doppler shift and, therefore, the maximum velocity component of the velocity profile. Usually this corresponds to velocity in the lumen centerline. As shown in Fig. 1, the complex and detailed information in a spectral recording is reduced to a waveform practically identical to a waveform recorded, for example, from an ABP catheter. For most monitoring and physiological response studies, such waveform recording is preferable to full spectral recording.

VOLUME FLOW CALCULATED FROM TCD RECORDINGS

Ideally, the signal power of a particular Doppler frequency is proportional to the number of blood cells having this velocity component. By using the signal power of each component of the Doppler spectrum, it would seem possible to determine the relative flow F_{mean} in the vessel insonated (4). However, this approach is valid only under the conditions that:

1. there are no vascular bruits or vessel wall movements
2. the signal is much stronger than the noise
3. the sample volume is centered on a straight segment of the artery
4. there are no branches or adjacent small vessels within the sample volume
5. there are only minimal sample volume sensitivity variations over the cross-section of the artery.

These conditions may be met by middle cerebral artery (MCA) recordings in normal young patients (Fig. 1) when using careful techniques to fix the transducer and position the sample volume. In typical clinical measurements, most of these conditions are violated. Using V_{max} as flow index also gives a considerably less noisy record than F_{mean}, as shown by the example in Fig. 1. However, use of velocity as a substitute for flow depends on the assumption that the cross-sectional area of the artery does not change to an extent that invalidates the recordings. The sudden blood pressure step in Fig. 1 was induced to test the autoregulatory response (7). In a new series of seven patients (12), we found that V_{max} and F_{mean} gave practically identical time courses when used as a flow index. Moreover, the step in arterial V_{max}

was the same as in the straight sinus on the venous side. These findings indicate that basal cerebral arteries are rather stiff and that diameter changes do not invalidate the use of V_{max} to assess changes in flow during moderate variations in blood pressure. An earlier study using electromagnetic flowmetry as the "gold standard" came to the same conclusion (13).

The recent development of a laser Doppler method (14) for cerebral perfusion measurements might give new data on the accuracy of the TCD method during ABP changes, and such investigations are underway.

The cerebral vascular bed is extremely sensitive to changes in arterial Pa_{CO_2}, and the so-called vasomotor reactivity was traditionally measured by tracer methods. Angiographic studies have demonstrated that the larger human basal cerebral arteries are unresponsive (at least within the tolerances of measurement) to changes in Pa_{CO_2} (15), while arteries that had diameters less than 1 mm responded. This is consistent with the assumption that the large basal cerebral arteries are not significantly involved in regulation of blood flow and act as mere conductance channels between the central circulation and the periphery. If this assumption is correct, then vasomotor reactivity measured by TCD should give the same values (percent change in CBF per mm Hg Pa_{CO_2}), as has been reported previously with regional cerebral blood flow (rCBF) methods. This has been confirmed in normal patients (16), and TCD is widely used to measure CO_2 reactivity. However, the long-term effects of Pa_{CO_2} on basal cerebral artery diameters has not been clarified.

Thiopentone and metaraminol bitartrate do not seem to influence MCA diameters because flow and velocity remain proportional (13) during administration. On the other hand, nitroglycerine seems to dilate the MCA significantly, as shown in a recent study using single photon emission computed tomography (SPECT) and TCD measurements (17). This finding underlines the importance of validating the relationship between changes in velocity and changes in volume flow for each intervention that is used for investigational or clinical purposes.

CALCULATION OF CHANGES IN CEREBROVASCULAR RESISTANCE FROM TCD RECORDINGS

Many indices have been proposed for use with Doppler measurements to calculate changes in resistance of the cerebrovascular bed. These are based on the changes in the pulsatile waveform due to changes in resistance. The pulsatility index (9):

$$PI = (V_{systolic} - V_{diastolic})/V_{mean}$$

and the resistance index (10):

$$RI = (V_{systolic} - V_{diastolic})/V_{systolic}$$

are the most widely used, but methods based on Fourier analysis also have been applied. Pulsatility and resistance indices were originally suggested for evaluation of the peripheral circulation. Quantitatively, the flow in the cerebral circulation is characterized by a very low resistance, and the pulsatile waveform of the flow is practically identical to that of the arterial blood pressure (Fig. 1). When the blood pressure waveform changes, the velocity will follow. Central cardiovascular factors therefore influence PI and RI more than local cerebral factors under certain conditions; an extreme example is shown in Fig. 2 in a patient with irregular heart rhythm. Between the first and the second box heart rate changed, resulting in an increase in PI from 0.82 to 2.2. (The RI also changed in a similar fashion.) But mean blood pressure divided by mean velocity decreased slightly, indicating that

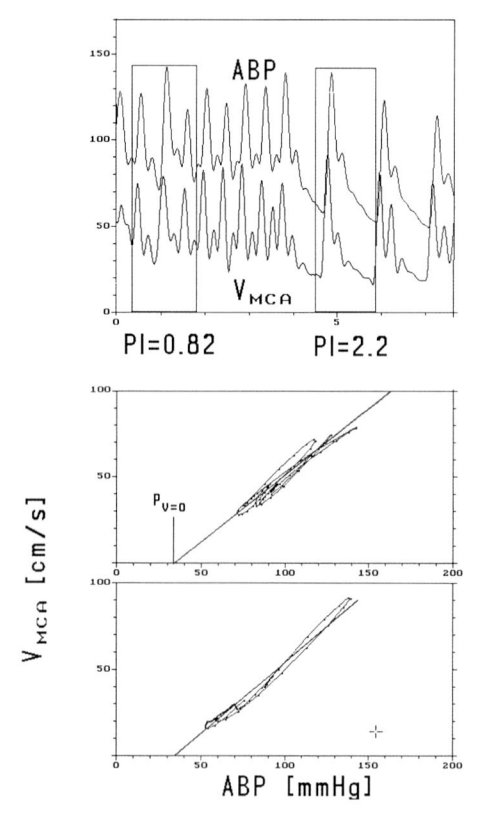

FIG. 2. Top: Recordings of arterial blood pressure (ABP) and middle cerebral artery velocity (V_{MCA}) in a patient with irregular heart rhythm. The Gosling pulsatility index (PI) is calculated for the two sections marked by rectangles. It increases due to decrease in heart rate and not due to an increase in resistance. **Middle and bottom:** Velocity plotted against ABP for the two sections marked in *top* panel. The regression line intercepts the pressure axis at the critical closing pressure $P_{V=0}$.

cerebrovascular resistance did not change much, and certainly did not increase dramatically as would mistakenly have been concluded from the indices based on the velocity waveform. In circumstances where central cardiovascular factors may change—as, for example, during a migraine attack—the type of waveform analysis by simple pulsatility indices is virtually useless to assess changes in cerebrovascular resistance. The use of PI and RI in the cerebral circulation should therefore be discouraged.

The only application of PI and RI would be to assess different relative responses in different vascular territories. For this the pulsatility transmission index can be used (18):

$$PTI = PI / PI_{ref}$$

This index compares the PI in the artery under consideration to the PI_{ref} of the reference artery. Central cardiovascular factors would affect both PIs similarly, and their effect can thus be minimized. However, the solution is not entirely satisfactory because in many situations we need to assess global cerebral vascular changes, and then there is no reference artery.

As mentioned above, changes in the ABP waveform caused by the central cardiovascular system is the main reason why PI and RI are useless. If the ABP waveform could be measured accurately, the pulsatility of ABP could possibly be used as PI_{ref}. Such accurate measurements of ABP waveforms are now possible by a new noninvasive method based on a servo cuff on the upper arm (19); the measurements shown in Fig. 1 were made with such a device. However, a more physiological approach than simple pulsatility analysis is possible and will be discussed.

PRESSURE-FLOW RELATIONSHIP OF THE CEREBRAL CIRCULATION

The formula:

$$CBF = CPP/CVR$$

is widely used in both investigational and clinical work to explain the relationship between cerebral blood flow (CBF), cerebral perfusion pressure (CPP), and cerebrovascular resistance (CVR). But this approach disregards the fact that flow and pressure are not proportional even if the vasomotor tone does not change. Like in the coronary circulation, the instantaneous pressure–flow relationship of the cerebral circulation is a linear function (20), but the line does not go through the origin. It intercepts the pressure axis at what is normally called the critical closing pressure or the $P_{F=0}$ (20). Using Doppler we could call it the $P_{V=0}$. In Fig. 2, velocity has been plotted against ABP for the two sections of the record. Even if pulsatility changes dramatically, the intercept as calculated by regression analysis remains constant. In a preliminary series we found excellent linear relationships between

ABP and velocity. When vascular tone changes, both the slope (CVR) and the intercept changed (20), indicating the need for a more comprehensive model of the cerebral circulation than that based only on CVR. Because $P_{V=0}$ is an absolute quantitative measurement of a key aspect of the circulation, it is a promising concept to apply to studies of the cerebral vascular bed. It also has the advantage that it can be determined by completely noninvasive means.

REFERENCES

1. Satomura S and Kaneko Z. Ultrasonic blood rheograph. In: Proceedings of the 3rd International Conference on Medical Electronics 1960; 254–258.
2. Kaneko Z. First steps in the development of the Doppler flowmeter. *Ultrasound Med Biol* 1986;12:187–195.
3. Aaslid R, Markwalder T-M, and Nornes H. Noninvasive transcranial Doppler ultrasound recording of flow velocity in basal cerebral arteries. *J Neurosurg* 1982;57:769–774.
4. Aaslid R, Huber P, and Nornes H. Evaluation of cerebrovascular spasm with transcranial Doppler ultrasound. *J Neurosurg* 1984;60:37–41.
5. Aaslid R. Visually evoked dynamic blood flow response of the human cerebral circulation. *Stroke* 1987;18:771–775.
6. Droste DW, Harders AG, and Rastogi E: A transcranial Doppler study of blood flow velocity in the middle cerebral arteries performed at rest and during mental activities. *Stroke* 1989;20:1005–1011.
7. Aaslid R, Lindegaard K-F, Sorteberg W, and Nornes H. Cerebral autoregulation dynamics in humans. *Stroke* 1989;20:45–52.
8. Kontos HA. Validity of cerebral arterial blood flow calculations from velocity measurements. *Stroke* 1989;20:1–3.
9. Gosling RG and King DH. Arterial assessment by Doppler shift ultrasound. *Proc R Soc Med* 1974;67:447–449.
10. Pourcelot L. Application cliniques de l'examen Doppler transcutane. Coloques de l'Institut Nationale de la Santé et de la Recherche Medicale. *Inserm* 1974;34:213–240.
11. The Doppler standards and nomenclature committee of the American Society of Echocardiography: recommendations for terminology and display for Doppler echocardiography. In: Kisslo J, Adams D, Mark DB eds. *Basic doppler echocardiography*. New York: Churchill Livingstone, 1986.
12. Aaslid R, Newell DW, Stooss R, Sorteberg W, Lindegaard K-F, and Nornes H. Assessment of cerebral autoregulation dynamics by simultaneous arterial and venous transcranial doppler 1991, *in press*.
13. Lindegaard K-F, Lundar T, Wiberg J, Sjoberg D, Aaslid R, and Nornes H. Variations in middle cerebral artery blood flow investigated with noninvasive transcranial blood velocity measurements. *Stroke* 1987;18:1025–1030.
14. Haberl RL, Heizer ML, and Ellis EF: Laser-Doppler assessment of brain microcirculation: Effect of local alterations. *Am J Physiol* 1989;256:H1255–1260.
15. Huber P and Handa J: Effect of contrast material, hypercapnia, hyperventilation, hypertonic glucose and papaverine on the diameter of the cerebral arteries—angiographic determination in man. *Invest Radiol* 1967;2:17–32.
16. Markwalder T-M, Grolimund P, et al. Dependency of blood flow velocity in the middle cerebral artery on end-tidal carbon dioxide partial pressure. A transcranial Doppler study. *J Cereb Blood Flow Metab* 1984;4:368–372.
17. Dahl A, Russell D, Nyberg-Hansen R, and Rootwelt K: Effect of nitroglycerin on cerebral circulation measured by transcranial Doppler and SPECT. *Stroke* 1989;20:1733–1736.
18. Lindegaard K-F, Bakke SJ, Grolimund P, Aaslid R, Huber P, and Nornes H: Assessment

of intracranial hemodynamics in carotid artery disease by transcranial Doppler ultrasound. *J Neurosurg* 1985;63:890–898.
19. Aaslid R and Brubakk AO: Accuracy of an ultrasound Doppler servo method for noninvasive determination of instantaneous and mean arterial blood pressure. *Circulation* 1981;64:753–759.
20. Dewey RC, Pieper HP, and Hunt WE: Experimental cerebral hemodynamics: Vasomotor tone, critical closing pressure, and vascular bed resistance. *J Neurosurg* 1974;41:597–606.

*Migraine and Other Headaches:
The Vascular Mechanisms,*
edited by Jes Olesen.
Raven Press, Ltd., New York © 1991.

43

Transcranial Doppler Studies During Migraine and Other Headaches

Andreas Thie

Department of Neurology, University of Hamburg, D-2000 Hamburg 20, Germany

Transcranial Doppler (TCD) has become an established method in clinical practice for a variety of problems (1) reflected by a growing body of literature, but there is a remarkable paucity of data concerning headache. Vascular abnormalities are features of migraine and cluster headache (2), although their role in pathophysiology remains incompletely understood. To use TCD, which is a noninvasive and economic method, and to study vascular features in selected headache syndromes is appealing.

MIGRAINE: INTERVAL FINDINGS

First case reports of TCD findings in migraine during the headache-free period (3) have focused on elevated flow velocities (FVs) and have raised the question of prolonged vasospasm. Systematic study of TCD features in migraineurs has yielded different results (4). The sample of Thie et al. consisted of 100 consecutive patients with common (n = 61) or classic (n = 39) migraine according to the criteria of the Ad Hoc Committee on Classification of Headache (5). Forty age-matched healthy volunteers served as controls. Since FVs decrease with age (6), it is essential to compare groups of similar age. Mean flow velocities (MFVs) (7) and pulsatility indices (PIs) were recorded. PI indicates systolic minus diastolic FV divided by MFV (8).

Flow Velocity

In the migraine sample, intracranial MFVs were significantly higher in all arteries, that is, middle cerebral artery (MCA), anterior cerebral artery (ACA), posterior cerebral artery (PCA), and basilar artery (BA), when compared with the control group (Table 1). MFV in the internal carotid artery

TABLE 1. *TCD findings in migraineurs vs. controls*

	Migraine (n = 100)	Controls (n = 40)	Significance/ p value
ICA			
MFV	48 ± 10	46 ± 8	n.s.
PI	0.82 ± 0.17	0.98 ± 0.17	$p < 0.001$
MCA			
MFV	76 ± 16	68 ± 9	$p < 0.001$
PI	0.74 ± 0.14	0.83 ± 0.13	$p = 0.003$
ACA			
MFV	64 ± 14	57 ± 10	$p = 0.001$
PI	0.76 ± 0.15	0.84 ± 0.14	$p = 0.005$
PCA			
MFV	52 ± 10	43 ± 6	$p < 0.001$
PI	0.70 ± 0.14	0.78 ± 0.12	$p = 0.005$
BA			
MFV	49 ± 10	44 ± 7	$p = 0.002$
PI	0.75 ± 0.12	0.81 ± 0.15	$p = 0.05$

From ref. 4, with permission.

MFV, mean flow velocities (cm/sec), PI, pulsatility indices (mean ± SD); ICA, internal carotid artery; MCA, middle cerebral artery; ACA, anterior cerebral artery; PCA, posterior cerebral artery; BA, basilar artery; n.s., not significant.

PI in migraine sample are based on n = 49 (BA), n = 47 (ICA), n = 45 (MCA, ACA, PCA).

(ICA) in the neck insonated 4–5 cm cranially of the mandibular angle did not show any significant difference between groups. PIs were significantly lower in migraineurs than in controls in all insonated arteries extracranially and intracranially. Marked increases of MFV above 3 SD of control values in at least one artery were found in 16% of migraineurs, but not in controls ($p < 0.0001$). These investigators were unable to detect differences in MFVs or PIs between common and classic migraine.

Yet, controversy exists regarding FV in migraineurs (Table 2). Recently, Abernathy et al. (9) confirmed the results of Thie's group in a study of 37 headache-free migraineurs and 31 controls. FVs of migraineurs were significantly higher in the MCA, ACA, PCA, BA ($p < 0.0001$), and the intracranial vertebral arteries ($p < 0.001$). In the ICA insonated at the level of the carotid siphon and in the ophthalmic artery MFV did not differ between groups. Other investigators (10–13) have not detected differences in FV between migraineurs and healthy controls (Table 2), but most control groups were not age-matched.

Drugs like ergotamine, calcium entry blockers, or sumatriptan do not appear to affect FV markedly in migraineurs, neither in acute trials during interval or attack nor with chronic treatment, but data are scanty (3,14).

From these findings it may be concluded that FVs are higher in some migraineurs than in age-matched healthy controls, but excessively high only in a small portion of patients. Possibly, increased FVs in migraineurs reflect slightly elevated vasotonus of the insonated large basal cerebral arteries.

TABLE 2. *Flow velocities in headache-free migraine*

Author	Type	n	Artery	Age	Difference
Rosa	CO	75	MCA, ACA, BA	Unmatched	n.s.
	CL	15			
	Cts	50			
Haring	CO	23	MCA, ACA, PCA	Unmatched	n.s.
	CL	17			
	Cts	20			
De Benedittis	CO	20	MCA	Unmatched	n.s.
	Cts	10			
Pavy-le-Traon	CO	18	MCA	Matched	n.s.
	CL	10			
	Cts	28			
Abernathy	MI	37	MCA, ACA, PCA,	Unmatched	higher
	Cts	31	BA, VA		in mi.
			Siphon, OphA		n.s.
Thie	CO	69	MCA, ACA, PCA, BA	Matched	higher
	CL	31			in mi.
	Cts	40			

CO, common migraine; CL, classic migraine; MI, mi, migraine unspecified; Cts, controls; MCA, middle cerebral artery; ACA, anterior cerebral artery; PCA, posterior cerebral artery; BA, basilar artery; VA, vertebral artery; OphA, ophthalmic artery; n.s., not significant.

With regard to normal regional cerebral blood flow (rCBF) studies in headache-free migraineurs (18) (i.e., lack of global hypoperfusion), one would have to assume concomitant slight vasodilatation of arterioles to be associated with relative vasoconstriction of large arteries to result in normal CBF. Proof for this assumption awaits simultaneous measurement of FV and rCBF in migraineurs with markedly elevated FV.

Flow Asymmetries

In studies of rCBF, flow asymmetries during the headache-free period have been described (15), presumably representing instability of CBF control. Slight side differences of FV are commonly detected in normal persons (6).

Thie and coworkers (4) counted differences of MFV in paired intracranial arteries above 20 cm/sec somewhat arbitrarily as "flow asymmetries," provided that adequate Doppler signals could be obtained on both sides. They found asymmetric MFV in 12% of migraineurs and 1 of 40 (2.5%) controls (not significant).

Bruits

Another important and common finding in this sample was the detection of noises (bruits), most often of low frequency (Fig. 1). On the directional

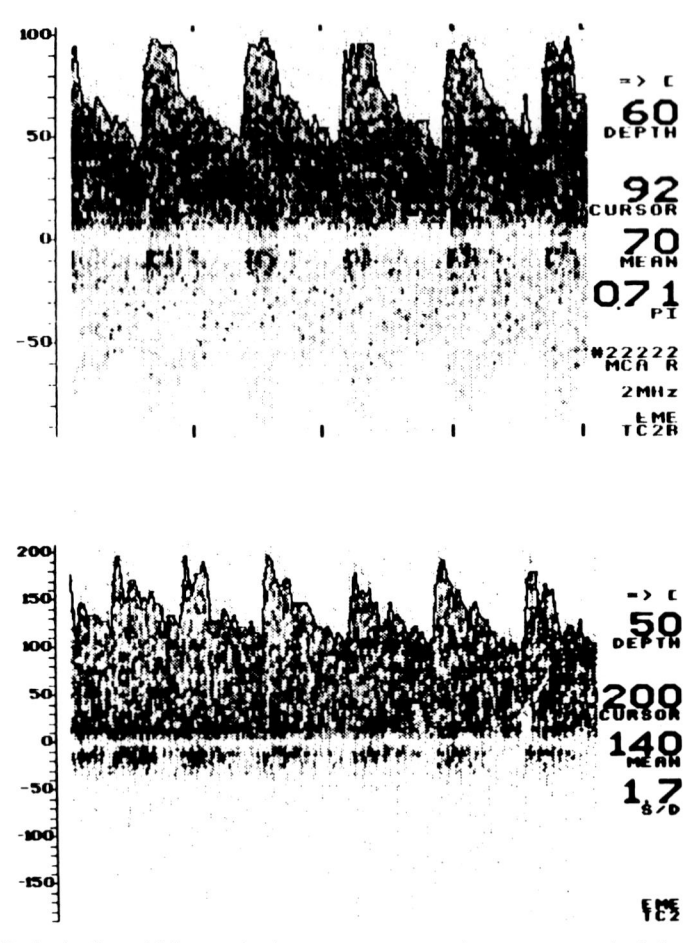

FIG. 1. Bruits in the middle cerebral artery, represented as a symmetrical dense pattern shown above and below the zero frequency baseline. Bruits may be associated with normal flow velocity (*top*), or with markedly increased flow velocity (*bottom*). (From ref. 4, with permission.)

Doppler spectrum, bruits are represented as symmetrical pattern shown above and below the zero frequency baseline (16). These bruits may have a musical or harmonic character, commonly sound like "boots in the snow," and some patients have low frequency bruits on one side and high pitched bruits (like "cries of a sea gull") on the other. The predilecting site of these acoustic phenomena is the intracranial branching of the ICA into MCA and ACA, but other segments may be involved, with a distribution similar to that of bruits in vasospasm after subarachnoid hemorrhage (17). The detection of bruits was significantly more frequent in migraineurs (56%) compared with healthy controls (7.5%) ($p < 0.0001$).

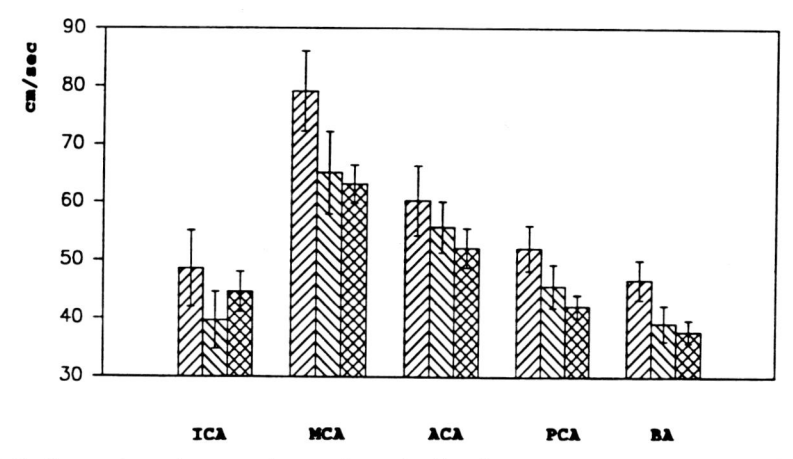

FIG. 2. Comparison of averaged mean flow velocities (in cm/sec with 95% confidence limits) of 31 classic migraineurs with bruits (*left bars*) or without bruits (*middle bars*) and 40 controls (*right bars*) for different arteries. ICA, internal carotid artery; MCA, middle cerebral artery; ACA, anterior cerebral artery; PCA, posterior cerebral artery; BA, basilar artery.

Bruits of this type are nonspecific, but may occur in subarachnoid hemorrhage, atherosclerotic stenosis, vasculitis, or without any known abnormality especially in the young (Thie et al., unpublished results).

Bruits were usually associated with normal FVs, yet FVs in patients with bruits were generally higher than in those without. This was demonstrated by comparing a subgroup of 31 patients with classic migraine and controls (Thie et al., unpublished results). Migraineurs with bruits had significantly higher MFV in most arteries than those without bruits (Fig. 2). Furthermore, only migraineurs with bruits exhibited significantly higher MFV compared with controls, although migraineurs without bruits also had a tendency toward higher MFV than controls.

Bruits are presumably produced by turbulent flow through arterial narrowing or increased blood flow through normal arteries, and arterial wall motion secondary to turbulent flow (16, 19). Since bruits are usually associated with normal or only slightly elevated FV, one may speculate that bruits in migraineurs are produced by increased or unstable vasotonus and consecutive turbulence.

Clinico-Ultrasonic Correlation

So far no major correlation between TCD abnormalities and clinical findings emerged; in particular, FVs and bruits did not correlate with side of headache or aura (4).

Most recent sporadic observations suggest that in some cases MFVs are markedly higher during a period of clinical instability, for example, frequent attacks or change of migrainous features (first aura in a common migraineurs, first prolonged aura), but may normalize subsequently over months to years (Thie et al., unpublished results).

Cerebrovascular Reactivity

Altered vasoreactivity in migraineurs concerning extracranial and intracranial vessels has been described previously (2). Thomas et al. (20) reported excessive vasomotor reactivity to 5% CO_2 inhalation in migraineurs. MFV in the MCA increased by 47 ± 15% in 10 migraineurs but by 28 ± 14% in 10 controls (p = 0.026). Since end-expiratory pCO_2 was not measured, correlation of FV with achieved change of pCO_2 was not possible, making the results hard to interpret. The same group (21) claimed that excessive CO_2 reactivity normalized after successful prophylactic therapy with propranolol in a few cases.

Reinecke and coworkers (22) extended this approach to discriminate migraine from other headaches by means of TCD vasoreactivity testing. They submitted 103 patients with different headache syndromes and 26 normal controls to a standardized Valsalva maneuver. FVs in the MCA, blood pressure, and end-expiratory pCO_2 were monitored simultaneously. During the straining phase, migraineurs showed a significantly steeper rise of FV and a higher ratio of flow acceleration divided by rise of blood pressure. Using both ratios, accuracy of migraine diagnosis was about 74%.

Recently, Thie et al. (23) studied cerebrovascular reactivity in a somewhat different approach with a variety of stimuli in 11 migraineurs and 12 age-matched normal controls. Increase of MFV in the MCA during a cognitive task that required patients to write down a literary text projected on a slide was greater in migraineurs than in controls, but this difference failed to be statistically significant (p = 0.06). Two tests of motor activation produced similar increases of MFV in both groups. CO_2 reactivity was no different between the groups either for hypocapnia, hypercapnia, or total reactivity when end-expiratory pCO_2 was monitored, and change of MFV was correlated with achieved change of end-expiratory pCO_2. Thus, these investigators were unable to confirm the results of Thomas et al.

Thie and colleagues used photic stimulation and had the patients observe complex images to test vasoreactivity (VR) in the PCA. Increase of MFV in both tests for PCA reactivity was significantly greater in migraineurs than in controls: about 20% versus 10%, respectively, for both tests. Due to overlap of individual results, however, the discriminative value of both tests is low.

What may be striking in some migraineurs is the extent of spontaneous fluctuations of FV. Significantly greater variability of MFV in the PCA for migraineurs compared to controls was calculated during rest and stimulation phases.

These studies suggest that cerebral vasoreactivity may be abnormal in migraine, but not with every test or at any particular time. It is of special interest that abnormalities may be demonstrated in tests of autonomic function, and that they might be more pronounced in the posterior than in the anterior vascular territory.

MIGRAINE: FINDINGS DURING ATTACKS

With regard to changes of FV during migraine attacks, major controversy, even confusion, is reflected by the literature (11, 13, 24–27) (Table 3).

In Thie et al.'s study (27), rather uniform changes of MFV apparently depending on the type of migraine were found. TCD examination was performed in 18 patients, within 6 hr after start of symptoms in 7, within 7–12 hr in 2, within 13–24 hr in 4, and within 25–36 hr in 5. All patients with classic migraine were examined during the headache phase.

All patients with common migraine exhibited a decrease of MFV in the intracranial cerebral arteries and the extracranial ICA and an increase of PI. Bruits tended to be less frequently detectable than during the interval (Table 4). Reduction of MFVs in common migraineurs were slight, and ranged from 13.7% for both ICAs to 18.75% for the right ACA.

All patients with classic migraine showed just the opposite: increase of MFV, decrease of PI, and greater prominence of bruits (Table 5). Elevation of MFV in classic migraineurs averaged 20–25%. In individual patients, MFV changed by more than 10 cm/sec in at least one artery on either side; in most patients two or more arteries showed FV alterations of this degree.

TABLE 3. *TCD findings during spontaneous migraine attacks*

Author	Type	n	Artery	Change of FV	Timing of TCD
Haring	CO	7	MCA, ACA, PCA	n.s.	?
	CL	3	MCA, ACA, PCA	n.s.	
Liboni	CL	13	MCA	Increase	−36 hr (?)
	CO	5	MCA	n.s.	
Zwetsloot	CL	27	MCA, ACA	(Decrease)	?
	CO	4	MCA, ACA	n.s.	
Formisano	CO	12	MCA, ACA, PCA	Increase 9	?
				Decrease 1	
				n.s. 3	
Pavy-le-Traon	CO	19	MCA ↘	Increase 9	−34 hr
	CL	2	MCA ↗	Decrease 7	
				(Decrease) 4	
				n.s. 1	
Thie	CO	13	MCA, ACA, PCA	Decrease 13	−36 hr
	CL	5	MCA, ACA, PCA	Increase 5	

CO, common migraine; CL, classic migraine; MCA, middle cerebral artery; ACA, anterior cerebral artery; PCA, posterior cerebral artery; n.s., not significant; ( ), tendency without significance.

TABLE 4. *Common migraine: TCD findings interval vs. attack (n = 13)*

	Right			Left		
	Int	Att	p	Int	Att	p
ICA						
MFV	51 ± 13	44 ± 11	**	51 ± 10	44 ± 9	*
PI	0.75 ± 0.22	0.84 ± 0.27	n.s.	0.74 ± 0.20	0.85 ± 0.22	*
Dec		4			4	
MCA						
MFV	79 ± 18	66 ± 19	**	79 ± 19	66 ± 18	***
PI	0.76 ± 0.17	0.82 ± 0.23	n.s.	0.74 ± 0.15	0.81 ± 0.19	n.s.
Bruits	7	3		6	2	
Dec		7			8	
ACA						
MFV	64 ± 20	52 ± 13	*	68 ± 14	58 ± 12	**
PI	0.76 ± 0.14	0.78 ± 0.19	n.s.	0.65 ± 0.14	0.73 ± 0.13	*
Bruits	6	3		3	1	
Dec		7			6	
PCA						
MFV	53 ± 17	45 ± 7	n.s.	51 ± 7	43 ± 8	***
PI	0.71 ± 0.16	0.83 ± 0.27	n.s.	0.75 ± 0.15	0.84 ± 0.20	n.s.
Bruits	2	1		—	—	
Dec		5			5	

From ref. 27, with permission.
MFV, mean flow velocities (cm/sec); PI, pulsatility indices (mean ± SD); Att, attack; Int, interval; ICA, internal carotid artery; MCA, middle cerebral artery; ACA, anterior cerebral artery; PCA, posterior cerebral artery; n.s., not significant.
p: p value; *, $p < 0.05$; **, $p < 0.01$; ***, $p < 0.005$.
Dec, number of arteries in which MFV decreased by >10 cm/sec. Bruits, number of arteries in which bruits appeared.
MFV and PI of both ICAs and right PCA based on 11 patients.

Flow reduction in one artery and flow elevation of this extent in another in the same patient was never detected. No correlation was found between side of headache or aura and change of FV. Timing of the examination had no apparent effect on general findings.

With regard to their results, Thie and coworkers concluded that reduction of FV in common migraine attacks was compatible with slight vasodilatation of large cerebral arteries and intact autoregulation in the view of normal rCBF findings, very similar to cluster headache attacks (see below). Slight increase of arteriolar tonus, that is, interpretation of TCD findings as being secondary to increased peripheral resistance, would also be possible. Increase of FV during classic attacks is harder to conceive. It might be caused by an inverse vascular reaction: slight vasoconstriction of large vessels contributing to the known decrease of rCBF during the initial phase of the attack. Unfortunately, this increase of FV was also found during a period when rCBF might have been in the hyperemia phase.

When results from different groups are compared, no clear picture emerges. To resolve this confusion we need repeated or serial examinations in the same patients by the same examiners or a fixed head probe, and be

TABLE 5. *Classic migraine: TCD findings interval vs. attack (n = 5)*

	Right			Left		
	Int	Att	p	Int	Att	p
ICA						
MFV	35 ± 10	43 ± 9	*	37 ± 8	45 ± 8	n.s.
PI	0.97 ± 0.20	1.01 ± 0.39	n.s.	0.88 ± 0.31	0.89 ± 0.39	n.s.
Inc		1			1	
MCA						
MFV	65 ± 9	72 ± 12	n.s.	65 ± 5	79 ± 9	*
PI	0.96 ± 0.10	0.80 ± 0.19	*	0.81 ± 0.08	0.85 ± 0.21	n.s.
Bruits	2	4		1	5	
Inc		2			3	
ACA						
MFV	50 ± 14	54 ± 19	n.s.	50 ± 12	62 ± 8	*
PI	0.86 ± 0.20	0.74 ± 0.06	n.s.	0.87 ± 0.17	0.80 ± 0.18	n.s.
Bruits	1	2		1	3	
Inc		1			3	
PCA						
MFV	46 ± 10	66 ± 33	n.s.	43 ± 10	54 ± 19	n.s.
PI	0.79 ± 0.26	0.76 ± 0.24	n.s.	0.87 ± 0.14	0.68 ± 0.13	**
Bruits	—	1		—	1	
Inc		3			2	

From ref. 27, with permission.
MFV, mean flow velocities (cm/sec); PI, pulsatility indices (mean ± SD); Att, attack; Int, interval; ICA, internal carotid artery; MCA, middle cerebral artery; ACA, anterior cerebral artery; PCA, posterior cerebral artery; n.s., not significant.
p: p value; *, $p < 0.05$; **, $p < 0.01$.
Inc, number of arteries in which MFV increased by >10 cm/sec. Bruits, number of arteries in which bruits appeared.
MFV and PI of both ICAs based on 3 patients.

prepared for only slight changes. There is urgent need to examine (a) the time course of FV during attacks, (b) rapid fluctuations of FV during attacks, (c) flow changes in different migraine types, in particular, migraine with prolonged aura and migrainous infarction, and (d) correlation of TCD with rCBF studies.

Recently, Wallasch and Goebel (28) demonstrated that during induced headache attacks by mechanical pressure stimulation of the forehead, MFV in the MCA increased with intensity of pain and PI decreased. This constellation is similar to what Thie et al. (27) have found during classic migraine attacks. End-expiratory pCO_2 was monitored to exclude effects of ventilation on FV. These investigators correctly pointed to the possibility that any head pain by itself could influence MFV.

MIGRAINE: CONCLUSIONS

TCD recordings during the headache-free period have disclosed that there are (a) high FV, (b) bruits, (c) asymmetry of FV, (d) fluctuations of FV, and (e) abnormal vasoreactivity in some migraineurs, possibly reflecting increase and instability of vasotonus of the large and/or small cerebral arteries. These findings might point to a disturbance in autonomic vessel supply. It will not be possible to delineate the pathophysiological basis of these findings by TCD alone. Clinical investigators should evaluate TCD for its ability to discriminate migrainous disease from related disorders. So far, no single test shows promise to reach sufficient sensitivity and specificity to diagnose migraine with a reasonable amount of certainty.

During attacks findings of vascular changes are controversial and need better characterization. What may be concluded at this point is that (a) flow changes measured by TCD appear to be slight, (b) there is no regular "vasospasm," (c) FV might be altered in a nonsystematic fashion, (d) there might be individual "vasodilators" and "vasoconstrictors," and (e) flow changes might not be relevant to pathogenesis at all.

CLUSTER HEADACHE

Gawel and Krajewski (29) examined 42 patients with cluster headache during the headache-free period and 41 controls. MFVs were similar but right–left asymmetry was significantly greater in patients. MFVs in patients were higher on the symptomatic side.

In spontaneous and nitroglycerin-induced attacks of cluster headache, Dahl and coworkers (30) demonstrated by TCD in combination with rCBF studies that FV in the MCA markedly decreased while rCBF remained unchanged. These findings clearly point to vasodilatation of the MCA in cluster attacks with preserved arteriolar function. The same could hold true in spontaneous attacks of common migraine.

ACKNOWLEDGMENTS

The author gratefully acknowledges the help of other investigators who made their own data available: H.C. Diener (Essen), H.P. Haring (Innsbruck), W. Liboni (Turin), M. Reinicke (Frankfurt), and T.M. Wallasch (Kiel).

REFERENCES

1. Caplan LR, Brass LM, DeWitt LD, et al. Transcranial Doppler ultrasound: present status. *Neurology* 1990; 40:696–700.
2. Meyer JS, Hata T, and Imai A. Evidence supporting a vascular pathogenesis of migraine and cluster headache. In: Blau JN, ed. *Migraine: clinical, therapeutic, conceptual and research aspects.* London: Chapman and Hall, 1987; 265–302.
3. Thie A, Spitzer K, Lachenmayer L, and Kunze K. Prolonged vasospasm in migraine detected by noninvasive transcranial Doppler ultrasound. *Headache* 1988; 28:183–186.
4. Thie A, Fuhlendorf A, Spitzer K, and Kunze K. Transcranial Doppler evaluation of

common and classic migraine. Part I. Ultrasonic features during the headache-free period. *Headache* 1990; 30:201–208.
5. Ad Hoc Committee on Classification of Headache. Classification of headache. *JAMA* 1962; 179:717–718.
6. Grolimund P and Seiler RW. Age dependence of the flow velocity in the basal cerebral arteries—a transcranial Doppler ultrasound study. *Ultrasound Med Biol* 1988; 14: 191–198.
7. Aaslid R, Markwalder T-M, and Nornes H. Noninvasive transcranial Doppler ultrasound recording flow velocity in basal cerebral arteries. *J Neurosurg* 1982; 57:769–774.
8. Gosling RG and King DH. Arterial assessment by Doppler-shift ultrasound. *Proc R Soc Med* 1974; 67:447–449.
9. Abernathy M, Wieneke J, Ramos M, et al. Transcranial Doppler: Intracranial blood flow velocities in headache-free migraineurs and non-headache-prone volunteers. *Neurology* 1990; 40 [Suppl 1]:213.
10. Rosa R, Bellini V, Filippi MC, Taddei MT, Vitali T, and Conigliaro S. Hemodynamic studies by transcranial Doppler in primary headache. *Cephalalgia* 1987; 7 [Suppl 6]:280.
11. Haring HP, Aichner F, Bauer G, Rainer J, Bangerl J, and Gerstenbrand F. Hemodynamic findings in migraine patients by means of 3-D TCD scanning. In: *Abstracts of the 2nd International Conference on Transcranial Doppler Sonography.* Salzburg, 1988.
12. DeBenedittis G, Ferrari C, Granata G, Lorenzetti A, Longostrevi GP, and Cabrini GP. CBF changes during headache-free periods and induced attacks in common and classic migraine: A TCD and SPECT comparison study. In: *Abstracts of the 2nd International Conference on Transcranial Doppler Sonography.* Salzburg, 1988.
13. Pavy-le-Traon A, Cesari JB, Fabre N, Morales MP, Géraud G, and Bès A. Contribution of transcranial Doppler to the study of cerebral circulation in the migraineur. In: FC Rose, ed. *New advances in headache research.* London: Smith-Gordon, 1989; 157–161.
14. Diener HC, Peters C, Rudzio M, et al. Action of ergotamine, flunarizine and sumatriptan on cerebral blood flow velocity in normal subjects and patients with migraine. (*submitted*)
15. Levine SR, Welch KMA, Ewing JR, Joseph R, and D'Andrea G. Cerebral blood flow asymmetries in headache-free migraineurs. *Stroke* 1987; 18:1164–1165.
16. Spencer MP. Vascular bruits. In: Spencer MP, ed. *Ultrasonic diagnosis of cerebrovascular disease.* Dordrecht: Martinus Nijhoff Publishers, 1987; 147–156.
17. Aaslid R and Nornes H. Musical murmurs in human cerebral arteries after subarachnoid hemorrhage. *J Neurosurg* 1984; 60:32–36.
18. Lagrèze HL, Dettmers C, and Hartmann A. Abnormalities of interictal cerebral perfusion in classic but not in common migraine. *Stroke* 1988; 19:1108–1111.
19. Spencer MP. Hemodynamics of arterial stenosis. In: Spencer MP, ed. *Ultrasonic diagnosis of cerebrovascular disease.* Dordrecht: Martinus Nijhoff Publishers, 1987; 117–146.
20. Thomas TD, Harpold GJ, and Troost BT. Cerebral vascular reactivity in migraineurs as measured by transcranial Doppler ultrasound. *Cephalalgia* 1990; 10:95–99.
21. Thomas D and Harpold G. Alteration of cerebrovascular reactivity in migraineurs treated with propanolol. *Neurology* 1988; 38 [Suppl 1]:108.
22. Reinicke M, Wallasch TM, and Langohr HD. Autonomic cerebrovascular reactivity in migraine and other headaches. *Cephalalgia* 1989; 9 [Suppl 10]:160–161.
23. Thie A, Carvajal-Lizano M, Schlichting U, Spitzer K, and Kunze K. Cerebrale Vasoreaktivitaet: Entwicklung einer multimodalen Testbatterie. In: Firnhaber W, Dworschak K, Lauer K, Nichtweiss M, eds. *Verh Dtsch Ges Neurol,* Vol. 6. Berlin: Springer Verlag (*in press*).
24. Liboni W, Castellano GC, Chianale G, Duca S, and Matra G. Middle cerebral artery hemodynamic changes assessed by TCD in migraine. *Abstracts of the Club Doppler,* Paris, 1989.
25. Zwetsloot CP, Caebeke JFV, Jansen JC, Odink J, and Ferrari MD. Flow velocity changes in migraine: a transcranial Doppler study. *Cephalalgia* 1989; 9 [Suppl 10]: 64–65.
26. Formisano R, Zanette E, Cerbo R, et al. Transcranial Doppler on spontaneous and induced attacks in migraine patients. *Cephalalgia* 1989; 9 [Suppl 10]:68–69.
27. Thie A, Fuhlendorf A, Spitzer K, and Kunze K. Transcranial Doppler evaluation of

common and classic migraine. Part II. Ultrasonic features during attacks. *Headache* 1990; 30:209–215.
28. Wallasch TM and Goebel H. The influence of experimental induced headache on cerebral hemodynamic parameters. *Pain (in press)*.
29. Gawel MJ and Krajewski A. Intracranial haemodynamics in cluster headache. *Headache* 1988; 28:484–487.
30. Dahl A, Russell D, Nyberg-Hansen R, and Rootwelt K. Cluster headache: transcranial Doppler ultrasound and rCBF studies. *Cephalalgia* 1990; 10:87–94.

44

Transcranial Doppler Measurement of Blood Flow Velocity Changes in the Middle Cerebral Artery During Experimentally Induced Headache

Thomas-Martin Wallasch and Hartmut Göbel

Department of Neurology, Christian-Albrechts University, D-2300 Kiel, Germany

Headaches are among the most prevalent yet poorly understood problems in clinical neurology. Studies of regional cerebral blood flow (rCBF) using the xenon-133 methodology have shown conflicting data and controversial interpretations in migrainous headaches. It remains unclear whether changes in rCBF are caused by ischemia/hyperemia of brain tissue or correspond to vasodilation of cerebral arterioles. Technical limitations like the effects of Compton scatter may be partly responsible for these problems. The small number of transcranial Doppler ultrasound studies (TCD) performed during migraine attacks revealed controversial data (1, 2). Furthermore, the relationships between blood flow (velocity) changes and pain-inducing mechanisms are yet to be clarified. However, no findings are reported to explain whether blood flow (velocity) changes are of pathophysiological relevance or a secondary pain-induced epiphenomenon of headache attacks. Accordingly, our study examines TCD values of middle cerebral artery (MCA) during experimentally induced headache.

METHODS

Twenty-nine healthy volunteers recruited from students and the hospital staff were examined. There were 17 men and 12 women between 20 and 27 years of age (23.1 ± 1.9 years). Use of analgetics, alcohol, caffeine, and nicotine was forbidden over a period of 36 hr before testing. No female volunteer was pregnant or used birth control pills.

The volunteers were seated for experimental pain induction. Their heads were fixed to a head-rest ensuring a constant head position during the examination. An adjustable weight of 341.3 g was attached by a spindle to a lever, which was mounted to a brass cylinder with a circular contact area of 2.56 mm^2. The latter was applied to the head (F_z). To start the test the lever was lowered and a constant mechanical pressure of 1.316 Megapascal was applied (3). The induced pain intensity was assessed by the volunteers using the category subdividing procedure, as described elsewhere (4).

A 2-MHz Doppler instrument (TC 2-64, EME, Überlingen, Germany) was used for TCD examinations. During testing the Doppler probe was fixed to the heads of the volunteers. Insonation of the MCA was performed through the "temporal window" at a depth of 45–60 mm. The resistance index (RI) was calculated as described by Pourcelot (5). Blood pressure (bosomat II, Bosch, Jungingen, Germany) and end-tidal pCO_2 concentration measurements (CO_2-Monitor, Dräger, Lübeck, Germany) were also performed and monitored on-line on a chart recorder.

Analysis of MCA blood flow velocity, blood pressure, and end-tidal pCO_2 concentration measurements was done before pain induction, at "very weak," "average," and "very strong" pain intensities. Control readings were gathered by repeating the study sequence without pain stimulus (crossover design).

RESULTS

MCA mean blood flow velocities were found to increase significantly with elevation of "experimentally induced headache intensities," whereas Pourcelot indices decreased (Table 1). No significant side differences were observed. Studies without mechanical pain stimulus (control measurements) revealed no significant changes in analyzed parameters. Systolic blood pressure increased continuously with stronger pain intensities from 119.3 ± 3.0 (mean ± SEM) to 123.9 ± 3.2 mm Hg, but without a significant difference. End-tidal pCO_2 concentrations remained constant within a range of 40.0 ± 2.0 mm Hg.

CONCLUSIONS

Elevation of "experimental headache" sensitivities using the mechanical pressure stimulation method (3) produced an increase of MCA mean blood flow velocities and simultaneously a decrease of Pourcelot indices. Blood pressure effects or changes of end-tidal pCO_2 concentrations were ruled out as main causes for these changes on cerebral hemodynamic parameters. The observed changes in MCA flow patterns during "experimental headache" may be due to a sympathetic-induced vasodilatation of peripheral resistance vessels. The findings provide evidence that abnormalities on cerebral blood

TABLE 1. Values of mean blood flow velocities (MFV) and Pourcelot indices (PI)

	Before pain induction	Very weak	Average pain intensity	Very strong
MFV				
Controls	58.0 ± 2.1	57.2 ± 2.0	56.4 ± 2.0	56.8 ± 2.0
Pain induction	57.5 ± 2.0	60.2 ± 2.1	60.4 ± 2.0	60.6 ± 2.1
	n.s.	*	**	**
PI				
Controls	0.585 ± 0.01	0.594 ± 0.01	0.591 ± 0.01	0.587 ± 0.01
Pain induction	0.589 ± 0.01	0.568 ± 0.01	0.558 ± 0.01	0.559 ± 0.01
	n.s.	**	***	***

Mean ± SEM for control readings (controls) and measurements during "experimentally induced headache" (cross-over).
* $p \leq 0.05$.
** $p \leq 0.01$.
*** $p \leq 0.001$.
(t - test).

flow parameters during headache attacks could reflect a secondary adjusted pain-induced phenomenon.

Accordingly, cerebral blood flow changes during headache attacks should be interpreted carefully as an etiological factor.

REFERENCES

1. Thie A, Fuhlendorf A, Spitzer K, and Kunze K. Transcranial Doppler evaluation of common and classic migraine. Part II. Ultrasonic features during attacks. *Headache* 1990;30:209–215.
2. Pavy-Le Traon A, Cesari JB, Fabre N, Morales MP, Geraud G, and Bes A. Contribution of transcranial Doppler to the study of the cerebral circulation in the migraineur. In: Rose FC, ed. *New advances in headache research*. London: Smith-Gordon and Company 1989; 1:157–161.
3. Göbel H and Schenkl S. Post-lumbar puncture headache: the relation between experimental suprathreshold pain intensity and a quasi-experimental clinical pain syndrome. *Pain* 1990; 40:267–278.
4. Heller O. Theorie und praxis des verfahrens der kategorien-unterteilung (KU). In: O. Heller, ed. *Forschungsbericht 1981*, Institute of Psychology, University of Würzburg, 1982.
5. Pourcelot L. Diagnostic ultrasound for cerebral vascular diseases. In: Donald I, Levi S, eds. *Present and future of diagnostic ultrasound*. New York: John Wiley, 1976:141–147.

*Migraine and Other Headaches:
The Vascular Mechanisms*,
edited by Jes Olesen.
Raven Press, Ltd., New York © 1991.

45

Cerebrovascular Reactivity During Valsalva Test in Migraine

*Thomas-Martin Wallasch and †Martin Reinecke

*Department of Neurology, Christian-Albrechts University, D-2300 Kiel,
†Praxisgemeinschaft Nordwest Zentrum, D-6000 Frankfurt/Main, Germany*

Recently we described a new transcranial Doppler ultrasound method (TCD) as an auxiliary test in the clinical evaluation of headache patients (H) (1,2). Simultaneous noninvasive TCD, blood pressure, and end-tidal pCO_2 recordings were performed during a Valsalva maneuver. In this study, the accuracy of the method for migraine diagnosis and the results in other forms of headache are described using the following criteria: straining phase: amount of the difference of left minus right measurements for end-diastolic flow acceleration and the ratio of end-diastolic flow acceleration to the corresponding end-diastolic blood pressure acceleration, and overshoot phase: end-diastolic flow acceleration. Finally, the Valsalva ratio was examined as a parameter for parasympathetic heart rate control.

METHODS

One hundred and three H including 48 with migraine (Mig) and 55 with other headaches (OH) aged 15–44 years were evaluated. An age-matched group of 32 headache-free control subjects (Ctl) was recruited from the medical staff. As far as possible the diagnosis of H was made in accordance with the criteria of the New International Headache Classification (IHS) (3) from the case histories without knowledge of the result of the TCD test.

A 2-MHz pulsed Doppler device was used for TCD (TC 2–64, EME, Überlingen, Germany). The middle cerebral artery (MCA) was insonated with a fixed Doppler probe at a depth of 45–55 mm. The Finapres system (4) was used for noninvasive blood pressure measurement. A continuous recording of the end-tidal pCO_2 concentration was also performed (Capnolog, Dräger,

TABLE 1.

	n	Valsava straining dv/dt dp/dt (| left–right)	p	ratio > 1.0
Migraine	38	0.61 (0.26–1.27)	0.01 **	15/38
Other headaches	37	0.27 (0.13–0.61)	0.002 **	5/37
Control	18	0.27 (0.09–0.38)	0.27	1/18

Median and 25th–75th percentiles (brackets) of criteria as described above during a Valsalva maneuver. Number of subjects with double-sided test (n). Results of group comparisons using the Mann-Whitney U test (p).

Lübeck, Germany) and all curves were monitored simultaneously on a chart recorder.

A standardized Valsalva maneuver was performed as described by Ewing (5). Briefly, the subjects blew into a mouthpiece connected to a modified shygmomanometer and maintained a pressure of 40 mm Hg for a duration of at least 10 sec.

At the steepest part of the rise of end-diastolic flow velocity and pressure during straining and during the overshoot phase, end-diastolic flow acceleration (dv/dt) and pressure rise per second (dp/dt) were determined in cm/sec^2 and mm Hg/sec, respectively. Only double-sided tests were used for analysis and the mean of left and right side measurements was employed for the determination of end-diastolic flow acceleration during the overshoot phase and for the calculation of the Valsalva ratio. For further analysis the amount of the result of the difference of left minus right measurements (| left − right) was computed. The Valsalva ratio was calculated from the longest R-R interval shortly after the maneuver to the shortest R-R interval during straining. The pCO_2 retention was determined by computing the difference between values present before and after the experiment.

Group comparisons were carried out using the Mann-Whitney U test. All p values greater than 0.05 were reported as not significant.

TABLE 2.

	n	Valsava straining dv/dt (| left–right)	p	
Migraine	38	1.73 (0.66–4.05)	0.21	
Other headaches	37	1.15 (0.71–2.36)	0.73	0.13
Control	18	1.00 (0.33–2.47)		

TABLE 3.

	n	Valsava overshoot dv/dt	p	> 10
Migraine	26	11.98 (5.7–14.8)	0.004 **	15/26
Other headaches	24	5.47 (3.0–8.6)	0.007 **	5/24
Control	27	5.95 (3.7–8.6)	0.69	3/27

RESULTS

Mig (n = 38) exhibited a higher (| left − right) ratio of dv/dt / dp/dt in comparison with OH (n = 37) or Ctl (n = 18) during the straining phase of a Valsalva maneuver. Ctl and OH were not different (Table 1). There was no correlation between flow acceleration and CO_2 retention during the maneuver. A ratio of >1.0 was present in 15 of 38 Mig, 5 of 37 OH, and 1 of 18 controls. Thus the accuracy of the migraine diagnosis was 39.5 to 94.4%.

No significant differences were seen for (| left − right) dv/dt during straining (Table 2).

Mig (n = 26) showed a higher dv/dt for the mean of left and right MCA recordings during the overshoot phase than OH (n = 24) or Ctl (n = 27). Ctl and OH were not different (Table 3). A ratio of >10 was found in 15 of 26 Mig, 5 of 24 OH, and 3 of 27 Ctl. Accordingly, the accuracy of the migraine diagnosis was 57.7 to 88.9%.

In all groups investigated, no significant differences were found for the Valsalva ratio (Table 4).

CONCLUSIONS

There is an increased ratio of end-diastolic flow acceleration to the corresponding blood pressure acceleration (amount of the difference of left minus right side measurements) during straining of a Valsalva maneuver in patients with Mig in comparison with OH or Ctl. Neither alterations in CO_2 retention nor an exaggerated blood pressure rise explain these findings.

TABLE 4.

	n	Valsava ratio	p
Migraine	33	1.67 (1.35–2.08)	0.40
Other headaches	31	1.61 (1.36–1.79)	0.72
Control	25	1.57 (1.40–1.78)	0.95

Likewise, Mig showed a steeper rise of end-diastolic flow acceleration in the overshoot phase. The reported criteria have a relatively high specifity and a moderate sensitivity and can be used as individual parameters for migraine diagnosis. The Valsalva ratio was examined as a parameter for parasympathetic heart rate control. No differences were found between all groups, which were investigated.

Our results provide evidence for a disturbance of the autonomic neuronal cerebrovascular innervation in patients with Mig. However, the parasympathetic system does not seem to be affected. Moreover, a disturbance of the sympathetic perivascular neuronal net or the trigeminovascular system can be assumed.

REFERENCES

1. Reinecke M, Wallasch TM, and Langohr HD. Abnormal autonomic cerebrovascular reactivity in migraine: clinical experience with a new transcranial Doppler ultrasound method. *Neurology* 1989; 39 [Suppl 1]: 324 (abst).
2. Reinecke M, Wallasch TM, and Langohr HD. Autonomic cerebrovascular reactivity in migraine and other headache. *Cephalalgia* 1989; 9 [Suppl 10]:160–161.
3. Headache Classification Committee of the International Headache Society. Classification and diagnostic criteria for headache disorders, cranial neuralgias and facial pain. *Cephalalgia* 1988; 8 [Suppl 7]:1–96.
4. van Lieshout JJ, Wieling W, van Montfrans GA, Settels J, Speelman JD, Endert E, and Karemaker JM. Acute dysautonomia associated with Hodgkin's disease. *J Neurol Neurosurg Psychiatry* 1987; 50:503–504 (in reply to a letter of the authors).
5. Ewing DJ. REcent advances in the non-invasive investigation of diabetic autonomic neuropathy. In: Bannister R, ed. *Autonomic failure*. 2nd ed. Oxford: Oxford University Press 1988; 667–689.

46

Orthostatic Cerebrovascular Reactivity in Migraine

*Martin Reinecke, †Thomas-Martin Wallasch, ‡M. Schütz, and §H. D. Langohr

*Praxisgemeinschaft Nordwest Zentrum, D-6000 Frankfurt/Main, †Department of Neurology, Christian-Albrechts University D-2300 Kiel, ‡Psychiatrische Universitätsklinik, D-3550 Marburg, §Klinik für Neurologie und Neurophysiologie, D-6400 Fulda, Germany

The function of the autonomic nerve supply to the cerebral arteries is not completely known. Since sympathetic and parasympathetic reflexes are known to have a latency and a time constant in the range of seconds, all methods of evaluating the cerebral circulation using a temporal resolution in the range of minutes do not allow a complete study of the autonomic innervation of the cerebral vasculature. Compared to other methods of evaluating the cerebral circulation, transcranial Doppler (TCD) ultrasound measurements have the advantage of reporting changes in the real time mode.

During straining or rising from the sitting to standing position, regular changes of median cerebral artery flow velocity (MCAFV) can be observed. These changes are similar to the changes of arterial blood pressure during a Valsalva maneuver or during early orthostatic adaptation.

During straining, there is a steeper maximum end-diastolic middle cerebral artery (MCA) flow acceleration in migraine compared to other headache patients or controls. This exaggerated flow velocity response cannot be explained by an exaggerated pressure rise and is not due to an enhanced CO_2 reactivity in migraine. Thus, a disturbed autonomic cerebrovascular reactivity in migraine can be inferred from this finding (1).

The cause of the exaggerated MCAFV response in migraine is not clear. There may be a stronger sympathetic activation of the cerebral vessels in this disease, which may lead to an enhanced constriction of the MCA and/or an enhanced dilation of the cerebral arterioles during straining. Since the temporal sequence of parasympathetic and sympathetic influences during early orthostatic adaptation is known (2), we now report the results of TCD and pressure measurements during rising from the sitting to standing position.

METHODS

A 2-MHz pulsed Doppler instrument was used for transcranial Doppler ultrasound measurement of MCAFV (TC 2–64, EME). The Finapres system (Ohmeda, Puchheim bei München, FRG) was used for continuous noninvasive blood pressure measurement. The envelope curve of the Doppler frequency spectrum of the MCA and the pressure curve were reported simultaneously on a chart recorder. A continuous recording of the end-expiratory CO_2 concentration of the respiratory air (Capnolog, Dräger) was included in some probands. There were no consistent CO_2 changes during rising.

The results of examination of 31 left or right MCAs in 16 female and 4 male migraineurs (7 with aura and 13 without aura) aged 16–43 (median 28) years and of 41 left or right MCAs in 11 female and 13 male healthy volunteers aged 22–44 (median 30) years were compared. Group comparisons were carried out using the Mann-Whitney U test. All p values greater than 0.05 were reported as not significant.

The blood pressure and MCAFV response to rising from the sitting to standing position is characterized by an immediate rise followed by a striking fall and a quick recovery. During the immediate rise of pressure and MCAFV there is an initial heart rate increase, which is followed by an inconstant decrease during the fall of pressure and a further increase during the recovery phase. Finally, after the peak of pressure is reached a relative bradycardia can be observed.

During the initial rise of blood pressure and MCAFV the flow acceleration (dv/dt_{INIT}) and the pressure rise per second (dp/dt_{INIT}) were determined in cm/sec^2 and mm Hg/sec, respectively. The flow deceleration (dv/dt_{FALL}) and acceleration (dv/dt_{RECOV}) and the rate of end-diastolic pressure fall (dp/dt_{FALL}) and rise (dp/dt_{RECOV}) during the fall of MCAFV and arterial pressure and during the recovery phase were determined accordingly (Fig. 1). The distance between systolic peaks of the pressure curve were used to calculate the heart rates.

RESULTS

The acceleration of MCAFV during the initial rise of flow velocity was reduced in the migraineurs compared to controls. The deceleration of flow velocity was exaggerated in the migraine group. In addition, there was an enhanced flow acceleration during the recovery phase in migraine patients compared to controls. The rates of pressure change were not different between both groups. Since the pressure rise per second during the recovery

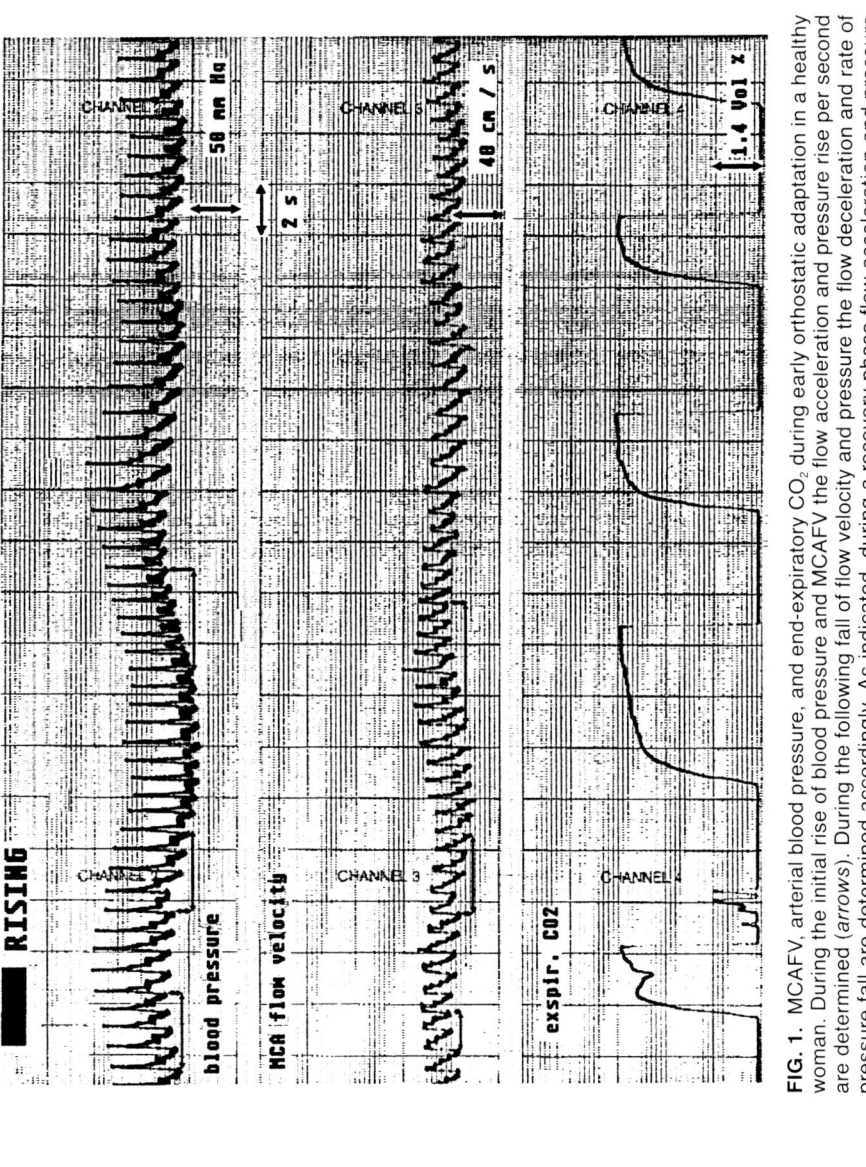

FIG. 1. MCAFV, arterial blood pressure, and end-expiratory CO_2 during early orthostatic adaptation in a healthy woman. During the initial rise of blood pressure and MCAFV the flow acceleration and pressure rise per second are determined (arrows). During the following fall of flow velocity and pressure the flow deceleration and rate of pressure fall are determined accordingly. As indicated, during a recovery phase flow acceleration and pressure rise per second can be evaluated.

TABLE 1. *Flow acceleration (dv/dt) within the MCA and rate of pressure change (dp/dt) during different phases of early orthostatic adaptation in healthy subjects (n = 24) and migraineurs (n = 20)*

	Healthy subjects (n = 24) median (25th–75th percentile)	Migraine (n = 20) median (25th–75th percentile)	p Mann-Whitney U test
dv/dt (INIT) (cm/sec^2)	3.67 (2.86–5.47)	2.67 (1.53–4.73)	0.02
dv/dt (FALL) (cm/sec^2)	2.34 (1.69–3.10)	3.57 (2.44–4.39)	0.002
dv/dt (RECOV) (cm/sec^2)	3.23 (2.02–5.00)	4.08 (2.72–5.82)	0.03
dp/dt (INIT) (mm Hg/sec)	4.61 (3.75–6.71)	3.48 (1.44–6.07)	0.16
dp/dt (FALL) (mm Hg/sec)	3.59 (2.46–4.81)	4.89 (3.23–5.95)	0.09
dp/dt (RECOV) (mm Hg/sec)	4.20 (3.16–5.00)	3.62 (2.51–4.85)	0.12
Ratio dt/dt (RECOV) / dp/dt (RECOV) (cm/mm Hg/sec)	0.76 (0.41–1.07)	1.15 (0.80–1.97)	0.003

INIT, initial rise of flow velocity and pressure; FALL, drop of flow velocity and pressure; RECOV, recovery phase.

phase tended to be reduced in migraine, the ratio $dv/dt_{RECOV}/dp/dt_{RECOV}$ was clearly higher in the migraine group (Table 1). Heart rates at rest, during the initial and second heart rate peak, and during the secondary heart rate valley and after an early steady state was reached were not different between migraineurs and controls.

DISCUSSION

The rate of end-diastolic flow velocity changes in the MCA during early orthostatic adaptation is different in migraineurs compared to controls. Since there is a similar blood pressure regulation in migraineurs and controls and CO_2 changes do not occur during rising from the sitting to standing position, we interpret this finding as a further sign of a disturbed autonomic neural control of the cerebral vasculature in migraine. The initial phase of early orthostatic adaptation is due to an abrupt withdrawal of parasympathetic influences to the circulation. Because of a longer latency period the sympathetic system appears to be active mainly during the recovery phase of early orthostatic adaptation. Our finding may therefore be the result of a decreased local parasympathetic influence and an increased local sympathetic influence on the cerebral circulation in migraine.

REFERENCES

1. Reinecke M, Wallasch TM, and Langohr HD. Autonomic cerebrovascular reactivity in migraine and other headaches. Results of transcranial Doppler, blood pressure and CO_2 recordings during a Valsalva maneuver. *Cephalalgia* 1989; 9 [Suppl 10]:160–161.
2. Wieling W. Standing, orthostatic stress, and autonomic function. In: Bannister R, ed. *Autonomic failure*, 2nd ed. Oxford: Oxford University Press 1988; 308–320.

47

Blood Flow Velocity Changes and Vascular Reactivity During Migraine Attacks Without Aura: A Transcranial Doppler Study

*C. P. Zwetsloot, *J. F. V. Caekebeke, †J. C. Jansen, ‡J. Odink, and †M. D. Ferrari

Departments of *Clinical Neurophysiology and †Neurology, University Hospital, 2300 RC Leiden, and ‡Department of Clinical Biochemistry, TNO-CIVO Institutes, 3700 AJ Zeist, The Netherlands

Vascular mechanisms in migraine attacks without aura (MO) are still controversial (1). Partly this may be because of logistic problems studying patients during migraine attacks. The transcranial Doppler technique offers a noninvasive tool to determine blood flow velocities (BFV) as representation of flow in intracranial vessels (2). We therefore determined BFVs in the carotid arteries and their intracranial branches of MO patients with lateralized headache, during and outside an attack. We also studied vascular reactivity to decrease of arterial CO_2 in a group of MO patients during and outside an attack and in healthy controls.

METHODS

BFV Changes During Attacks

BFV was determined as the mean flow velocity using a transcranial Doppler device (EME TC2-64B) in the common carotid (CCA), internal carotid (ICA), external carotid (ECA), medial cerebral (MCA), and anterior cerebral (ACA) arteries on both sides. Blood pressure and end-tidal CO_2 were determined before Doppler examination. Statistical analysis was done by ANOVA, type split-plot. Because of multiple comparisons, significance levels were set at 0.01.

Vascular Reactivity

End-tidal CO_2 volume percentage was recorded by an infrared CO_2 analyzer. BFV was determined in the MCA just before voluntary hyperventilation and after 1 min of hyperventilation, when a constant CO_2 volume percentage was reached of at least 1 vol%. Vascular reactivity was determined (a) as change in BFV per CO_2 vol% and (b) the vascular reactivity index as vascular reactivity percentage of the prehyperventilation BFV. Measurements outside an attack were done on the side of the pain during the last attack before examination, during an attack on the side of the head pain, and in the controls on the right side. Statistical analysis was done by Kruskal-Wallis one-way ANOVA.

Patients

The first part of the study was performed in 22 patients with lateralized headache (mean age 44 years; M:F, 4:18), both during and outside the attack. A subgroup of 11 patients had head pain on the same side in >75% of their attacks. These were compared with the group who had the head pain on the same side in <75%. The second part of the study, determining vascular reactivity, was performed in 28 patients (mean age 43 years; M:F, 7:21) outside an attack, in 9 patients (mean age 42 years; M:F, 1:8) during an attack, and in 17 normal controls (mean age 36 years; M:F, 7:10).

RESULTS

No differences were found between the groups who had the head pain in more or less than 75% of their attacks on the same side. Therefore, results of these groups were taken together and are presented in Table 1. There were

TABLE 1. Blood flow velocities during and between migraine attacks

Vessel	Period	n	Headache side	Nonheadache side	p1	p2	p3
CCA	Attack-free	22	25.6	28.6	0.03	0.49	0.009
	Attack	22	22.4	23.6			
ICA	Attack-free	21	33.9	33.1	0.86	0.39	0.46
	Attack	21	32.2	32.3			
ECA	Attack-free	20	18.3	18.1	0.18	0.35	0.97
	Attack	20	18.7	17.6			
MCA	Attack-free	22	62.6	60.4	0.32	0.65	0.24
	Attack	22	64.6	63.8			
ACA	Attack-free	15	46.1	46.8	0.75	0.96	0.54
	Attack	15	47.9	48.8			

p1, difference between headache and nonheadache side.
p2, interaction between side and difference between attack and attack-free.
p3, difference between attack-free and attack.

TABLE 2. *Vascular reactivity (median and range)*

	Attack-free	Attack	Normal controls
n	28	9	17
VR[a]	13.5	11.3	12.0
	(5.0–33.3)	(6.7–20.0)	(5.6–27.1)
VRI[b]	0.19	0.19	0.19
	(0.08–0.48)	(0.03–0.25)	(0.11–0.37)

[a]VR, vascular reactivity (BFV change in cm/sec, per vol% CO_2).
[b]VRI, vascular reactivity index (vascular reactivity as percentage of the prehyperventilation BFV).

no differences between the BFVs on the headache and nonheadache side. During attacks, BFV was lower in the CCAs compared to the attack-free registration; no differences were found for the other vessels (Table 1).

Results of the vascular reactivity study are presented in Table 2. None of the investigated measures for vascular reactivity significantly differed between the three groups.

DISCUSSION

During MO attacks no prominent changes or asymmetries of the BFV were found in the large cranial vessels, aside from an isolated and mild symmetrical reduction of the BFV in the CCA during the attack. Vascular reactivity to CO_2 decrease due to voluntary hyperventilation was normal, both between and during attacks.

Reduction of the BFV in the CCA may be due to vasodilatation of the CCA, increase of the cerebrovascular resistance, notably at the level of arterioles, rise of the intracranial pressure, higher blood viscosity, reduction of the arterial blood pressure, or changes in the collateral flow (2). Under physiological conditions, most of these factors are counteracted by adequate autoregulatory responses and compensatory changes in cerebral blood flow (CBF). Because within-subject changes of the BFV in the MCA and CCA are well correlated with within-changes in blood flow (3), we must assume that blood flow has decreased in the CCA, without a compensatory CBF increase in the MCA territory. This would suggest a disturbance in the autoregulatory mechanisms in MO attacks. However, vascular reactivity to hyperventilation was found to be normal, but this does not exclude abnormalities in other parts; an excessive reaction to increase of CO_2 in migraineurs is described (4).

In conclusion, MO attacks are not associated with prominent changes or asymmetries of the BFV of the large cranial vessels. The isolated symmetrical reduction of the BFV in the CCA is novel and still unexplained. Reactivity to hyperventilation is normal in the MCA territory of MO patients, both during and between attacks.

REFERENCES

1. Skyhoj Olsen T and Olesen J. Regional cerebral blood flow in migraine and cluster headache. In: Olesen J, Edvinsson L, eds. *Basic mechanisms of headache*. Amsterdam–New York: Elsevier Science Publishers BV, 1988; 377–391.
2. Aaslid R and Lindegaard KF. Cerebral hemodynamics. In: Aaslid R, ed. *Transcranial doppler sonography*. Wien–New York: Springer-Verlag, 1986; 60–85.
3. Bishop CCR, Powell S, Rutt D, and Browse NL. Transcranial doppler measurement of middle cerebral artery blood flow velocity: a validation study. *Stroke* 1986; 17:913–915.
4. Thomas TD, Harpold GJ, and Troost BT. Cerebrovascular reactivity in migraineurs as measured by transcranial doppler. *Cephalalgia* 1990; 10:95–99.

48

Transcranial Doppler Studies: Discussion Summary

Rolf Nyberg-Hansen

Most studies of cerebral hemodynamics in migraine patients have been carried out by measurements of cerebral blood flow (CBF) with tracer techniques, mainly by intraarterial or intravenous injection, or by inhalation of xenon-133. Transcranial Doppler ultrasound (TCD) is a relatively new method that enables the measurement of blood flow velocities in the basal intracranial arteries. Although TCD does not directly measure flow, there is a linear relationship between flow and velocity in a particular artery if the diameter of the vessel remains constant. The relationship between velocity and volume flow in a defined cerebral artery system is, however, more complex. Velocity depends not only on the diameter of the inflow vessel, but also on the regional cerebral blood flow (rCBF) in its perfusion territory and the size of the territory in question. Changes in velocity will reflect changes in rCBF only as long as the vessel diameter and the perfusion territory both remain constant.

The TCD method has several practical advantages compared to tracer methods for the assessment of cerebral hemodynamics. It is inexpensive, relatively simple to perform, and therefore well suited for dynamic measurements of the cerebral circulation in migraine patients. It should be emphasized that when direct comparison is made between TCD and rCBF studies, it is essential that the measurements are performed under conditions identical with regard to pCO_2, preferably with simultaneous recordings.

TCD studies have been performed in migraine patients both during attacks and in headache-free periods. There is, however, some controversy and confusion with regard to the results. Some studies report abnormal cerebral vasoreactivity in headache-free periods, indicating instability of the vasomotor tone of cerebral vessels.

During headache attacks in patients with migraine with aura, an increase in velocity has been reported by some authors. This could be due to vasoconstriction of large vessels leading to the decrease in rCBF demonstrated by tracer methods. However, a recent study reported at the symposium demonstrated a decrease in blood velocity in the middle cerebral artery

(MCA) on the symptomatic (headache) side in migraine patients with unilateral headache. This probably indicates vasodilation of the MCA. It is indeed interesting to note that the same findings were observed in patients with and without aura. This could indicate a common pathophysiological factor in these two types of migraine. Furthermore, the decrease in velocity was normalized after sumatriptan administration.

In patients with cluster headache, TCD studies and rCBF measurements with single photon emission computed tomography (SPECT) have shown that spontaneous and nitroglycerin-provoked attacks are accompanied by bilateral decrease in MCA blood velocity. However, mean hemispheric CBF and rCBF in the MCA perfusion territory were both within normal limits during provoked attacks, and similar to those found when the patients were free of attacks. These findings strongly suggest vasodilation of the MCA in attacks of cluster headache.

The possibility that velocity changes during attacks of migraine and cluster headache are a consequence of pain should seriously be considered. Generalized changes may in part be a secondary phenomenon caused by a stress reaction. Any pain in the head could thus influence blood flow velocity.

There is an urgent need for studies correlating TCD and rCBF measurements in migraine with and without aura, with particular emphasis on the time course of velocity changes during the attacks. It is necessary, however, to standardize the TCD examination. It should be performed by an experienced examiner, preferably with fixed head probes during the headache attacks. For repeated examinations, the same acoustic window should be used and the same insonation depth should be employed for comparison. The patients should be investigated in the supine position with eyes closed in a quiet room with no activation from external sources. The blood pressure, heart rate, and end-tidal pCO_2 should be monitored. Finally, the examiner should be blinded without knowing the history of the patients examined.

The noninvasive TCD method represents a rapid and easily repeatable technique that is well suited for dynamic measurements of the cerebral circulation in migraine patients. However, so far the results obtained are somewhat confusing, and controversy exists between different studies. This seems, at least in part, to be due to lack of standardization of the examination and patient selection. Recent studies reported are promising, however, and it may be expected that future TCD studies will contribute to a better understanding of cerebral hemodynamics in migraine patients.

PART IX
Cluster Headache

49

^{99m}TC-HMPAO Study During Cluster Headache Period and in Acute Attacks

Rachel Hering, E. G. M. Couturier, Paul T. G. Davies, and T. J. Steiner

The Princess Margaret Migraine Clinic, Charing Cross Hospital, London W6 8RF, England

Regional cerebral blood flow (rCBF) during cluster headache periods and in cluster-free intervals has been studied by several authors using ^{99m}Tc-hexamethyl-propylene-amine-oxime (HMPAO). In one study a marked regional hypoperfusion was found in two patients during the cluster period, in contrast to normal perfusion in seven patients in the cluster-free interval (1). In another, during an attack of cluster headache, abnormal tracer uptake in the territories of the superficial temporal arteries was the most conspicuous finding (2).

AIMS

Identification or exclusion of rCBF abnormalities in cluster headache patients during cluster periods.

MATERIAL

Fourteen patients were investigated, 13 male and 1 female, of mean age 29 years (range 20–60 years), and attending The Princess Margaret Migraine Clinic for treatment of episodic cluster headache. All were in the cluster period, two during an acute attack. Diagnoses of cluster headache were according to the International Headache Society Classification of Headache, 1988 (3).

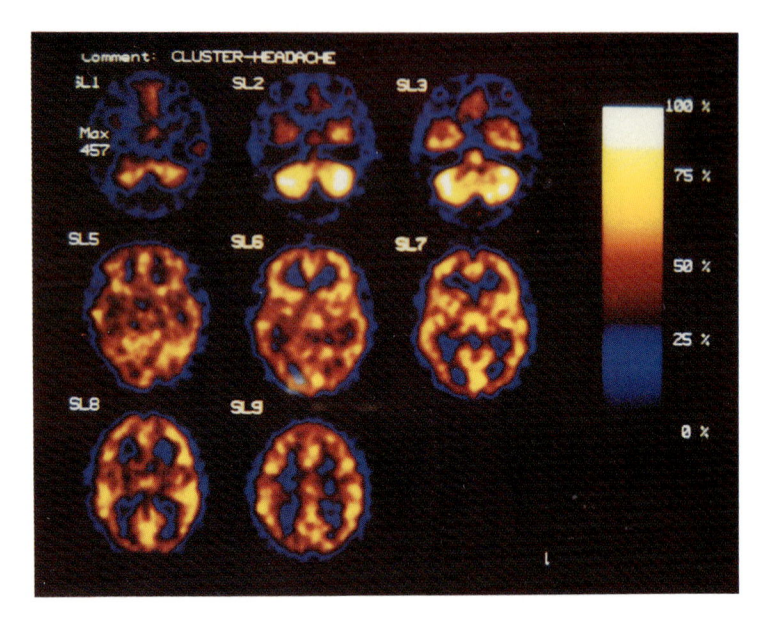

FIG. 1. A CBF-SPECT study carried out during a cluster headache period, 15 min after the onset of headache, after iv injection of 740 MBq (20mCi) ^{99m}Tc-HMPAO, using the NOVO 810 SPECT scanner. Normal distribution of CBF.

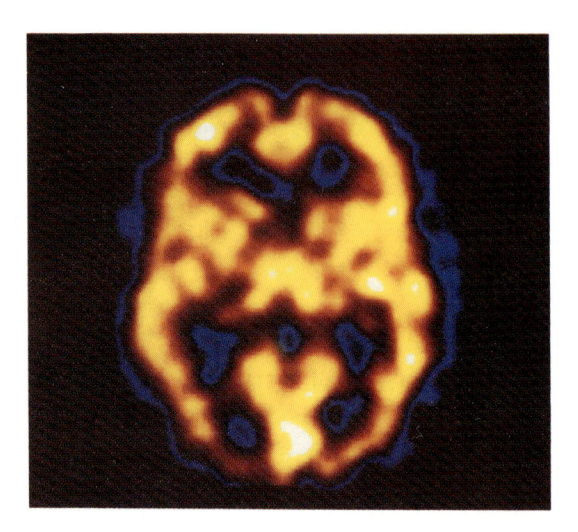

FIG. 2. A transverse HMPAO-SPECT image taken from Fig. 1. In this slice the gray cortical matter, internal capsule, head of caudate nucleus, and thalamus are well demonstrated.

METHODS

All patients were clinically assessed and informed of the nature, purpose, and hazards of the project. ^{99m}Tc-HMPAO, 7–10 MBq/kg, was administered intravenously under standard conditions. Imaging began 10–20 min after injection using the Novo 810 SPECT scanner. Ten transverse brain slices of 10 mm thickness were obtained in each case. When needed (in two patients), symptomatic treatment was given after the injection, on the assumption that the distribution of the tracer was fixed, within 2 min.

RESULTS

Scans of high quality and high resolution were obtained with ^{99m}Tc-HMPAO and single photo emission computed tomography (SPECT) (Figs. 1 and 2). No intracranial or extracranial blood flow abnormalities were found during the course of a cluster headache period, either within or between attacks. Normal images of tracer uptake were observed in all 14 patients.

DISCUSSION

The cluster headache patients showed normal cerebral perfusion with an imaging technique giving the highest spatial resolution available so far. These results need to be confirmed by advanced image analysis. If they are, they will suggest that there is no involvement of cerebral blood flow in the pathophysiology of cluster headache. This does not rule out changes in vessel calibre, or of perfusion pressure in regional vascular beds.

CONCLUSION

These results give no support to a vascular hypothesis of cluster headache, but do not preclude vascular involvement as a factor in its aetiopathogenesis.

REFERENCES

1. Schlake HP, Bottger IG, Grotemeyer KH, et al. Tc-99m HM-PAO-SPECT during the pain-free interval of migraine and cluster headache. *Cephalalgia* 1989; 9[Suppl 10]:33–34.
2. Wessely P, Suess E, Koch G, Wober C, and Deecke L. SPECT (99m)Tc-HMPAO findings in acute headache and during symptom free interval. *Cephalalgia* 1989; 9[Suppl 10]: 62–63.
3. Headache Classification Committee of the International Headache Society. Classification and diagnostic criteria for headache disorders, cranial neuralgias and facial pain. *Cephalalgia* 1988; 8[Suppl 7]:1–96.

Migraine and Other Headaches:
The Vascular Mechanisms,
edited by Jes Olesen.
Raven Press, Ltd., New York © 1991.

50

Brain Imaging with ^{99m}Tc-HMPAO and SPECT in Episodic Cluster Headache: An Interictal Study

*Hans-Peter Schlake, †Ingolf G. Böttger, *Karl-Heinz Grotemeyer, *Ingo W. Husstedt, and †Otmar Schober

*Departments of *Neurology and †Nuclear Medicine, Westfälische Wilhelms-Universität, D-4400 Münster, Germany*

Cluster headache is usually considered to be of vascular origin, but only few and rather inconclusive results have been reported on its cerebral hemodynamics until now (1–3). On the other hand, the strictly unilateral localization of pain and its concomitant symptoms suggest a regional alteration of vascular and/or neuronal structures to be involved in the pathogenic process.

We investigated pain-free patients suffering from episodic cluster headache (during and between cluster episodes) by means of single photon emission computed tomography (SPECT) and the flow tracer ^{99m}Tc-HMPAO (hexamethyl-propylene-amino-oxime).

In contrast to radiopharmaceuticals used in conventional brain scintigraphy, this lipophilic agent is able to cross the intact blood-brain barrier; it shows a high first-pass extraction into the brain proportional to blood flow with a maximum of cerebral uptake after 1–2 min and a nearly constant maintenance of the regional distribution over several hours (4,5).

MATERIAL AND METHODS

Twenty-three male patients, aged 20–57 years, during (n = 15) and between (n = 8) cluster episodes were studied. At the time of investigation all patients were headache-free and had not taken any medication for at least 2 weeks.

SPECT investigation of regional cerebral flow (rCBF) was performed under standardized environmental conditions (quiet room, dimmed light, eyes open). Fifteen min after intravenous (iv) administration of 400–600 MBq

^{99m}Tc-HMPAO, 64 single images were obtained within a 360° circle using a rotating gamma camera (General Electric 400 ACT). Imaging time per projection was 30 sec and 40 min per examination. Tomographic slices of 12.5 mm width were reconstructed in sagittal, coronal, and horizontal projections by filtered backprojection employing a Butterworth filter with a cut-off frequency of 0.2 cycles/pixel.

Interpretation was performed qualitatively and semiquantitatively by a specialist in nuclear medicine in a quasi-blinded way, as he only knew the diagnosis "cluster headache" but did not have any information on individual clinical stage or pain localization.

By visual inspection SPECT findings were divided into four categories:

1. symmetrical perfusion
2. inhomogeneous regional perfusion (bilateral)
3. slight hypoperfusion (regional side difference 2–4 of 16 steps on the color scale, representing a regional hypoperfusion of 14–28%)
4. marked hypoperfusion (regional side difference >4 of 16 steps on the color scale, representing a regional hypoperfusion of >28%)

According to ^{99m}Tc-HMPAO SPECT findings in healthy volunteers reported in the literature (5), a regional difference of cerebral tracer uptake exceeding two steps (approx. 14%) was considered to be significant.

RESULTS

Clinical neurological investigation revealed a normal result in all patients. There were no pathological findings in computed tomography (CT; n = 16) and magnetic resonance imaging (MRI; n = 5) of the brain. Electroencephalography (n = 23) revealed a normal result in all cases except one patient during cluster phase, in whom a focal dysrhythmic activity could be obtained in the left-sided frontal region, which corresponded to the side of hypoperfusion in SPECT, but was contralateral to pain localization. Table 1

TABLE 1. ^{99m}Tc-HMPAO SPECT findings of all patients (n = 23) in relation to clinical state and pain localization

Results of ^{99m}Tc-HMPAO SPECT	During cluster episodes (n = 15)	Between cluster episodes (n = 8)
Normal perfusion	4	4
Bilaterally inhomogeneous or reduced perfusion	1	4
Unilateral hypoperfusion	8 (6)[a]	0
Unilateral hyperperfusion	2 (1)[a]	0

[a]Brackets, number of patients in whom side of cluster headache corresponded to side of hypoperfusion/hyperperfusion.

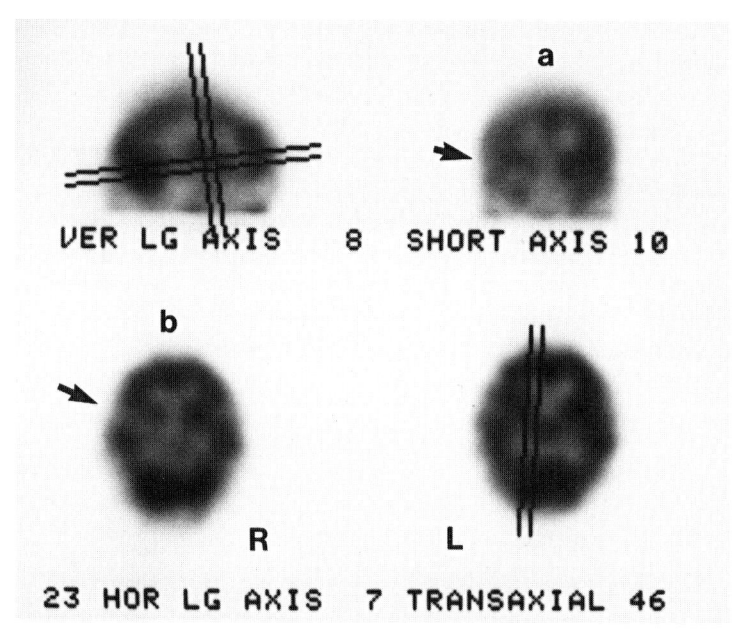

FIG. 1. Results of SPECT with ⁹⁹ᵐTc HMPAO in a 33-year-old man suffering from right-sided cluster headache attacks; the investigation was performed during a cluster episode. Coronal (**a**) and horizontal (**b**) projections showed a marked hypoperfusion in the right-sided temporobasal region (*arrow*), corresponding to the side of cluster headache. From Schlake, ref. 6, with permission.

gives a survey on ⁹⁹ᵐTc-HMPAO SPECT findings in all patients in relation to clinical state and localization of cluster headache.

Between cluster episodes (n = 8), SPECT with ⁹⁹ᵐTc-HMPAO showed a normal cerebral perfusion in four patients and four other patients revealed a bilaterally inhomogeneous or reduced tracer uptake.

During cluster phase, only 5 of 15 (headache-free) patients showed a normal (n = 4) or bilaterally reduced (n = 1) perfusion. A unilateral reduction of rCBF was obtained in seven patients, whereas two patients revealed a regional hyperperfusion. From these 10 patients, in whom rCBF was unilaterally altered, 7 showed a definite relation of the areas of hypoperfusion/hyperperfusion to pain localization during cluster headache attacks.

DISCUSSION

In the present study cerebral perfusion was investigated in 23 headache-free patients suffering from episodic cluster headache during (n = 15) and between (n = 8) cluster episodes by means of SPECT and the tracer ⁹⁹ᵐTc-HMPAO. Our results show a unilateral alteration of rCBF—a regional cerebral hypoperfusion or hyperperfusion—in 10 of 15 (headache-free) cluster headache patients during cluster episodes, whereas rCBF was normal or altered unspecifically in all eight patients who were investigated during the cluster interval. Although no consistent alterations of rCBF during cluster phase could be detected, pain localization corresponded to the side of rCBF changes in 7 of 10 patients.

These regional changes of cerebral perfusion in interictal cluster headache were only slight, but clearly exceeded the values that have been reported in the literature (5) for healthy persons, ranging between $0.42 \pm 2.45\%$ (SD) and $5.57 \pm 3.11\%$ in different cerebral regions. In addition, the intraindividual instability of regional tracer distribution was found to be 3.6% at most in one healthy volunteer in six ^{99m}Tc-HMPAO SPECT investigations (5).

Altogether, it appears that cluster episodes are characterized by a greater instability of cerebral perfusion as compared to the cluster interval. It requires further investigation as to whether or not these alterations of regional cerebral perfusion are of epiphenomenological nature or are part of the primary pathogenic process in cluster headache.

REFERENCES

1. Nelson RF, du Boulay GH, Marshall J, Russel RWR, Symon L, and Zilkha E. Cerebral blood flow studies in patients with cluster headache. *Headache* 1980; 20:184–189.
2. Norris JW, Hachinski VC, and Cooper PW. Cerebral blood flow changes in cluster headache. *Acta Neurol Scand* 1976; 54:371–374
3. Sakai F and Meyer JS: Regional cerebral hemodynamics during migraine and cluster headache measured by the ^{133}Xe inhalation technique. *Headache* 1978; 18:122–132.
4. Sharp PR, Smith FW, Gemmell HG, et al. Technetium.99m stereoisomers as potential agents for imaging regional cerebral blood flow: Human volunteer studies. *J Nucl Med* 1986; 27:171–177.
5. Podreka E, Suess E, Goldenberg G, et al. Initial experience with Technetium-99m brain SPECT. *J Nucl Med* 1987; 28:1657–1666.
6. Schlake H-P, Böttger IG, Grotemeyer K-H, Husstedt IW, Schober O. Brain imaging with ^{99m}Tc-HMPAO in episodic cluster headache during and between cluster episodes. *Headache Quarterly* 1990; 1:303–306.

51

CT-CBF and [133]Xe Inhalation Cerebral Blood Flow Studies in Cluster Headache

John Stirling Meyer, Jun Kawamura, and Yasuo Terayama

Cerebral Blood Flow Laboratory, Veterans Affairs Medical Center and Department of Neurology, Baylor College of Medicine, Houston, Texas 77030

Cluster headache is recognized as a clinically identifiable form of vascular headache despite the fact that its etiology is unknown. Clinical observations of cephalic vascular changes, including conjunctival hyperemia of the affected eye, accompanying cluster attacks have been consistently reported. However, reports concerning changes in cephalic perfusion during cluster headaches have been less consistent.

The present study was designed to elucidate changes in cerebral blood flow (CBF) among patients with spontaneously occurring cluster headaches and to study their cerebral vascular responses to 5% CO_2 and 100% oxygen inhalation.

SUBJECTS

Subjects studied included 29 patients with chronic cluster headache and 22 normal volunteers. Diagnosis of cluster headache met criteria required for Classification and Diagnosis Criteria for Headache Disorders, Cranial Neuralgias, and Facial Pain recommended by the Headache Classification Committee of the International Headache Society. All patients were asked to discontinue medication for at least 48 hr before CBF measurements.

METHODS

Regional cerebral blood flow (rCBF) was measured in 16 of the 29 patients with cluster headache by a modification of the ^{133}Xe inhalation method described by Obrist et al. (1). In brief, ^{133}Xe gas mixed with room air (5–7 mCi) was inhaled through a face mask and clearance of isotope from the head was monitored by 16 detectors mounted over both hemispheres. Each head curve was deconvoluted by a computer using Obrist's two-compartment model in which the faster clearing compartment (F_1) is considered to represent primarily gray matter flow (Fg). Cerebrovascular responsiveness to 5% CO_2 inhalation was tested in 6 of 16 patients examined by the ^{133}Xe inhalation method.

In 13 patients, local cerebral blood flow (LCBF) values were measured by the xenon CT-CBF method described previously (2). After obtaining baseline computed tomography (CT) scans, inhalation of 27% xenon gas was begun and seven serial CT scans were made at 1-min intervals from the second to the eighth minute after beginning inhalation of xenon gas. Calculation of LCBF values was performed by a series of computer programs based on Kety's formula.

Cerebral vasoconstrictive responses to 100% oxygen inhalation were examined in 10 of 16 patients measured by ^{133}Xe inhalation method and in 5 of 13 patients measured by the CT-CBF method.

RESULTS

Studies by ^{133}Xe Inhalation Method

As shown in Fig. 1, mean Fg values measured by the ^{133}Xe inhalation method among seven patients during typical cluster headaches (94.8 ± 12.4

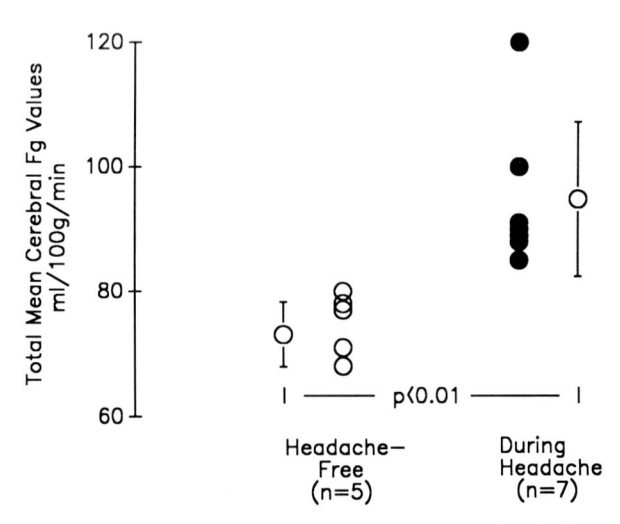

FIG. 1. Mean Fg values in two groups of patients with cluster headache compared when headache-free and during typical attacks of cluster headache. Three patients included in both groups were studied during headache and headache-free intervals.

ml/100 g brain/min) were significantly higher than measured in five patients when headache-free (73.1 ± 5.2), as shown in Fig. 1.

Hemispheric CO_2 responsiveness was impaired particularly on the side of headache (0.1 Δ%Fg/mm Hg $PECO_2$) in some patients studied during an attack and was less impaired on the non-headache side (1.7 Δ%Fg/mm Hg $PECO_2$). Immediately after the cluster headaches had subsided, impaired CO_2 responsiveness rapidly returned to normal (4.0 ± 0.5) within 24–48 hr and there were no longer any significant differences between the side of the headache (4.5 ± 0.5) and the nonheadache side (3.7 ± 0.9).

Fg values showed diffuse and excessive reductions during inhalation of 100% oxygen in patients during their cluster attacks by −33.0% ± 10.6% compared with normals (−9.4% ± 5.4%) (Fig. 2). One hundred percent oxygen inhalation also provided prompt and notable relief of headache. Another six patients with cluster headache were examined when headache-free, and at this time they showed Fg reductions of −6.7% ± 2.7%, which were not significantly different from values measured in normals.

Studies by Xe CT-CBF Method

Pooled mean LCBF values for nine cerebral regions compared between normal volunteers and patients with cluster headache while headache-free

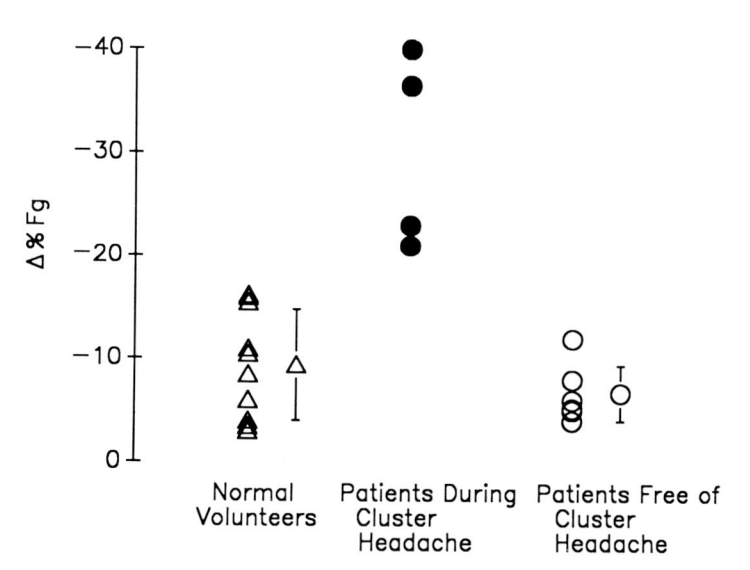

FIG. 2. Mean hemispheric Fg changes during 100% oxygen inhalation in patients during cluster headache are displayed. There are diffuse and excessive reductions of mean hemispheric Fg values that are more than three times those seen in normals. An additional six patients with cluster headache were tested when they were free of head pain. All six showed normal cerebral vasoconstrictive responses to 100% oxygen inhalation.

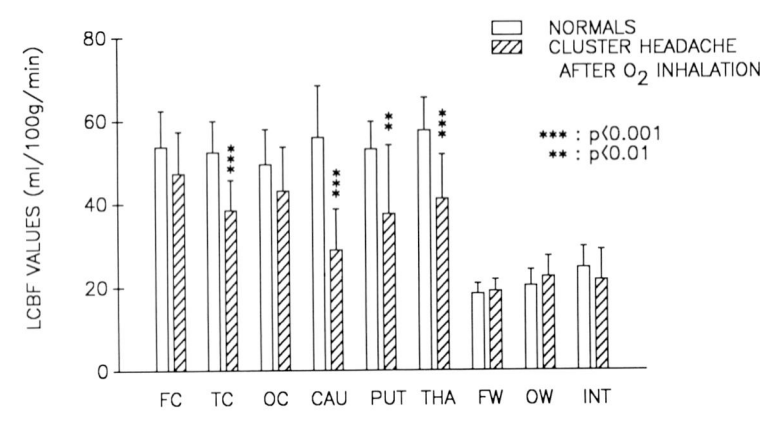

FIG. 3. LCBF values measured among nine representative regions of the brain obtained from patients with cluster headache immediately after terminating typical headaches by administration of 100% oxygen inhalation. LCBF values are significantly decreased for temporal cortex, caudate nucleus, putamen, and thalamus in patients compared to age-matched normals. FC, frontal cortex; TC, temporal cortex; OC, occipital cortex; CAU, caudate nucleus; PUT, putamen; THA, thalamus; FW, frontal white matter; OW, occipital white matter; INT, internal capsule.

were normal. LCBF values in three patients with spontaneously occurring cluster headache were increased significantly in temporal cortex, putamen, thalamus, and frontal white matter on the headache side and temporal cortex and basal ganglia and frontal and occipital white matter of the opposite (nonheadache side) hemisphere. There were no significant differences in the increased hemispheric LCBF values between the headache and nonheadache sides in patients during cluster headaches.

Figure 3 displays LCBF values for patients during cluster headache immediately after administration of 100% oxygen inhalation compared to normal volunteers. LCBF values became significantly reduced compared to normals during 100% oxygen inhalation in temporal cortex, caudate nucleus, putamen, and thalamus among patients with cluster headache, which resulted in prompt termination of the head pain. Percentage changes for LCBF values after oxygen inhalation compared to those in normals were $-9.5\% \pm 7.7\%$ in cortical gray matter and $-19.6\% \pm 10.5\%$ in subcortical gray matter.

DISCUSSION

Although the pathogenesis of cluster headache remains unknown, there is little doubt from clinical observations that there are cephalic vascular changes in both the intercranial and extracranial vascular systems that contribute to the classical signs and symptoms of cluster headaches (3–5). The pathogenesis of these changes in the cephalic circulation has not been investigated to the same degree in patients with cluster headache as it has been in migraine, and the few results reported of cerebral hemodynamic changes measured in patients during typical attacks of cluster headache have not been consistent (6–12).

In the present study, increased cerebral blood flow was observed in both ipsilateral and contralateral hemispheres to the side of head pain in patients with spontaneously occurring cluster headache by means of both the ^{133}Xe inhalation and the CT-CBF methods. Hyperperfusion of both cortical and subcortical brain regions disclosed by the CT-CBF method cannot be explained entirely by changes of cortical neuronal activities secondary to the head pain itself, since they were extensive and not limited to the contralateral thalamus and parietal cortex.

Cerebral vasoconstrictive responses to 100% oxygen inhalation were excessive in patients with cluster headache during attacks using both ^{133}Xe inhalation method and CT-CBF method. The vasoconstrictive action of 100% oxygen inhalation may be explained by excessive activity of the sympathetic nervous system, which is modulated by other neurotransmitter systems (13). Therefore, excessive CBF responses to inhaled oxygen supports the role of abnormalities of autonomic and/or other neurotransmitter systems in the pathogenesis of cluster headache.

In summary, results indicate unique cerebrovascular responses during cluster headache and their termination by 100% oxygen inhalation which may provide clues to the pathogenesis of this painful disorder.

REFERENCES

1. Obrist WD, Thompson HK, Wang HS, and Wilkinson E. Regional cerebral blood flow estimated by ^{133}Xe inhalation. *Stroke* 1975; 6:245–256.
2. Meyer JS, Shinohara T, Imai A, Kobari M, Sakai F, Hata T, Oravez WT, Timpe GM, and Solomon E. Imaging local cerebral blood flow by xenon-enhanced computed tomography—Technical optimization procedures. *Neuroradiology* 1988; 30:283–292.
3. Kudrow L. Cluster headache. *Mechanism and management.* Oxford: Oxford University Press, 1980.
4. Ekbom KA. Pathogenesis of cluster headache. In: Blau JN, ed. *Migraine: clinical, therapeutic, conceptual and research aspects.* London: Chapman and Hall, 433–448.
5. Meyer JS, Hata T, and Imai A: Evidence supporting a vascular pathogenesis of migraine and cluster headache. In: Blau JN, ed. *Migraine: clinical, therapeutic, conceptual and research aspects.* London: Chapman and Hall, 265–302.
6. Broch A, Horven I, Nornes H, Sjaastad O, and Tonjum A. Studies on cerebral and ocular circulation in a patient with cluster headache. *Headache* 1970; 10:1–8.
7. Norris JW, Hachinski VC, and Cooper PW. Changes in cerebral blood flow during a migraine attack. *Brit Med J* 1976; 3:676–677.
8. Sakai F and Meyer JS. Regional cerebral hemodynamics during migraine and cluster headache measured by the ^{133}Xe inhalation method. *Headache* 1978; 18:122–132.
9. Sakai F and Meyer JS. Abnormal cerebrovascular reactivity in patients with migraine and cluster headache. *Headache* 1979; 19:257–266.
10. Nelson RF, du Boulay GH, Marshall J, Russell RWR, Symon L, and Zilhka E. Cerebral blood flow studies in patients with cluster headache. *Headache* 1980; 20:184–189.

11. Krabbe AAE, Henriksen L, and Olesen J. Tomographic determination of cerebral blood flow during attacks of cluster headache. *Cephalalgia* 1984; 4:17–23.
12. Kobari M, Meyer JS, Ichijo M, and Kawamura J. Cortical and subcortical hyperperfusion during migraine and cluster headache measured by Xe CT-CBF. *Neuroradiology* 1990; 32:4–11.
13. Nakajima S, Meyer JS, Amano T, Shaw T, Okabe T, and Mortel KF. Cerebral vasomotor responsiveness. During 100% oxygen inhalation in cerebral ischemia. *Arch Neurol* 1983; 40:271–276.

52

Cerebral Blood Flow Response to Oxygen in Cluster Headache

*Jan Erik Hardebo and †Erik Ryding

*Departments of *Neurology, Medical Cell Research, and †Clinical Neurophysiology, University Hospital of Lund, S-221 85 Lund, Sweden*

Inhalation of 100% oxygen, usually at 6–7 1/min, has been known to be effective and rapid in relieving pain during attacks in most cluster headache sufferers (1). This is in contrast to migraine patients, who obtain no relief from pain by O_2 inhalation and have a normal response to O_2 in cranial vessels (2).

Oxygen inhalation constricts large and small extracranial and small cerebral vessels in humans (1–3). Also agents with α-adrenergic properties like adrenaline, noradrenaline, and ergotamine induce a constriction of large cranial vessels and are effective in alleviating pain of an attack. Substantial evidence has been obtained for an ipsilateral dilation of the anterior and middle cerebral arteries, and of the ophthalmic, supraorbital, and supratrochlear arteries with microvessels during attacks (4–6). Accordingly, it would be tempting to assume that the direct vasoconstrictor action of oxygen is responsible for the pain relief during attacks, by reducing distension in the vessel wall and in the bony channels of the skull. However, apart from an alleviating effect of O_2 inhalation on ischemic heart pain, no such effect of O_2 on pain of various origin and location has been reported. The craniovascular action of O_2 inhalation was evaluated by regional cerebral blood flow (rCBF) measurements in cluster headache sufferers, and correlated with the degree of benefit by the treatment. It was also evaluated whether the symptoms of autonomic dysfunction accompanying an attack were influenced.

When measuring regional CBF response to O_2 in sufferers an enhanced reduction in flow has been observed during attacks as compared to controls (2). These patients also received prompt and notable relief from headache. However, the O_2-induced reduction occurred from an elevated flow level as compared to flow values from sufferers between attacks and controls (7).

Hence, it is reasonable to assume that the enhanced flow values during attacks is caused by pain perception. Therefore, part of the flow reduction during curative O_2 inhalation probably results from pain relief, and the remaining lowering of flow may well be within normal limits of an O_2-induced flow reduction. Thus, measurements of CBF during attacks may not be representative for evaluating vascular O_2 reactivity. A study has indicated that an enhanced response might also persist between periods of attacks (8). Therefore, measurements of O_2 reactivity were made within a period when one or more attacks per day occurred, but with a delay of 2–12 hr after the last attack, and compared to the reactivity outside the period.

METHODS

Fourteen patients with cluster headache (13 men, 1 woman; mean age 37.2 years) and five normal volunteers (men; mean age 34.6 years) were studied with rCBF measurements at rest. CBF measurements were made during inhalation of 100% oxygen at 7 l/min and at normoventilation before and after the inhalation. The rCBF measurements were made by recording the clearance of intravenously administered xenon-133 with 30 extracranial detectors over each hemisphere. The gray matter flow values were calculated by monoexponential analysis of the 1–2 min segment of the clearance curves. During the rCBF measurements the end-tidal PCO_2 was continuously recorded.

RESULTS

The resting CBF was within normal limits in all sufferers and controls. No regional or asymmetrical differences were found in the O_2 response in sufferers or controls. End-tidal PCO_2 values in sufferers were 37.8 ± 1.1 (mean ± SEM) before and 37.7 ± 1.1 after O_2, and 36.0 ± 0.8 during O_2 inhalation. Corresponding values in controls were 41.4 ± 1.1 before, 40.8 ± 0.8 after, and 39.6 ± 0.9 during O_2 inhalation.

Four of the cluster headache sufferers had an O_2 response (27–44% reduction in CBF; mean ± SEM 35.2 ± 3.1) that exceeded that of any of the controls (8% increase to 23% reduction in CBF; mean 14.9 ± 2.9). In the remaining 10 patients a response within normal limits was obtained (6% increase to 21% reduction; mean 8.4 ± 2.1). Thus, it appears that an enhanced O_2 response between attacks is present only in a subgroup of patients. All these four patients had the episodic type of cluster headache and did not differ from the other patients in location of pain, duration of disease, response to other therapies, and so forth.

In two of these four patients the response was also tested outside a period, and was found to be normalized (1–14% reduction). One of these four patients, tested when pain-free by retro-Gasserian glycerol injection but still within the usual length of an ongoing period, maintained a strong CBF response to O_2 (28% reduction).

The effect on pain and autonomic symptoms by the O_2 inhalation was evaluated during at least five individual attacks by the patients after careful instruction. It was found that patients with abnormally high CBF reactivity responded best to the inhalation. In these patients autonomic symptoms disappeared simultaneously with the pain. Also, in six of the patients with a normal CBF response an effect on pain, although less marked, was obtained. This indicates that the vasoconstriction induced by O_2 may not be the only factor responsible for pain relief. Only patients with best effect on pain showed a marked effect also on autonomic symptoms. It thus appears as if the autonomic symptoms are coupled to the intensity of pain, perhaps as a reflex phenomenon secondary to activation of pain fibers. Such an assumption is supported by the observation that pain precedes extracranial skin flow changes (3). As many as five of the patients reported return of an attack within 30–60 min; due to the short length of these attacks, three of these patients clearly meant it was the end of the original attack that returned.

DISCUSSION

Available data on flow and diameter changes in intracranial and extracranial vessels during attacks of cluster headache do not indicate a widespread dilation. Rather, segments with dilatations and possibly edema in the vessel wall may be present in some large cranial vessels, together with a reduced lumen (due to constriction, edema, or vasculitis) in the internal carotid artery and retroorbital veins (4–6). Dilatation of cerebral microvessels does not contribute to pain, since brain flow is not enhanced during attacks more than may be explained by pain perception, and inhalation of CO_2, which enhances brain flow, does not provoke an attack as in migraine patients (2). This adds further doubt about a vasoconstrictor action of oxygen as being solely responsible for the effect on pain, also in patients with an enhanced response.

The unique enhanced responsiveness of the vasculature to O_2 in some sufferers does not seem to be confined to the cerebral circulation. Extracranial vessels are also found to be hyperresponsive, particularly on the symptomatic side and during attacks (1). However, the scalp flow was reduced during attacks from a preinhalation level that was more than double that between attacks (2). The present findings indicate that the enhanced cerebrovascular responsiveness to O_2 is uniformly represented in the right and left hemispheres, despite the striking unilaterality of pain and autonomic symptoms.

Further, it seems to be a temporary phenomenon since it did not persist during a remission period.

The precise pathophysiological mechanism behind the enhanced responsiveness in some sufferers to O_2—peripherally located in this vessel wall or centrally at a possible chemoreceptor in the brain stem—remains unknown. Not only hypoxemia but also a reduced CBF reactivity to hypoxemia is present during the build-up of an attack (9). Via unknown steps, this eventually leads to the pain and autonomic symptoms of the attack. Therefore it is not surprising that sufferers with a strong CBF response to O_2 also are best relieved from their symptoms by the inhalation.

REFERENCES

1. Drummond PD and Anthony M. Extracranial vascular responses to sublingual nitroglycerin and oxygen inhalation in cluster headache patients. *Headache* 1985; 25:70–74.
2. Sakai F and Meyer JS. Abnormal cerebrovascular reactivity in patients with migraine and cluster headache. *Headache* 1979; 19:257–266.
3. Drummond PD and Lance JW. Thermographic changes in cluster headache. *Neurology* 1984; 34:1292–1298.
4. Jensen K. Headache and extracerebral blood flow. In: Olesen J, Edvinsson L, eds. *Basic mechanisms of headache*. Amsterdam: Elsevier, 1988; 313–320.
5. Hannerz J, Hellström G, Klum T, and Wahlgren NG. Cluster headache and "dynamite headache": Blood flow velocities in the middle cerebral artery. *Cephalalgia* 1990; 10: 31–38.
6. Dahl A, Russell D, Nyberg-Hansen R, and Rootvelt K. Cluster headache: Transcranial Doppler ultrasound and rCBF studies. *Cephalalgia* 1990; 10:87–94.
7. Sakai F and Meyer JS. Regional cerebral hemodynamics during migraine and cluster headaches measured by the ^{133}Xe inhalation method. *Headache* 1978; 18:122–132.
8. Nelson RF, du Boulay GH, Marshall J, Russell RWR, Symon L, and Zilkha E. Cerebral blood flow studies in patients with cluster headache. *Headache* 1980; 20:184–189.
9. Kudrow L and Kudrow DB. Association of sustained oxyhemoglobin desaturation and onset of cluster headache attacks. *Headache* 1990; 30:474–480.

53
Cluster Headache: Discussion Summary

Jes Olesen

Opposing results were presented in this section. One group using hexamethyl-propylene-amine-oxime (HMPAO) found no abnormalities in cluster headache patients during a cluster period, and regional flow distribution was normal even during actual cluster headache attacks. This finding was supported by two previous single photon emission computed tomography (SPECT) studies that revealed no definite abnormalities of regional cerebral blood flow (rCBF) during cluster headache attacks. Another group, which had previously described interictal abnormalities in migraine with aura and migraine without aura, also described interictal rCBF abnormalities in cluster headache. In some, they were related to the localization of symptoms. The findings were not supported by a control group and evaluation of results was only by visual inspection, which in another report has been demonstrated to be unreliable. Using ^{133}Xe inhalation and stationary detectors as well as stable xenon computed tomography, a global hyperperfusion was described during cluster headache attacks, a finding contrasting with the published SPECT studies. Reaction to breathing of 100% oxygen was excessive during but not outside of attack, even in periods with frequent cluster headache attacks. Another group suggested that the excessive response during an attack was in fact not due to hyperreactivity of blood vessels but secondary to amelioration of pain, pain activation being responsible for the increased blood flow during attacks.

Transcranial Doppler studies have indisputably shown decreased velocity in the middle cerebral artery simultaneously with unaltered brain blood flow, which strongly indicates a dilatation of the middle cerebral artery during attacks. At present it seems most likely that cluster headache is associated with changes in the large arteries whereas changes in brain blood flow are inconspicuous or absent.

PART X
Other Headaches and Effects of Antimigraine Drugs

54

Regional Cerebral Blood Flow in Chronic Tension-Type Headache

*Allan R. Andersen, Michael Langemark, and †Jes Olesen

*Department of Neurology, Rigshospitalet, DK-2100 Copenhagen Ø, and †Department of Neurology, Gentofte Hospital, University of Copenhagen, DK-2900 Hellerup, Denmark

Regional cerebral blood flow (rCBF) changes have been demonstrated in the course of attacks of migraine with aura, although no clear-cut changes have been found during attacks of migraine without aura. Considering chronic tension-type headache, the literature is rather limited. We have studied rCBF in such patients and compared the results to an age-matched control group using xenon-133 and ^{99m}Tc-hexamethyl-propylene-amine-oxime (HMPAO) and single photon emission computerized tomography (SPECT). The preliminary data are given.

PATIENTS

Forty-one patients with chronic tension-type headache were included. Fourteen had less than one migraine attack per month, leaving 27 without any migraine symptoms. Nineteen were male, 22 female. Age: 42.6 ± 14 years (mean ± SD); frequency of headache: 28.8 days/month; duration of headache: 8.0 years (6 months–18 years); medication: paracetamol 1–2 g/day. The headache was monolateral in 11 patients. Five had right-sided, six left-sided predilection of symptoms, whereas 30 had bilateral symptoms. Patients with known brain disease, hypertension, or other common causes of symptomatic headache were excluded.

METHODS

The patients were studied during a period of habitual headache. Resting conditions without headache could not be achieved. All subjects were re-

TABLE 1. Cerebral blood flow in tension-type headache

	Headache patients	Controls
Number	41	33
Age	43 ± 14	41 ± 7
Global CBF[a]	58 ± 7	54 ± 9
Asymmetry (%)	−0.6 ± 3.3	−0.5 ± 2.6

[a] ml/100 g/min.

cumbent with eyes closed. CBF was measured by SPECT after ^{133}Xe inhalation (six slices parallel to the canthomeatal line) in all cases and also after injection of 0.7–1.0 GBq ^{99m}Tc-HMPAO intravenously (nine slices parallel to the canthomeatal line) in 25 of the cases.

Cerebral computed tomography (CT) scan was performed and normal in all cases. The control population comprised normal volunteers investigated on the same SPECT device.

RESULTS

By visual evaluation the rCBF patterns of the tension headache patients was without focal abnormalities using both tracers and could not be separated from the normal cases. The ^{133}Xe data are given in Table 1. The rCBF values were corrected to a pCO$_2$ of 36 mm Hg (4.8 kPa). The mean hemispheric CBF was normal and no abnormal (> 9%) side-to-side asymmetry was noted. No correspondence was seen between laterality of headache and laterality of rCBF (Table 2), but the numbers evaluated were few and type 2 error is possible. The 14 patients who sometimes, but not frequently, had migraine did not differ from the other patients with respect to rCBF pattern or level (Table 3). Only two of these patients had, however, had migraine attacks with aura.

The regional pattern of CBF was normal.

TABLE 2. Laterality of headache vs. laterality of CBF

Headache	CBF Right	CBF Left
Right	2	3
Left	1	5

TABLE 3. *CBF in patients with tension headache and migraine compared to patients without migraine*

Tension headache	With migraine (n = 14)	Without migraine (n = 27)
ml/100 g/min	60 ± 6	58 ± 6

COMMENT

Regional and global CBF is normal in tension-type headache in the chronic disease state when the patients are treated with paracetamol. This is in agreement with earlier results.

55

Decrease of Pourcelot Index in the Middle Cerebral Artery During Post–Lumbar Puncture Headache

Hartmut Göbel and Thomas-Martin Wallasch

Department of Neurology, University of Kiel, D-2300 Kiel, Germany

AIM OF INVESTIGATION

The pathogenesis of post–lumbar puncture headache is a topic of controversial discussion (1,2). It is assumed that position-dependent headache is caused by a reduction of cerebrospinal fluid pressure with subsequent dilatation of intracranial vessels (puncture-hold seepage theory). Today it is not possible to obtain absolute statements about vessel diameters of cerebral arteries *in vivo*. Using transcranial Doppler sonography it is possible to compute the Pourcelot Index of cerebral arteries (3), a parameter for the peripheral vessel resistance (*index de resistance*) This index gives information about reactive changes in peripheral vessel diameters. Therefore it was of particular interest to see if patients with and without post–lumbar puncture headache differ in the Pourcelot Index of the middle cerebral artery before and 48 hr after lumbar puncture.

METHODS

Design

A prospective study was done on 36 neurological inpatients who required lumbar puncture. The first reading of cerebral flow velocities (transcranially using Doppler ultrasonography) was taken on the day before lumbar puncture. Puncture was performed after a standard protocol. On the day of lumbar puncture and on seven consecutive days, the intensity of position-dependent headache was registered quantitatively using a verbal pain rating scale on an hourly basis. The physicians performing the ultrasound examination were not informed of the algesimetric results (double-blind set up). Forty-eight hours after lumbar puncture, the second transcranial Doppler ultrasound reading was taken.

Patients

The 36 patients entered the study in the order in which they were admitted to the hospital. There were 13 women and 23 men. The mean age was 40.5 ± 14.1 years. Each patient's treatment as well as other diagnostic measures were performed independently of this study.

Transcranial Doppler Ultrasonography

The readings were taken using a TC-64 by Eden (Überlingen, Germany). During the readings, the patients lay supine on the examining cot. The Doppler signal was evaluated using a frequency analysis based on the Fast Fourier Transformation principle. Readings of flow velocities in the middle cerebral artery were taken on both sides. The systolic velocity (sv), the diastolic velocity (dv), and the mean velocity (mv) were evaluated. Pourcelot Index (RI) was computed according the equation RI = (sv − dv)/sv.

Lumbar Puncture

Lumbar puncture was performed between the spinous processes of L3 and L4 with the patient in a sitting position. Disposable spinal cannulas cut according to Quincke (0.9 × 86 mm), Spinocan (Braun Melsungen, Germany), were used.

Analysis of Data

The Student's t test for independent and dependent samples was used to determine the significance of the differences in Pourcelot Index between and within the subject groups.

RESULTS

About 31% of the patients were shown to suffer from strong or very strong post–lumbar puncture headache. There proved to be no significant differences in the expression of post–lumbar puncture headache between men and women. Figure 1 shows Pourcelot Indices in relationship to the time of transcranial Doppler ultrasonography and to occurrence of post–lumbar punc-

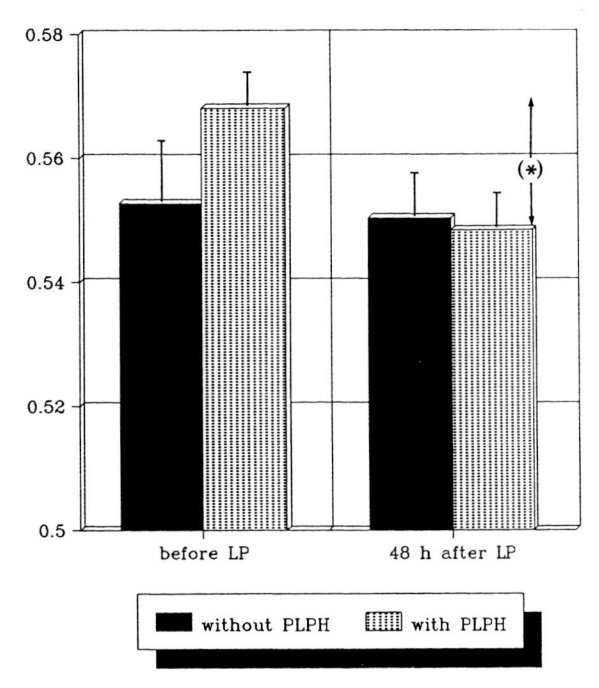

FIG. 1. Vessel resistance (pourcelot indices) in relationship to the time of transcranial Doppler ultrasonography and to occurrence of post–lumbar puncture headache for the middle cerebral artery. Student's *t* test: (*) $p \leq 0.10$.

ture headache for the middle cerebral artery. Patients with post–lumbar puncture headache showed a nearly significant ($p < 0.10$) reduction of Pourcelot Index (before lumbar puncture: 0.5681 ± 0.064; after lumbar puncture: 0.5484 ± 0.056). In contrast, patients without post–lumbar puncture headache showed no significant changes of Pourcelot Index (before lumbar puncture: 0.5527 ± 0.096; after lumbar puncture: 0.5504 ± 0.073).

DISCUSSION

These findings suggest that during post–lumbar puncture headache a decrease of peripheral vessel resistance in the middle cerebral artery occurs. This decrease might be a consequence of low pressure of cerebrospinal fluid and reactive dilatation of intracranial vessels. Low pressure of cerebrospinal fluid caused by a dura defect produced by lumbar puncture and consequent dilatation of intracranial vessels has been postulated as being the critical pathogenetic principle of post–lumbar puncture headache. The observation described here favors this puncture-hole seepage theory as a pathogenetic principle of post–lumbar puncture headache. Alternatively, the decrease of

Pourcelot Index during post–lumbar puncture headache might be a consequence of pain-induced dilatation of peripheral cerebral vessels (see Wallasch and Göbel).

REFERENCES

1. Göbel H, Klostermann H, Lindner V, and Schenkl S. Changes in cerebral haemodynamics in cases of post-lumbar puncture headache: A prospective transcranial Doppler ultrasound study. *Cephalalgia* 1990; 10:117–122.
2. Göbel H and Schenkl S. Postpunktionelles Kopfschmerzsyndrom. *Psycho* 1990; 16:590–606.
3. Pourcelot L. Diagnostic ultrasound for cerebral vascular diseases. In: Donald J, Levi S, eds. *Present and future of diagnostic ultrasound*. Rotterdam: Kooyker, 1976.

56

Nitroglycerin-Induced Headache and Intracranial Hemodynamics

*Helle K. Iversen, †Søren Holm, and †Lars Friberg

*Department of Neurology, Gentofte Hospital, University of Copenhagen, DK-2900 Hellerup, and †Department of Clinical Physiology and Nuclear Medicine, Bispebjerg Hospital, DK-2400 Copenhagen, Denmark

Nitroglycerin (NTG)-induced headache is an interesting experimental model for investigation of the nature of "vascular" headache (1). There are reportedly three different forms of NTG-induced headache. One is immediate, bifrontal or bitemporal, pulsating, and short lasting (1). The other is delayed several hours and described as occurring only in migraine patients and those with a family history of migraine. It often resembles previous migraine attacks (2). A third is cluster headache attacks, which can be induced during cluster periods but not at other times (3).

In an experimental model of vascular headache was found a dose-related headache response during intravenous (iv) infusions of glyceryl trinitrate. Nine of 10 healthy individuals experienced headache. The day-to-day variation of the headache intensity was low. Headache occurred rapidly after start of infusion, and no further increase in headache intensity was seen when infusion rates increased above 0.5 µg/kg/min NTG (1). Sublingual NTG can induce a reduction in mean blood velocity in the middle cerebral artery (MCA), without changes in the regional cerebral blood flow (rCBF) in the corresponding perfusion territory (4). This suggests a NTG-induced dilation of the large intracranial arteries with no effect on the arterioles. If a dilatation of the large arteries occurred, cerebral blood volume (CBV) would increase. Furthermore, CBV contributes with information about the venous system. In order to examine more closely the intracerebral hemodynamic response during NTG infusion, CBV, rCBF, and MCA velocity were measured simultaneously during intravenous NTG infusion.

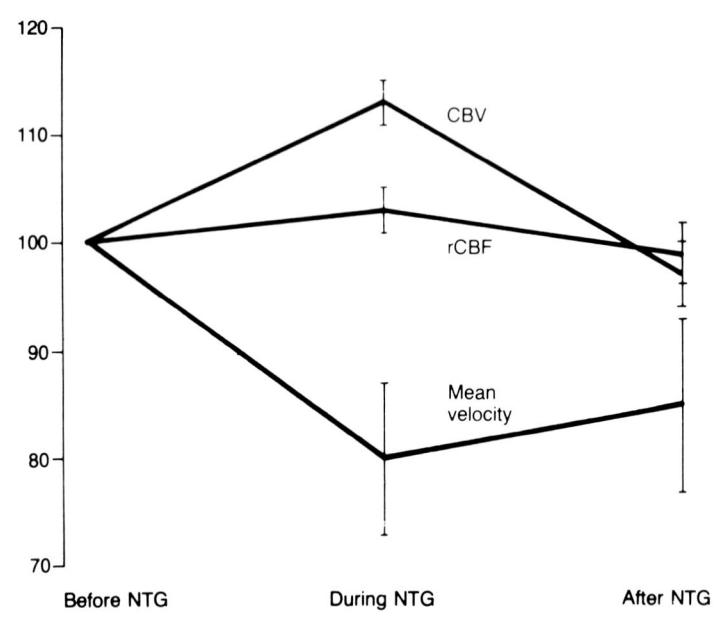

FIG. 1. Changes in mean velocity of MCA, CBV, and CBF in percent of baseline. Values are mean ± SEM.

METHODS

Six healthy volunteers, age 23–33 years, F:M ratio 3:3, with no history of migraine and who never or seldom suffered from headache (<1/month), were studied. Each investigation lasted 2 hr. CBV and velocity in the right MCA were recorded continuously. rCBF was measured in the supine position after 30 min of rest, during infusion of NTG 0.5 µg/kg/min after 15 min of preceding infusion, and 60 min after termination of infusion. The volunteers scored headache intensity on a scale from 0–10, 1 representing a very mild headache (including feeling of pressing or pulsation), 5 a headache of medium severity, and 10 the worst possible headache. rCBF and CBV were measured simultaneously with fast rotating single photon emission computerized tomography (SPECT) equipment (Tomomatic 232) with dual energy window facilities enabling separation of peak energies from ^{99m}Tc and ^{133}Xe (5,6). rCBF was measured after ^{133}Xe inhalation and with 4½ min data sampling. CBV was recorded after iv injection of ^{99m}Tc-labeled erythrocytes (7) and data were corrected for physical and biological decay. Mean rCBF and CBV values from the MCA perfusion territory were calculated from a transverse section of the brain obtained 50 mm above the orbitomeatal plane. Mean blood velocity in the MCA was recorded with a 2-MHz transcranial Doppler equipment (EME TC28) and the signals were stored on video tape. The averaged mean velocity obtained over 1-min sample periods before, during, and after NTG infusion were used (Fig. 1).

RESULTS

In five volunteers headache developed within 10 min, with a median maximal headache score of 4. One volunteer did not experience headache. All volunteers were headache-free 60 min after termination of NTG infusion.

Before NTG infusion the mean velocity in the MCA was 68 cm/sec, SEM 3. During infusion velocity decreased to 55 cm/sec, SEM 5 ($p < 0.05$) and 60 min after terminating the infusion the velocity was still reduced below the control value 56 cm/sec, SEM 5 ($p < 0.05$). Changes in CBV were calculated as percent deviation from the pre–NTG-infusion period. During infusion a mean CBV increase of 13%, SEM 2 ($p < 0.05$) was found. Sixty minutes after terminating the infusion mean CBV had returned to the control value -0.3%, SEM 3. rCBF values from the second and third measurements were corrected 2% per mm Hg; the end-tidal pCO_2 deviated from the control value. There were no significant changes in rCBF during and after NTG infusion.

DISCUSSION

Five of the six volunteers experienced headache. The cerebral hemodynamic response, however, was the same in all volunteers. Brain tissue perfusion was unchanged (no rCBF changes) and mean velocity in the MCA was decreased. Therefore, MCA must have been dilated. Furthermore, intracerebral blood volume was increased. This suggests that the cerebral resistance vessels (arterioles) were unaffected by NTG whereas the larger arteries and the venous system were dilated. Sixty minutes after NTG termination headache had disappeared in all volunteers. Mean flow velocity of MCA was still 15% below baseline, CBV was decreased to baseline values, and rCBF remained normal. The venous system contains the majority of the cerebral blood volume, whereas arterioles regulate CBF. A longer lasting effect on the arteries than on the venous system and no effect on the arterioles are thus indicated.

Contrasting with these findings, we have observed a close temporal relationship between dilatation of the radial artery and headache intensity during NTG 0.5 μg/kg/min infusion. After termination of the infusion, the induced headache decreased rapidly, in parallel with normalization of the arterial diameter (8). These differing responses between cerebral and peripheral arteries could be due to differences in the sensitivity to NTG or differing counterregulatory mechanisms, differences of the endothelial cell response, or of smooth muscle cells in the artery wall. It could also be due to an increased release of perivascular pain sensitizing vasodilatory peptides as CGRP, substance P, and neurokinin A from trigeminal nerve endings surrounding the vessels (9). These peptides are found in greater amounts around cerebral blood vessels than around peripheral arteries. During migraine attacks an increased level of CGRP has been found in blood from the external jugular vein on the headache side (10). The differences in cerebral hemodynamic response are important as any difference between peripheral and cerebral arteries may lead us to the answer of the question: Why do NTG and other vasodilatory compounds induce headache and not pain in other parts of the body?

REFERENCES

1. Iversen HK, Olesen J, and Tfelt-Hansen P. Intravenous nitroglycerin as an experimental headache model. Basic characteristics. *Pain* 1989; 38:17–24.
2. Sicuteri F, Bene ED, Poggioni M, and Bonnazzi A. Unmasking latent dysnociception in healthy subject. *Headache* 1987; 27:180–185.
3. Ekbom K. Nitroglycerin as a provocative agent in cluster headache. *Arch Neurol* 1968; 19:487–493.
4. Dahl A and Russell D. Cluster headache: middle cerebral artery velocities following the administration of glyceryl nitrate. *Cephalalgia* 1987; 7:323–324.
5. Lassen NA, Sveinsdottir E, Kanno I, Stokely EM, and Rommer P. A fast rotating single photon emission tomograph for regional cerebral blood flow studies in man. *J Comput Assist Tomogr* 1978; 2:661–662.
6. Holm S, Friberg L, Iversen HK, and Lassen NA. Dual energy brain SPECT—methods and applications. In: Schmidt HAE and Chambron J, eds. *Nuclear medicine: quantitative analysis in imaging and function*. Stuttgart–New York: Schattauer, 1990; 11–13.
7. Kelkaek H. Technetium-99m labeling of red blood cells: In vitro evaluation of a new approach. *J Nucl Med* 1989; 27:1770–1773.
8. Iversen HK, Nielsen TH, Tfelt-Hansen P, and Olesen J. Headache and changes in the diameter of the radial artery during 7 hours intravenous nitroglycerin infusion. *Cephalalgia* 1989; 9 [Suppl 10]:82–83.
9. Edvinsson L, MacKenzie ET, McCulloch J, and Uddmann R. Nerve supply and receptor mechanisms in intra- and extracerebral blood vessels. In: Olesen J and Edvinsson L, eds. *Basic mechanisms of headache*. Amsterdam: Elsevier, 1988; 129–144.
10. Goadsby PJ, Edvinsson L, and Ekman R. Vasoactive peptide release in the extracerebral circulation of humans during migraine headache. *Ann Neurol* 1990; 2:183–187.

57

Sumatriptan Increases the Cranial Blood Flow Velocity During Migraine Attacks: A Transcranial Doppler Study

*Jo F. V. Caekebeke, *C. P. Zwetsloot, *J. C. Jansen,
†‡Pramod R. Saxena, and *‡Michel D. Ferrari

*Department of Neurology, University Hospital, 2300 RC Leiden,
†Department of Pharmacology, Erasmus University, Rotterdam, and
‡Dutch Migraine Research Group, The Netherlands

Sumatriptan, a selective 5-hydroxytryptamine$_1$ (5-HT$_1$)–like receptor agonist, is a highly effective new drug in the acute treatment of migraine attacks (1). In animals, sumatriptan mediates a selective vasoconstriction of cephalic arteries and arteriovenous shunts, redirecting the blood flow to the capillary bed (2). Sumatriptan shares this "serotonergic/ergotamine-like" vasoconstriction with other effective antimigraine drugs, but lacks their systemic pharmacological actions (3). In humans, however, little is known about the pathological role of cerebral arteriovenous shunts, the localization of 5-HT$_1$–like receptors, and the mechanism of action of sumatriptan. Because of its high efficacy rate and remarkably selective pharmacological profile, studying the mechanism of action of sumatriptan may help to elucidate the pathophysiology of migraine. To understand better the effect in humans, we studied the blood flow velocity (BFV) in the common carotid (CCA), external carotid (ECA), internal carotid (ICA), and middle cerebral artery (MCA) during migraine attacks before and after treatment with sumatriptan. We therefore used a transcranial Doppler device, a noninvasive, relatively easy tool to repeatedly determine BFV (4).

METHODS

This study was performed as a part of two double-blind, placebo-controlled randomized clinical trials with various doses of sumatriptan during spontaneous migraine attacks. Patients presented at the clinic as soon as possible after the onset of an attack. On arrival in the hospital, the BFV were measured with the EME TC2-64B transcranial pulsed Doppler system (EME, Uberlingen, Germany), using a hand-held 2-MHz probe for the MCA and 4-MHz probe for the CCA, ECA, and ICA. The systolic peak flow velocity and time-mean velocity (over a period of 5 sec) were quantified bilaterally. In addition, blood pressure, heart rate, and respiratory frequency were measured and severity of the migraine symptoms was assessed on a 0–3 score. All patients were investigated during a severe attack, before treatment, and 65–90 min after the first dose of sumatriptan or placebo.

PATIENTS

Patients were classified according to the criteria of the International Headache Society Headache Classification Committee. Inclusion and exclusion criteria were the same as for the clinical trials (1). Exclusion criteria included the abuse of ergot-containing preparations ($\geq$ 10 mg/week) or other drugs, the use of migraine prophylaxis within the 2 weeks before the study, and the use of ergot-containing preparations within 24 hr, or simple analgesics or nonsteroidal antiinflammatory drugs within 6 hr before the study treatment. The study was approved by the local ethical committee and patients gave written, informed consent.

Three groups of patients were included:

1. 24 migraineurs (mean age of 44.9 ± 9.9 years, 8 men, 16 women), who were treated with 3–6 mg sumatriptan sc in one or two gifts (low-dose group)
2. 20 migraineurs (mean age of 46.0 ± 8.9 years, 2 men, 18 women), who received 6–12 mg sumatriptan sc in one or two gifts (high-dose study).
3. 7 migraineurs (mean age of 41.9 ± 12.8 years, 3 men, 4 women), who received placebo.

STATISTICS

Repeated measurement ANOVA was used to evaluate differences in blood flow velocities due to treatment and side of measurement. The low dose, high dose, and placebo group were analyzed separately. Patients were crossed with the repeated factors "time" (pre- and posttreatment) and "side" (right or left).

RESULTS

Blood pressure, heart rate, and respiratory frequency did not differ significantly between the two measurements, before and after treatment. Results

TABLE 1. *Peak and mean blood flow velocities (group means, SD) in CCA, ECA, ICA, and MCA before and after treatment with sumatriptan*

	Pretreatment	Posttreatment	p
Low-dose group (n = 24):			
CCA: Peak	51.8 (12.9)	47.8 (10.5)	0.05
Mean	22.4 (4.6)	21.4 (4.1)	0.2
ECA: Peak	49.2 (11.7)	45.7 (10.5)	0.1
Mean	18.5 (3.9)	18.2 (4.0)	0.7
ICA: Peak	52.6 (9.2)	58.2 (10.3)	<0.001
Mean	32.0 (5.7)	35.5 (6.6)	<0.01
MCA: Peak	93.2 (18.9)	96.2 (19.1)	0.06
Mean	60.8 (13.4)	63.2 (14.0)	0.04
High-dose group (n = 20):			
CCA: Peak	55.6 (11.0)	55.7 (9.9)	1.0
Mean	25.8 (5.9)	27.3 (5.4)	0.06
ECA: Peak	51.2 (10.3)	51.2 (11.0)	1.0
Mean	20.8 (4.3)	22.3 (5.4)	0.07
ICA: Peak	59.0 (12.7)	71.6 (17.0)	<0.001
Mean	40.0 (9.9)	49.4 (12.5)	<0.001
MCA: Peak	99.7 (20.4)	111.2 (18.3)	<0.001
Mean	68.6 (15.7)	75.0 (12.7)	<0.001
Placebo group (n = 7):			
CCA: Peak	54.7 (21.7)	53.6 (19.7)	0.6
Mean	22.4 (5.8)	22.6 (4.6)	0.9
ECA: Peak	54.4 (11.2)	50.5 (5.8)	0.2
Mean	22.0 (5.2)	19.1 (4.2)	0.09
ICA: Peak	56.3 (13.2)	51.8 (8.5)	0.4
Mean	34.4 (7.6)	32.9 (5.1)	0.5
MCA: Peak	102.8 (18.3)	94.1 (20.3)	0.04
Mean	65.4 (12.2)	59.5 (11.1)	0.05

of BFV measurements are summarized in Table 1 and presented as group means (and SD) of the mean and peak BFV.

There were no significant interactions between the factors "time" and "side" and no significant differences between the right and left side. Therefore, only the effect of treatment is given. "High-dose" sumatriptan produced a statistically highly significant increase of the BFV in the ICA and MCA. The low-dose group shows a similar tendency, but only the BFV increase in the ICA was statistically significant. No significant changes were observed for the BFV in the CCA and the ECA. In contrast, placebo gave a mild reduction of the BFV in the MCA and did not alter the BFV in the other vessels.

DISCUSSION

This study disclosed that during migraine attacks, sumatriptan induces a selective and probably dose-dependent increase of the BFV in the internal carotid arterial bed without changing the BFV in the external carotid artery. After placebo treatment, cranial BFVs are not altered or even decreased. These findings suggest that during migraine attacks, sumatriptan either constricts the ICA and MCA or reduces the peripheral vascular resistance in the ICA/MCA outflow tract. Reduction of the peripheral vascular resistance appears to be an unlikely mechanism in view of animal studies that show that sumatriptan constricts arteriovenous (AV) shunts, redirects the blood flow to the cranial capillary circulation, and slightly reduces the total carotid flow consequently (2). This constriction of AV shunts would result in opposite BFV changes and therefore cannot explain our findings. Thus, constriction of the ICA and large basal arteries remains the most likely mechanism of action of sumatriptan in curing migraine attacks.

These results are unexpected in view of observations on 5-HT and ergotamine in man, suggesting that these two "mother compounds" of sumatriptan primarily give a vasoconstriction in the ECA vascular bed (5).

In conclusion, our findings suggest that sumatriptan constricts the large basal arteries to the brain during migraine attacks. For definite conclusions we must await the findings in the same patients outside attacks.

ACKNOWLEDGMENTS

This study was supported financially by the Dutch Migraine Foundation, Glaxo Group Research, Greenford, England and Glaxo BV, Nieuwengein, The Netherlands.

REFERENCES

1. Ferrari MD, Melamed E, Gawel MJ, et al. Effective treatment of migraine attacks with subcutaneous sumatriptan. A randomized placebo-controlled clinical trial (submitted).
2. Perren MJ, Feniuk W, and Humphrey PPA. The selective closure of feline carotid arteriovenous anastomoses by GR43175. *Cephalalgia* 1989; 9[Suppl 9]:41–46.
3. Saxena PR and Ferrari MD. 5-HT$_1$-like receptor agonists and the pathophysiology of migraine. *TIPS* 1989; 10:200–204.
4. Aaslid R, ed. *Transcranial doppler sonography*. Vienna–New York: Springer-Verlag, 1986.
5. Puzich R, Girke W, Heidrich H, and Rischke M. Assessment of extracranial cerebral vessels in patients with migraine after administration of ergotamine tartrate using Doppler ultrasound. *Deutsche Medizinische Wochenschrift* 1983; 108:457–461.

58

Effect of Sumatriptan on Pial Vessel Diameter *In Vivo*

Patrick P. A. Humphrey, H. E. Connor, C. M. Stubbs, and W. Feniuk

Department of Neuropharmacology, Glaxo Group Research Ltd., Ware, Hertfordshire SG12 0DP, England

Sumatriptan, a selective 5-hydroxytryptamine$_1$ (5-HT$_1$)–like receptor agonist, which is effective in the acute treatment of migraine (1), causes contraction of large isolated cerebral arteries from many species including humans (2). In this study, the effect of sumatriptan on pial vessel diameter has been compared *in vivo* after local (perivascular) or intravenous administration to anesthetized cats.

MATERIAL AND METHODS

Cats (either sex, 2.4–3.5 kg) were anesthetized (chloralose 80 mg/kg i.p. and pentobarbitone 10 mg/kg i.p.) and artificially ventilated with room air so that arterial pH, pCO$_2$, and pO$_2$ were maintained within normal physiological limits. Blood pressure and heart rate were measured via a cannula in the left femoral artery. Left common carotid blood flow was measured using a Doppler flow probe; carotid vascular resistance was calculated as mean blood pressure divided by carotid blood flow. An open pial window (approx. 2.0 × 1.5 cm) was prepared above the left parietal cortex, as described by Wahl et al. (3). Pial blood vessel diameter was measured via a video microscaler (For-A) linked to a camera and microscope. Sumatriptan, dissolved in artificial cerebrospinal fluid (CSF; pH 7.25) (3), was injected perivascularly in a volume of 1–2 µl over 30 sec, via a glass micropipette (tip diameter 8–10 µm). Normal reactivity of pial vessels was checked at the beginning of each experiment by their response to CSF containing 10 mM K$^+$: this produced a dilatation of about 30–40%. In other animals, saline vehicle (0.5 ml/min for 10 min) followed about 30 min later by sumatriptan (6.4 µg/kg/min for 10 min) was infused via the left femoral vein. These animals also received sumatriptan (1 µM) perivascularly at the beginning and end of the experiment.

RESULTS

Sumatriptan (0.1–10 µM) caused a concentration-related decrease in pial artery diameter (Fig. 1); the maximum effect, produced by 1 µM, was −19 ± 2% (n = 15 in six cats). This effect was immediate in onset but relatively transient with pial artery diameter returning to basal level within 2–5 min after the injection. Small (80–120 µm) and large (120–240 µm) diameter pial arteries were constricted similarly. In contrast, sumatriptan (1–10 µM) had no effect on the diameter of pial veins (resting diameter 130–380 µm).

In other animals, intravenous infusion of saline (0.5 ml/min for 10 min) had no effect on resting parameters. However, intravenous infusion of sumatriptan (6.4 µg/kg/min for 10 min), while having no significant effect on blood pressure or heart rate, caused a decrease in carotid blood flow and an increase in carotid vascular resistance (maximum change of −20 ± 7% and

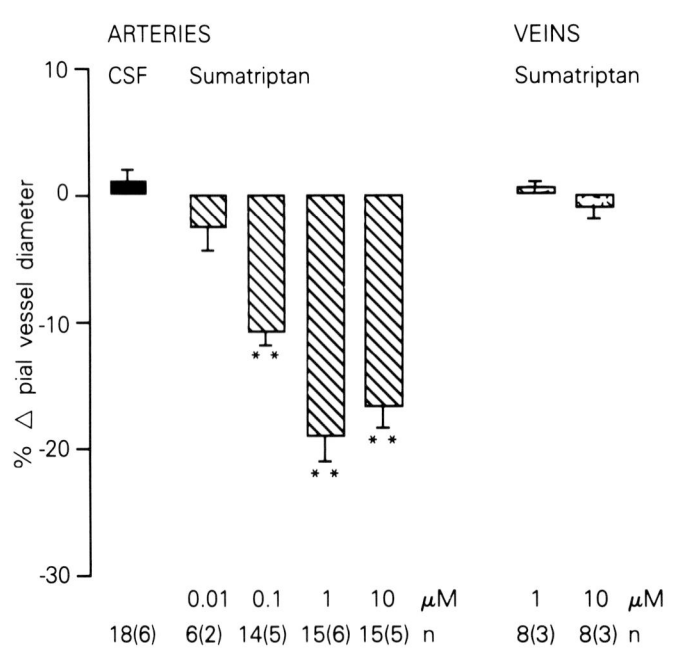

FIG. 1. Effect of CSF or sumatriptan on pial vessel diameter after perivascular injection in anesthetized cats. Responses are expressed as percent change from preinjection diameter. Each value is the mean ± SEM of n observations (shown beneath the bars with the number of animals used given in parentheses). **$p < 0.01$ compared to CSF, unpaired Student's t test.

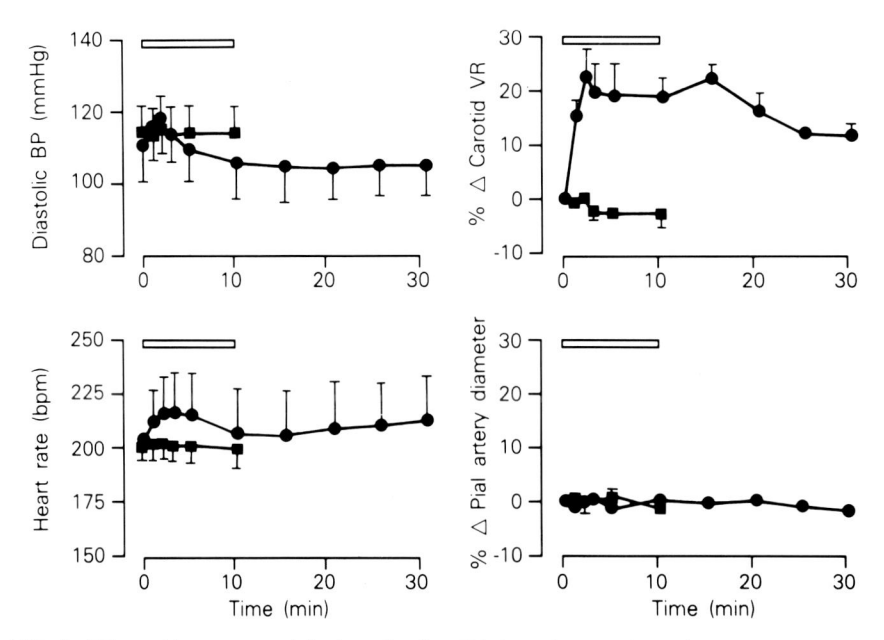

FIG. 2. Effect of intravenous infusion of saline (■, 0.5 ml/min) followed by sumatriptan (●, 6.4 μg/kg/min) for 10 min in anesthetized cats. Infusion time is shown by the bar. Resting carotid vascular resistance and pial artery diameter were 5.8 ± 1.4 mm Hg min/ml and 165 ± 23 μm, respectively, before saline infusion and 5.6 ± 1.0 mm Hg min/ml and 158 ± 24 μm respectively, before sumatriptan infusion. Values are means ± SEM from four animals.

+23 ± 5% respectively, n = 4). However, there was no change in pial artery diameter (Fig. 2). Perivascular injection of sumatriptan (1 μM) before and after the infusion caused pial artery constriction (−18 ± 2% and −16 ± 2%, respectively).

DISCUSSION

These results demonstrate that pial arteries can be constricted *in vivo* by perivascular administration of the selective 5-HT$_1$–like receptor agonist, sumatriptan, at the same concentrations that cause contraction of large cerebral arteries *in vitro* (2). However, intravenously administered sumatriptan, at a dose that has been shown to be clinically effective in the acute treatment of migraine (1), constricted the carotid vascular bed but did not modify pial vessel caliber in anesthetised cats. This is consistent with findings from a previous study using radiolabeled microspheres showing that sumatriptan, even at relatively high doses (up to 1 mg/kg iv), does not modify cerebral blood flow in anesthetized cats (4), and suggests that sumatriptan only poorly penetrates the cerebrovascular intima. This is in accordance with other studies that show that sumatriptan does not readily penetrate the blood-brain barrier (5,6).

REFERENCES

1. Perrin VL, Färkkilä M, Goasguen J, Doenicke A, Brand J, and Tfelt-Hansen P. Overview of initial clinical studies with intravenous and oral GR43175 in acute migraine. *Cephalalgia* 1989; 9[Suppl 9]:63–72.
2. Humphrey PPA, Feniuk W, Perren MJ, Connor HE, and Oxford AW. The pharmacology of the novel 5-HT$_1$-like receptor agonist, GR43175. *Cephalalgia* 1989; 9[Suppl 9]:23–33.
3. Wahl M, Schilling L, and Whalley ET. Cerebrovascular effects of prostanoids. *Naunyn Schmiedebergs Arch Pharmacol* 1989; 9:314–320.
4. Perren MJ, Feniuk W, and Humphrey PPA. The selective closure of feline carotid arteriovenous anastomoses (AVAs) by GR43175. *Cephalalgia* 1989; 9[Suppl 9]:41–46.
5. Sleight AJ, Cervenka A, and Peroutka SJ. *In vivo* effects of sumatriptan (GR43175) on extracellular levels of 5-HT in the guinea-pig. *Neuropharmacology* 1990; 29:511–513.
6. Humphrey PPA, Feniuk W, Perren MJ, Beresford IJM, Skingle M, and Whalley ET. Serotonin and migraine. *Ann NY Acad Sci* 1990; 600:587–598.

59

The Effect of Ergotamine on Human Cerebral Blood Flow and Cerebral Arteries

*Peer Tfelt-Hansen, †Bjørn Sperling, and ‡Allan R. Andersen

*Departments of *Neurology and †Clinical Physiology and Nuclear Medicine, Bispebjerg Hospital, DK-2400 Copenhagen, and ‡Department of Neurology, Rigshospitalet, DK-2100 Copenhagen, Denmark.*

The use of ergotamine (E), a potent constrictor of peripheral arteries (1) in the treatment of migraine with aura, where transient neurological symptoms form part of the attack, has been controversial for a long time since it was feared that E might increase the risk of ischemia by an effect on the cerebral vasculature and induce permanent neurological symptoms. Serious cases of reversible cerebral arteriopathy with segmental stenosis and even completed strokes have been reported after E was administered in inappropriately high doses (2). On the other hand, many patients have been treated with E during attacks of migraine with aura without any serious cerebrovascular side effects.

In the present series of studies, young healthy male volunteers were therefore challenged with the maximum intravenous (iv) dose of E in order to detect any vasoconstrictory effect of the drug on the cerebral vasculature. In a previously published study (3), the effect of E on resting and acetazolamide-stimulated cerebral blood flow (CBF) was investigated. Since no effect was observed, the effect of E on blood flow velocity in the middle cerebral artery recorded with transcranial Doppler (TCD) ultrasonography was investigated.

METHODS

The study consisted of two parts. In the first part the effect of E on CBF was studied (3). Second, when TCD became available to us later on, the effect of E on the blood flow velocity of the middle cerebral artery was investigated.

Part 1

Eight healthy medical students were studied. On the control study day CBF was measured before and 20 min after iv injection of 1 g acetazolamide. On the E study day (at least 1 week later) CBF was measured before and 210 min after iv injection of 0.5 mg ergotamine tartrate. CBF was measured again 20 min after iv injection of 1 g acetazolamide (240 min after E injection). CBF was measured by ^{133}Xe inhalation and single photon emission computerized tomography (SPECT). For details about the method and actually used equipment, see refs. 3 and 4.

On the E study day systolic blood pressures were measured simultaneously in triplicate on the left upper arm and big toes with strain-gauge plethysmography (1) before and 30, 120, and 240 min after E injection.

Part 2

Ten healthy male medical students were studied. Blood flow velocity in the left middle cerebral artery (MCA) was recorded by means of a TCD using a 2-MHz probe. Each measurement was the mean of four continuous 14-sec sweeps. During the investigation the probe position was held constant by a specially designed headband.

After a baseline recording, 0.5 mg ergotamine tartrate was injected iv, and blood flow velocities were repeated after 15, 30, 60, 90, 120, 240, and 360 min. For statistical evaluation of results, Friedman's two-way analysis of variance by ranks and Wilcoxon's test for paired data were used.

RESULTS

Part 1

E did not cause any changes in resting global CBF as measured after 210 min (Table 1). After acetazolamide similar increases in global CBF were observed independent of whether E was administered before (26%) or not

TABLE 1. *Effect of 0.5 mg ergotamine tartrate iv on resting and acetazolamide-stimulated global CBF (ml/100 g/ min) (n = 8)*

Min after administration		0	20	210	240
Acetazolamide (A)	Mean	54	69 (28%)	n.d.	n.d.
	SEM	2	1		
Ergotamine	Mean	57	n.d.	57	72 (26%)
(+ A at 220 min)	SEM	3		3	3

Note: n.d. denotes not done.

TABLE 2. *Middle cerebral artery blood flow velocity (cm/sec) after 0.5 mg ergotamine tartrate iv (n = 10)*

	\multicolumn{7}{c}{Min after administration}
	0	15	30	60	120	240	360
Mean	60	70[a]	75[a]	80[a]	76[a]	71[a]	67
SEM	3	4	5	6	3	5	4
Range	(46–71)	(46–87)	(52–105)	(62–107)	(59–90)	(50–100)	(54–88)
% Change		17	25	33	26	19	12

[a]Significant different changes ($p < 0.05$, Wilcoxon's test).

(28%) (Table 1). No changes were found in the regional distribution of CBF in the cerebellum or the hemispheres. In contrast, E caused a constriction of extremity arteries, as measured by a decrease in toe–arm systolic gradients (1). The mean decreases were 6 mm Hg after 30 min, 20 mm Hg after 120 min, and 23 mm Hg after 240 min ($p < 0.001$, Friedman's test).

Part 2

E caused an increase in blood flow velocity of the left MCA ($p < 0.001$, Friedman's test). The increases were statistically significant from 15 to 240 min and ranged from 17% (15 min) to 33% (60 min), whereas the 12% increase after 360 min was not statistically significantly different from baseline (Table 2).

DISCUSSION

The controversy of whether or not to use E in the treatment of migraine with aura was apparently solved when Hachinsky et al. (5) demonstrated that intramuscular injection of 0.2–1.0 mg ergotamine tartrate did not change CBF in 16 patients when measured before and 15–20 min after E administration. What was measured was, however, CBF, a function of the arterioles. It is more likely that the possible mechanism of ischemia in migraine with aura after E is vasoconstriction of cerebral arteries, as indicated by the observation of symptomatic arteriopathy with segmental stenosis in patients after high doses of E (2).

The cerebral arteries are not normally flow-limiting. Thus, even if a small to moderate constriction of arteries is present this will not result in a decrease in CBF, because such a constriction of the arteries will be counteracted by a dilatation of arterioles. In the first part of this study we therefore tried to optimize the conditions for detecting a possible effect of E on cerebral arteries. As demonstrated by the measurement of the vasoconstrictory effect of E on peripheral arteries, the decreases in toe–arm systolic gradients, the effect is slowly developing and only at maximum after hours. Similar results were found previously (1). We therefore measured the effect on CBF after 210 min. Furthermore, 1 g acetazolamide iv, which has been used to test flow limitation after occlusion of the carotid artery (6), and which increased CBF approximately 30%, was administered to reveal any flow limitation caused by arterial constriction. Even if acetazolamide was administered at a time of presumable maximum arterial effect of E, no effect of E on acetazolamide-stimulated CBF was found.

In contrast, blood flow velocity in the MCA measured with TCD increased after E. Preferably CBF should have been measured simultaneously, but based on results in the present study and earlier investigations (4) we assume that CBF was unchanged. If so, the increase in blood flow velocities indicates a constriction of the MCA after E. In this study the maximum iv dose of 0.5 mg ergotamine tartrate was administered, and the increase in blood flow velocity was a maximum of 30% after 60 min, corresponding to a decrease of 13% of the arterial diameter. Thus, even if the maximum iv dose of E was administered, only a small and presumably not flow-limiting vasoconstriction of the cerebral arteries was found.

The present study in young healthy male volunteers thus indicates a potential of E for constriction of cerebral arteries. The problem should be investigated further with simultaneous measurements of TCD and CBF after E administration in migraine patients during attacks, before one can give firm recommendations about the use of E in migraine with aura.

REFERENCES

1. Tfelt-Hansen P. The effect of ergotamine on the arterial system in man. *Acta Pharmacol Toxicol* 1986; 59 [Suppl 3]:1–30.
2. Henry PY, Larne P, Aupy M, Lafforgue JL, and Orgogozo JM. Reversible cerebral arteriopathy associated with the administration of ergot derivatives. *Cephalalgia* 1984; 4:171–178.
3. Andersen AR, Tfelt-Hansen P, and Lassen NA. The effect of ergotamine and dihydroergotamine on cerebral blood flow in man. *Stroke* 1987; 18:10–23.
4. Celsis P, Goldman T, Henriksen L, and Lassen NA. A method for calculating regional cerebral blood flow from emission computed tomography of inert gas concentrations. *J Comput Assist Tomogr* 1981; 5:641–645.
5. Hachinsky V, Norris JW, Edmeads J, and Cooper PW. Ergotamine and cerebral blood flow. *Stroke* 1978; 9;594–596.
6. Vorstrup S, Brun B, and Lassen NA. Evaluation of cerebral vasodilatory capacity by acetazolamide test before EC-IC bypass surgery in patients with occlusion of the internal carotid artery. *Stroke* 1986; 1:1291–1298.

60

Other Headaches and Effects of Migraine Drugs: Discussion Summary

Jes Olesen

Given the difficulties of studying spontaneous migraine attacks it was suggested to study headaches elicited by, for example, nitroglycerine or histamine. Studies of this nature were presented, but although such models are extremely useful in the further analysis of the mechanisms of migraine attacks, there is still reason to make a sharp distinction between experimental headaches and spontaneous attacks. It was pointed out that many published studies on experimental headaches suffer from a lack of sufficient clinical description. It must be required for future studies that, in each patient, the symptoms be so meticulously recorded that the studied attacks can be classified according to the operational diagnostic criteria for migraine without aura of the International Headache Society. The exact route of administration, dose, and timing of the provoking substance must obviously be given in any publication. The interesting findings of normal regional cerebral blood flow (rCBF) in tension-type headache and the possibility that large cerebral artery dilatation may be involved in post–lumbar puncture headache were not discussed further.

Large cerebral arteries were, however, believed to be a possible target for antimigraine drugs such as the novel 5-hydroxytryptamine (5-HT$_1$)-like receptor agonist sumatriptan and ergotamine. How sumatriptan could exert such action was not clear, since a study documented its inability to constrict pial arteries after systemic administration. When given to the adventitial side, it did, however, constrict pial arteries. New data were presented in the discussion, which seemed to demonstrate conclusively dilatation of the middle cerebral artery on the painful side during migraine attacks. These changes were reversed within 30 min after intravenous sumatriptan. Constriction of large cerebral arteries was therefore proposed as the mechanism of action of sumatriptan. This would imply that it had in fact crossed the endothelium of the affected large basal arteries. Some relatively old evidence in the literature indicates that the barrier in arteries is less tight than in capillaries, and changes in barrier function due to migraine is another possibility of explaining the passage of the drug into the arterial wall.

61
Conclusions and Prospects for the Future

Jes Olesen

As discussed in the introduction, headache disorders are heterogeneous and difficult to study with current methods for regional cerebral blood flow (rCBF) determination. Many of the results in this book seem mutually contradictive and many chapters may leave the readers more confused rather than the opposite. If one pays careful attention to the quality of description of the case material, the exactness of timing in relation to onset of attacks and the quality of the methodology applied to the studies, the picture does, however, become clearer. It also becomes clear that this is a fertile research field and that it is far from having been harvested completely.

The very early phase of migraine attacks can be studied only when attacks are induced by carotid angiography, and with the good temporal and spatial resolution of the intracarotid ^{133}Xe method. Most such studies have been from our group. They have described the so-called spreading oligemia or hypoperfusion, that is, an occipital area of low flow spreading gradually anteriorly and not respecting territories of supply of major branches of the middle cerebral artery. The low flow continued long after aura symptoms had disappeared and well into the headache phase. Other groups agree that a focal reduction of rCBF is seen in the early stages of migraine attacks with aura, but they have been unable to provide details. The previously hypoperfused area becomes hyperperfused after one to several hours in most cases but in other cases focal low flow just normalizes without an interposed hyperemic phase. The focal hyperperfusion has only been seen by our group, but is a consistent finding. It may have been overlooked by others because ^{133}Xe inhalation with external stationary detectors has a poor spatial resolution and easily might overlook focal changes, and because single photon emission computed tomography (SPECT) studies with hexamethyl-propylene-amine-oxime (HMPAO) are ill-suited to demonstrate hyperperfusion due to backdiffusion of the tracer. The most controversial issue is whether there is a global increase of blood flow in the headache phase of migraine with aura. This has been described by three groups, but three other groups, partially using the same methods and partially using SPECT, have been unable to demonstrate any global abnormalities of brain blood flow during migraine attacks with aura. Methods with good quantitation of brain blood flow must be applied to resolve the controversy. The big arteries function independently of brain blood flow, but techniques were previously not available for studying them. Transcranial Doppler (TCD) combined with brain blood flow measurements now allow an estimate of the diameter of the large basal arteries in man. So far, only a few patients with aura have been studied and the picture is as yet unclear, although a number of abnormalities have been described.

A detailed discussion of pain mechanisms in migraine with aura is possible today thanks to brain blood flow studies. It seems clear that both temporally and topographically the aura symptoms and the rCBF changes are closely linked. Most recently, it has been shown that the same pertains to the headache which, when unilateral, is virtually always located on the side of rCBF abnormalities. Quite often, however, unilateral rCBF changes are associated with bilateral headache. Although it seems reasonably clear that there is an association between the observable rCBF abnormalities and headache, the exact mechanism of pain activation is debatable. The animal experimental phenomenon of cortical spreading depression (CSD) of Leao has been proposed as the cause of migraine aura, and this was supported by several chapters and by the discussion. CSD and vascular mechanisms are not mutually exclusive. On the contrary, it appears that ischemia may elicit spreading depression and that spreading depression elicits marked abnormalities of brain blood flow and cerebrovascular reactivity. Furthermore, spreading depression is a graded phenomenon that may involve a differing number of cortical layers, a variable number of cortical regions, and that may be associated with more or less marked blood flow abnormalities. This variability fits well with the findings in migraine patients.

In migraine without aura no initial low flow areas have been described. One chapter focused on the onset of attacks induced by red wine, and these findings need to be confirmed using techniques with a good spatial resolution. Several studies have examined spontaneous attacks after one to several hours. Again, no focal abnormalities have been described. Focal hyperperfusion such as in migraine with aura has not been disclosed. There seems to be universal agreement about these findings. When it comes to global changes in brain blood flow, however, views are different. Some groups have described global hyperperfusion, others a perfectly normal global blood flow. This is identical to the discrepancies observed in migraine with aura.

Spreading depression seems to be a useful model of migraine aura and may explain the subsequent headache, but no such model is currently available for migraine without aura. The two forms of migraine respond to the same drugs. It is therefore likely that pain mechanisms are the same, just triggered by different mechanisms. Transcranial Doppler studies have shown decreased blood velocity in large cerebral arteries during attacks of migraine without aura. rCBF was not measured simultaneously, but since it is normal or perhaps globally increased during migraine attacks, it may be inferred that the large cerebral arteries are probably dilated during attacks. This is a possible mechanism of pain, but simple vasodilatation is not usually painful. Therefore, neurogenic inflammation has been suggested to occur, and it is extremely interesting that drugs effective in treating migraine attacks block experimental neurogenic inflammation in the dura mater. The novel 5-hydroxytryptamine ($5\text{-}HT_1$)–like receptor agonist, sumatriptan, is particularly interesting because it has such a highly selective mode of action. Unfortunately, $5\text{-}HT_1$–like receptor agonism does not only counteract neurogenic inflammation, but it also constricts large cerebral arteries. It is therefore uncertain whether it is one or the other or both of these mechanisms that account for the dramatic therapeutic effectiveness of this compound.

Despite all controversies, it is obvious that we are now at the heart of migraine pathophysiology. For the first time ever, we have at our disposal sufficiently advanced techniques for measuring rCBF, arterial blood velocity, and cerebral blood volume. Also, the diameter of the superficial temporal artery may now be measured accurately. When such techniques are combined with better classification and description of clinical features and with new and exciting pharmacological tools, we can be sure to make great advances in the future. There is no lack of worthy problems to study. It is rather the necessity of combining high-tech equipment and study methods with clinical expertise and a sufficient flow of patients that limits how much we can do. A few large academic research units with sufficient funding, devoted to the study of migraine, could greatly increase the pace of progress.

SUBJECT INDEX

A
Acetazolamide
 CBF effects, 38, 339–340, 342
 ergotamine reversal of, 339–340, 342
 as vasodilator, 35, 339
Aging
 cortical atrophy in, 25
 ISI in, 71–73, 214–216
 LCBF valves in, 32
 in migraine, 71–74, 213–216
 in MO, 213–216
 normal, 25–26, 71–74
 rCBF in, 2–26, 71–74, 213–216
Alzheimer's disease (AD)
 Tc-HMPAO, rCBF in, 25–26
Angiography
 migraine induction, 79, 95
 in migrainous stroke, 90
Anterior cerebral artery (ACA)
 in migraine, 263–265, 270–271
 in MO, 201, 289–291
 TCD recordings, 263–265, 270–271, 289–291
Antimigraine drugs
 actions of, 154–156, 196
 aspirin as, 155
 cephalic blood vessel effects, 153–159
 ergot alkaloids as, 154–155, 157
 plasma protein leakage and, 154
 rat studies of, 153–159
 serotonin receptors and, 153, 155, 196
Asparate, CSD and, 161–164
Asymmetry of CBF
 aging and, 214–216
 anterior-posterior, 57
 cause of, 58
 in interictal migraine, 56–58
 in MA, 56–58, 107–112, 214–216
 methodology and, 38–41
 in MO, 200–202, 204–206, 246–248
 in MO ictal, 232–233, 246–249
 rate of, 57–58
 in rCBF, 38–41, 214–216
 regional, 56–58
 sermatriptan effect, 245–248
 TCD studies, 289–291
 in tension headaches, 320
Auras
 CSD and, 167, 180
 hypoperfusion and, 128, 129, 131, 137–141

infection provoked, 8, 47, 79
 ischemia and, 82–87, 137–141
 late phase of, 127
 neuronal interpretation of, 82–83, 87
 onset of, 79
 rCBF in, 79–80, 124–125, 140
 timing of, 126–127, 140
 vascular interpretation of, 83–87, 102–103, 140
 visual, 47, 121, 124–125, 195
Autonomic nervous system
 in migraine, 282, 283, 286
 in MO, ictal, 234
 valsalva manuever and, 279, 282, 283, 286

B
Basal ganglia
 LCBF in, 107, 111
 in MA, 107, 111
 in MO ictal, 231, 240–241
Basilar artery (BA)
 MFVs in, 263–265, 267
 in migraine, 263
 TCD recordings in, 263–265
Blood-brain barrier (BBB)
 to sematriptan, 337–338
 to ^{99m}Tc-HMPAO, 24
Blood flow velocity (BFV)
 sermatriptan effects on, 331–334
 TCD studies, 331–334

C
Caudate nucleus
 LCBF in, 32, 230–233
 in MO ictal, 230–233
Cephalic blood vessels
 as nociceptive molecule source, 156–157
 ergot alkaloids action on, 154–155, 157
 headaches and, 156–157
Cerebral blood flow (CBF)
 aura onset and, 79–81, 138–141, 195
 in CSD, 171–174, 181–185
 ergotamine effects, 339–343
 hypercapnia effects, 183–185
 in ischemia, 11
 metabolism and, 177

351

Cerebral blood flow (CBF) (*contd.*)
  migraine symptoms onset and, 81–87, 185
  in migrainous stroke, 90–93
  neuronal theory and, 82–83
  pressure-flow relations in, 259–260
  TCD studies, 339–343
  vascular theory and, 83–87
  visual stimulation, 195
  ^{133}Xe methods, 5
Cerebral blood volume (CBV)
  in NTG headaches, 327–329
Cerebral cortex
  LCBF in, 32, 108–109, 230–233
  in MA, 108–112
  in MO ictal, 230–233, 240–243, 247
Cerebral perfusion pressure (CPP), CBF and, 259
Cerebrovascular reactivity
  autonomic system and, 282
  orthostatic, 283–286
  TCD studies of, 268–269, 283–286, 289–291
Cerebrovascular resistance (CVR)
  calculation from TCD, 257–259
  factors influencing, 258
Cluster-type headache
  CO_2 responsiveness in, 307
  CT in, 302
  EEG in, 302
  episodic, 269, 301–304
  Fg in, 306–307
  hyperfusion in, 302, 309
  hypoperfusion in, 302
  LCBF in, 306, 308
  MRI in, 302
  normal cerebral perfusion in, 297–299, 315
  oxygen response in, 307, 308, 309, 311–314
  pain relief and, 311, 313
  rCBF in, 99–103, 297–299, 301–304, 305–309, 311, 315
  TCD recordings, 272, 294, 315
  Tc-HMPAO-SPECT studies, 99–103, 297–299, 301–304
  unilateral CBF changes in, 302–304
  Xe-CT studies of, 305–309
Compton scatter
  in CBF determinations, 84–85, 86, 95–96, 138–139, 141, 145–146, 195
  in ischemia determination, 138–139, 141, 145–146, 195
Computed tomography (CT)
  LCBF image comparison, 31, 32
  in MA interictal, 62, 65
  in MO, 210, 227–234
  ^{133}Xe-CBF use, 29–33, 105–107, 227–234

CO_2 responsiveness, in migraine/aura, 117–118
Cortical spreading depression (CSD)
  aspartate and, 161–164
  auras and, 167, 180, 349
  blood flow in, 137, 145, 146, 348–349
  blood gas effects, 183
  in cats, 171–174, 177–180
  CBF in, 171–174, 181–185
  cerebrovascular reactivity and, 173–174
  characterization of, 181
  cortical dysfunction and, 148
  DC potential measurements in, 167–168
  EEG in, 139, 169
  glutamate and, 149, 161–164
  induction of, 161–162, 171, 178
  inhibition of, 149–150, 162–164
  ischemia and, 137, 195
  hyperemia in, 185
  hypercapnia and, 183–185
  K^+ induction of, 162–164
  LCBF in, 161
  laser Doppler studies of, 177–180, 181–185
  LAW and, 190, 192
  MA and, 137, 145, 147–150, 195
  magnetic field measurements in, 167
  MEG and, 147–148, 190–192
  NMDA antagonists and, 161
  NMDA induction of, 149–150, 161, 164, 195
  occipital cortex in, 177–180
  oligemia and, 171, 173, 177, 185
  in rats, 161–164, 167–170, 181–185
  skin DC recordings in, 169–170
  skull DC recordings in, 169–170
  taurine and, 162–164
  vasodilation and, 183–185

D
Dementia, ^{99m}Tc-HMPAO rCBF in, 25; *see also* Vascular dementia

E
Electroencephalogram (EEG)
  in CSD, 139, 169
  in MA, 69
  in MO ictal, 232
  in MO intrictal, 210
Epileptic seizures
  rCBF in, 26–27
  SPECT in, 27
  ^{99m}Tc-HMPAO use in, 26–27
Ergot alkaloids
  action of, 154–155, 157, 339

as 5-HT receptor agonists, 155
  vasoconstriction and, 157–158, 339
Ergotamine
  acetazolamide reversal, 339–340
  CBF effects, 339–343, 345
  MCA effects, 339–343
  TCD studies of, 339–343
External cartoid artery (ECA)
  in MO, 289–291, 331–334
  sumatriptan effects, 331–334
  TCD studies of, 289–291, 331–334

G
Glutamate, CSD induction and, 149, 161–164
Gray matter flow (Fg), in cluster headache, 306–307

H
Headaches, *see also specific types*
  induction of, 275–276
  MCA-MFV's in, 275–277
  nitroglycerin-induced, 327–330
  PI in, 277
  post-lumbar puncture, 323–326
  TCD studies of, 275–277
Hippocampus
  in MO ictal, 230–233
  in MO interictal, 205–206
  rCBF in, 205–206, 230–233
5-Hydroxytryptamine (5-HT) serotonin
  ergot alkaloids and, 155–345
  receptors for, 155, 196, 345
Hypercapnia
  cardiovascular response, 183–185
  CBF effects, 183–185
  vasodilation and, 183–185
Hyperemia
  in CSD, 185
  diagnosis of, 103
  HMPAO use and, 103, 131, 134, 249
  in MA, 103, 131, 132, 139
  in MO, 249
  Xe studies, 134, 249
Hyperperfusion
  in cluster headache, 302, 309
  in MA, 122–123, 124–128, 129, 347
  MA interictal, 67–69, 122–123
  in MO ictal, 232, 234
  in MO interictal, 204–206
Hypoperfusion
  aura and, 128, 129, 131, 137–141
  focal, 137
  in MA interictal, 62–64, 67–69, 122–123
  in MA, 122–123, 128, 129, 131
  in MO interictal, 204–206, 210–212

pain localization relations, 210–212
  in rats, 146
  rCBF and, 145, 146
  spreading depression and, 137

I
Initial slope index (ISI)
  aging and, 71–73, 214–216
  in rCBF determinations, 36–41, 71–73, 214–216
  in tomography vs. stationary detectors, 36–41
Internal cartoid artery (ICA)
  in migraine, 267, 270–271, 331–334
  in migrainous stroke, 90–92
  in MO, 289–291
  sermatriptan effects, 331–334
  TCD recordings, 263–265, 267, 270–271, 289–291, 331–334
^{123}I-Iodoamphetamine (^{123}I-IMP)
  in MA interictal studies, 123
  SPECT studies of, 123
Iodine-123 (^{123}I), SPECT use of, 23
Ischemia
  aura and, 82–87, 137
  CSD and, 137, 195
  hemispheric, 89–93
  in MA, 82–87, 133, 137–141
  in migraine, 83–87, 89–93, 342
  oligemia and, 133
  rCBF in, 35–41, 83–87, 95
  reversible, 89–93
  spreading depression and, 137
  transient, 35
  Xe-SPECT use in, 35–41
Ischemic strokes
  angiography in, 35–36
  rCBF in, 35–41
  Xe-SPECT use in, 35–41

L
Large amplitude waves (LAW)
  in CSD, 190–192
  MEG signals and, 192
  significance of, 192
Laser Doppler studies, *see also Transcranial Doppler studies*
  of cerebral perfusion, 257
  of CSD, 177–180, 181–185
  of occipital cortex LCBF, 177–180
Local cerebral blood flow (LCBF)
  age-related declines in, 32
  asymmetries in, 107
  brain region valves, 32, 108–112
  in cluster headache, 306, 308
  in CSD, 177–180

Local cerebral blood flow (LCBF) (*contd.*)
  in gray/white matter, 32
  on headache side, 108–112
  laser Doppler studies, 177–180
  in MA, 105–112
  in normals, 108–112
  in occipital cortex, 177–180
  in retinal stimulation, 178–180
  in vascular headaches, 29
  Xe CT determination, 29–33, 105–112

M

Magnetic resonance imaging (MRI)
  energy metabolism and, 147
  in MA, 62
  in migraine, 147
  in MO, 210
Magnetoencephalographic (MEG) signals
  applications for, 191–192
  in CSD, 147–148, 190–192
  LAW and, 190–192
  in MA, 187–192
  in MO, 187–192
Mean flow velocities (MFVs)
  in ACA, 263–265
  age and, 263
  in BA, 263–265
  bruits and, 267, 270–271
  in headaches, 275–277
  in MCA, 263–265, 276–277, 283–286
  in migraine, 263–265, 269–272, 283–286
  in migraine, headache free, 269–272
  in TCD studies, 263–272, 275–277
N-Methyl-D-aspartate (NMDA)
  antagonists of, 161
  CSD induction, 149–150, 161, 164, 195
  neuronal injury and, 158
Middle cerebral artery (MCA)
  bruits in, 266
  ergotamine effects, 339–343
  in migraine, 263–265, 267, 270–271, 279–282, 283–286, 293–294, 331–334
  in MO, 201
  in NTG headaches, 327–329
  in post-lumbar puncture headache, 323–325
  sumatriptan effects, 331–334
  TCD recordings, 255, 256, 257, 263–265, 270–271, 279–280, 331–334, 339–343
  Valsalva test effects, 279–282, 283–286
Migraine
  aura and, 51–75, 79–96
  blood vessel wall and, 156–158
  diagnostic criteria for, 1, 105–106, 345, 347
  drugs for, 153–159, 196, 345
  duration of, 2
  ergotamine for, 342–343
  food induction of, 237, 238
  infection induction of, 8, 47
  interictal, 51–75
  ischemia and, 83–87, 89–93, 342
  late phase of, 127
  neuronal theory of, 82–83
  onset of, 79–96
  pathogenesis of, 111, 349
  provocation of, 47–48
  stroke and, 89, 195
  study methods, 1–49
  symptoms during, 122–123, 126
  TCD study of, 263–272, 279–282
  timing of symptomology, 1, 2
  Valsalva test in, 279–282, 283–286
  vascular theory of, 83–87, 102–103
  visual symptoms in, 47–48, 144
Migraine equivalents (ME)
  aging and, 71–74
  rCBF in, 71–74
Migraine, injection provoked
  aura in, 8, 47, 79
  incidence of, 8
  mechanism of, 48, 79, 95
  symptoms in, 8, 47
Migraine with aura (MA)
  aging and, 213–216
  basal ganglia in, 107
  CBF in, 107–141
  cerebral cortex in, 108–112
  CO_2 responsiveness and, 117–118
  CSD and, 137, 145, 147–150, 195
  drugs for, 153
  energy metabolism in, 147
  in headache-free period, 66–69
  headache laterality in, 127–128
  hyperemia and, 103, 131, 132, 139
  hyperperfusion in, 122–123, 124–128
  hypoperfusion in, 122–123, 128, 129, 131
  ischemia and, 82–87, 103, 133, 137–141
  LCBF in, 105–112
  literature review, 121–126
  mechanisms of, 137–141
  MEG in, 187–192
  neural theory of, 82–83, 143–144
  oligemia and, 82–83, 86, 111, 112, 132–133, 140–141
  oxygen effect, 117
  pain and, 348
  PET in, 139
  rCBF in, 101–103, 115–118, 121–129, 145–146, 213–216
  spreading depression in, 137, 145, 147–150
  symptoms during, 122–123

SUBJECT INDEX

99mTc-HMPAO-SPECT in, 99–103
temporal events in, 127–128, 133, 143, 144
vascular hypothesis of, 83–87, 102–103, 137, 141, 143
133Xe-CT-CBF in, 105–112
133Xe-rCBF in, 115–118
Migraine with aura (MA) interictal
aging and, 71–77
CT findings in, 62, 65
EEG findings in, 69
headache side and, 67–69
hemiplegic subtypes, 62–64, 75
hyperperfusion, 67–69
hypoperfusion in, 62–64, 67–69
123I-IMP studies, 61
infection induction, 8, 47–48
ischemia and, 82–87, 103
ISI in, 71–73
LCBF in, 108–112
MEG in, 187–192
MRI findings in, 62
neurologic deficits in, 66
opthalmic subtypes, 62–64
parietooccipital area in, 101
rCBF in, 53–58, 61–64, 65–69, 71–74, 75, 101–103
99mTc-HMPAO-SPECT use in, 54–58, 61–64, 65–69, 99–103, 347
vascular defect in, 83–84, 102–103
133Xe-CT use in, 105–112
Migraine with aura (MA), onset of
aura onset and, 79–81
CBF in, 79–87
hemodynamic variables in, 239–241
injection provoked, 79
ischemia and, 83–85, 86, 87
neuronal theory of, 82–83
oligemia and, 82–83, 86
rCBF in, 99–103
99mTc-HMPAO method in, 99–103
vascular theory of, 83–87
133Xe intracarotid injection method in, 79–87
Migraine without aura (MO) ictal
asymmetry in, 246–247
autonomic nervous system in, 234
in bilateral headaches, 232–233
CBF in, 223–225
CBF regional difference in, 230–233, 240–243, 246–247
cerebral autoregulation in, 228–230, 232
cerebral vasomotor responsiveness in, 228–230, 232
cortical CBF in, 230–233, 240–242
CT studies of, 227–234
diagnostic criteria for, 237–238
EEG in, 232

headache side and, 228–234, 247
hemodynamic variables in, 239–241
hyperemia and, 249
hyperperfusion in, 232, 234
induction of, 237
interval headaches and, 238
LCBF in, 228–234
literature review, 237–243
onset of, 239
rCBF in, 223–224, 227–234, 238–243, 245–248, 249–250
sematriptan effects on, 246–248
TCD studies of, 289–291, 331–334
99mTc-HMPAO-SPECT studies, 221–225, 245–248, 250
temporal muscle tracer uptake in, 223
white/gray matter in, 231–233, 247
Xe-CT studies of, 227–234
Xe-SPECT studies of, 237–243
Migraine without aura (MO) interictal
abnormal perfusion in, 204–206
ACA in, 201
aging and, 213–216
asymmetry in, 200–202, 204–206, 214–216
CT in, 210
EEG in, 210
frequency of attack, 204
frontal cortex in, 205–206
hemodynamic variables in, 239, 241
hippocampus in, 205–206
hyperperfusion in, 204–206
hypoperfusion in, 204–206, 210–212
inhalation studies of, 200–202
intervenous studies of, 200–202
localization of, 203–204, 210–212, 217
MCA in, 201
MEG in, 187–192
MRI in, 210
occipital region in, 205–206
pain localization and hypoperfusion in, 210–212, 217
rCBF in, 199–202, 203–206, 209–212, 213–216, 217
sumatriptan in, 245–248
TCD studies, 289–291
99mTc-HMPAO-SPECT studies, 203–206, 209–212, 245–248
temporal area in, 205–206
visual evaluation in, 201
Migrainous stroke
angiography in, 90, 95
case report, 89–93
cause of, 89
CBF in, 90–93
ICA in, 90–92
neurological findings in, 89–90
PET in, 90–91
SPECT in, 90–91

N

Neuronal theory
  aura and, 82
  CBF in, 82–83
  of MA migraine, 82–83, 143–144
  oligemia and, 82–83
Nitroglycerin-induced (NTG) headaches
  CBV in, 327–329
  forms of, 327
  MCA in, 327–329
  pathogenesis of, 327, 329–330
  rCBF in, 327–330
Nociceptive molecules
  headaches and, 156–157, 158
  sources of, 156–157, 158

O

Occipital area
  in CSD, 177–180
  laser Doppler studies, 177–180
  LCBF in, 177–180
  in MA, 102
  in MO, 205–206
  in MO ictal, 230–233, 247
  rCBF in, 205–206, 230–233, 247
  in retinal stimulation, 178–180
Oligemia
  CDS and, 171, 173, 177, 185
  ischemia and, 133
  in MA, 82–83, 86, 111, 112, 132–133, 140–141
  in parietooccipital area, 132–133
  spreading, 111, 171, 173
Oxygen inhalation, rCBF effect, 117
Oxygen response
  in cluster headache, 307, 308, 309, 311–314
  in migraine, 311
  pain relief and, 311, 312
  rCBF in, 311
  vascular effects of, 311, 313, 315

P

Parietooccipital area
  in migraine/aura, 101, 132–133
  oligemia in, 132–133
Pial blood vessel
  diameter measurements, 335–338
  sumatriptan effects on, 335–338
Positron emission tomograph (PET)
  in migraine/aura, 139
  problems of, 12
Posterior cerebral artery (PCA)
  in migraine, 263–265, 270–271
  TCD recordings, 263–265, 270–271
Post-lumbar puncture headache
  incidence of, 324
  MCA in, 323–325
  pathogenesis of, 323, 325–326
  Pourcelot index in, 323–326
  TCD study of, 323–326
Pulsatility index (PI)
  in migraine, 264, 269
  in TCD, 258–259, 269
Putamen
  LCBF in, 32, 108–109
  in migraine/aura, 108–109
  in MO ictal, 230–233

R

Radiation exposure
  SPECT image quality and, 43–46
  ^{99m}Tc-Xe comparison, 43–46
  [128]Xe use and, 43–46
  [133]Xe use and, 7, 11, 43–46
Regional cerebral blood flow (rCBF)
  acetazolamide effects, 35, 38
  in aging/migraine, 71–74
  in aging, normal, 25–26, 71–74, 213–216
  asymmetrical, 56–58, 107–112, 200–202, 204–206, 214–216
  aura and, 115–118, 124–125
  aura onset and, 79–81
  best method for, 49
  in cluster headache, 99–103, 297–299, 301–304, 305–309, 311–314
  Compton scatter effect in, 84–85, 86, 95–96, 138–139, 141, 145–146
  CO_2 responsiveness and, 117–118
  data analysis, 55–56
  focal symptoms and, 145–146
  headache and, 95, 115–118, 228–234, 347
  headache absence and, 66–69, 115–118, 228–234
  headache laterality and, 126–128
  on headache side, 108–110, 117–118, 234
  hypoperfusion and, 145
  inconsistent changes in, 247
  in ischemia, 35–36, 83–85, 86, 87, 95
  ISI valves in, 36–41
  literature review, 121–126
  in MA, 53–58, 121–129, 145–146, 213–216, 217
  in MA interictal/migraine/aura, 53–58, 61–64, 65–69, 71–74, 99–103
  in ME, 71–74
  measurement of, 36–38, 48
  in migraine attack, 28, 108–112, 347
  in MO ictal, 237–243, 245–248, 249–250
  in MO interictal, 199–202, 203–206, 209–212, 213–216, 217, 237–243
  neuronal hypofunction and, 101
  in normal controls, 56, 62
  in NTG headaches, 327–330
  oxygen effect, 117

SUBJECT INDEX

post headache, 116–118
in rats, 146–147
regulation of, 95–96, 250
SPECT use in, 35–41
TCD correlation, 293–294
^{99m}Tc-HMPAO-SPECT studies, 61–64, 65–69, 203–206, 209–212, 245–248
^{99m}Tc-HMPAO-Xe SPECT comparison, 43–46
in tension headaches, 100–101, 319–321
by tomographic vs. stationary detectors, 36–41
in vascular theory of migraine, 83–87
Xe-CT method in, 105–112, 227–234
Xe-SPECT use in, 8, 23, 27, 35, 54–58, 71–74, 121–129

S

Single photon emission computer tomograph (SPECT)
cerebrovascular disease rCBF and, 35–41
in epileptic seizures, 26–27
image quality and, 43
^{123}I use in, 23
literature review, 121–126
static imaging with, 23
stationary detector comparison, 35–41
Tomomatic instrument and, 8
in ^{133}Xe CBF method, 8, 23, 35–41, 43–46, 121–129
Stroke
migraine correlation, 89, 195
migrainous, 89–93
rCBF in, 35–41
^{99m}Tc-HMPAO rCBF in, 25
Xe-SPECT use in, 35–41
Sumatriptan
asymmetry and, 246–247
BBB and, 337–338
BFV effects, 331–334
cephalic blood vessel binding, 153, 154, 155, 195–196
in cats, 335–338
effects of, 195–196, 245–248, 331, 337–338, 345, 349
headaches and, 153, 157–158
hemoclynamic effects of, 336–337
in MO ictal, 245–248
in MO interictal, 245–248
pial vessel diameter effects, 335–338
TCD studies, 331–334

T

^{99m}Tc-D, L-hexa-methyl-propylene-amine-oxime (^{99m}Tc-HMPAO)
advantages of, 23
BBB trapping of, 24
resolution with, 23
as retained tracer, 23, 43–46
^{99m}Tc-HMPAO rCBF method
in acute migraine, 99–103
in AD, 25–26
advantages of, 221, 224–225
in aging, 25–26
clinical applications, 25–28
in cluster headache, 99–103, 297–299, 301–304
in dementia, 25–26
in epileptic seizures, 26–27
in MA, 53–58, 99–103, 221–225
in MA interictal, 53–58, 61–64, 65–69
in migraine studies, 27–28, 47, 99–103, 221–223
in MO, 221–225
muscle uptake in, 225
in NTG headaches, 327–330
radiation exposure and, 43–46
shortcomings of, 27, 28, 221, 250
SPECT use and, 54–58, 99–103, 221–225, 297–299, 301–304
in stroke, 25
^{99m}Tc-HMPAO distribution in, 24
in tension headache, 100–101, 319–321
in tension-type headache, 99–103
^{128}Xe SPECT comparison, 43–46
^{133}Xe-SPECT comparison, 27, 43–46, 49
Tc-PmAO
radiation exposure and, 43–46
Xe comparison, 43–46
Temporal region
in MO ictal, 230–233, 247
in MO interictal, 205–206
rCBF in, 205–206, 230–233, 247
Tension-type headache
asymmetry in, 320
CT in, 320
migraine and, 319–321
paracetamol in, 321
^{99m}Tc-HMPAO-SPECT studies, 99–103, 221–225, 319–321
rCBF in, 100–101, 319–321
Thalamus
LCBF in, 32, 108–109
in MA, 108–109
Transcranial Doppler (TCD) principles
anterial/venous spectra in, 255
CPP and, 259
CVR calculation, 257–259
development of, 253
MCA recordings, 256
multichannel recordings, 254–255
physics of, 253–254
PI in, 258–259
pressure-flow relations of, 259–260
spectral analysis in, 256

Transcranial Doppler (TCD)
  principles (contd.)
  velocity profiles in, 254–256
  volume flow calculations in, 256–257
Transcranial Doppler (TCD) studies
  of ACA, 263–265, 267, 270–271,
    289–291
  advantages of, 293, 294
  in BA, 263–265
  of BFV, 331–334
  bruits and, 265–267, 270–271
  of CBF, 339–343
  cerebrovascular reactivity and,
    268–269, 293
  in cluster headache, 272, 294, 315
  of ECA, 289–291
  of ergotamine effect, 339–343
  of flow asymmetries, 265, 293
  of headaches, 275–277, 279–282
  of ICA, 267, 270–271, 289–291
  in induced headaches, 275–277
  of MCA, 263–265, 267, 270–272,
    275–277, 279–282, 283–286,
    289–291, 293–294, 323–326,
    331–334, 339–343
  MFV in, 263–272, 275–277, 283–286
  in migraine, 263–265, 269–272, 279–282,
    283–286, 331–334
  in migraine, headache free, 269–272,
    289–291
  in MO, 289–291
  of PCA, 263–265
  PI in, 264, 269, 270–271, 277
  of post-lumbar puncture headache,
    323–326
  rCBF correlation, 293–294
  of sumatriptan effects, 331–334
  Valsalva test and, 279–282, 283–286
  of vascular reactivity, 268–269,
    283–286, 289–291

V
Vascular dementia (VD)
  AD differentiation, 26
  Tc-HMPAO studies of, 26
Vascular headaches
  LCBF in, 29, 33
  Xe CT-CBF determination in, 29–33
Vascular theory
  CBF in, 83–87
  of migraine, 83–87, 102–103, 137, 141,
    143
  MRI findings and, 147
  pH changes and, 147
  rCBF in, 83–84

X
Xenon (Xe)
  cerebral circulation effects, 33
  CT-CBF use, 29–33
  image quality and, 43–46
  inhalation, 29, 44–46, 47
  IV infection, 36, 47
  properties of, 6–7, 29, 33
  radiation exposure and, 7, 11, 43–46
  SPECT use, 35–41
  ^{99m}Tc comparisons, 43–46
  ^{127}Xe as, 43–46
  ^{133}Xe as, 6–7, 29, 33, 43–46
^{133}Xenon-CBF method
  advantages of, 33
  air artifacts in, 19
  angiography in, 8
  asymmetry and, 48–49
  aural phase result, 10
  brain blood volume and, 6
  of cluster headaches, 305–309
  comparison to other methods, 12–13
  Compton scatter and, 17–18
  concepts in, 6, 7, 11, 29–30
  CT use in, 29–33, 105–107, 227–234
  diagrammatic representation of, 9, 10
  half-life of, 7
  inert gas concept, 6
  inhalation technique, 5, 8, 15, 29–33,
    48, 54, 106, 115, 347
  interictal studies, 53–58
  intraarterial technique, 7–8, 15, 48, 54,
    79–81
  ischemic flow and, 11
  literature review of, 237–243
  in migraine attack, 28
  in MA onset, 79–87
  in MA spontaneous, 105–112, 115–118
  in MO, 227–234
  in MO ictal, 237–243
  in NTG headaches, 328–330
  Obrist method and, 15–16, 305–306
  radiation exposure in, 7, 11, 43–46
  reproducibility of, 31
  shortcomings of, 11
  spatial resolution in, 17–18
  SPECT system in, 8, 23, 27, 35, 54–58,
    71–74, 121–129, 237–243
  stationary detector use in, 15–20
  ^{99m}Tc-HMPAO method and, 12, 27,
    43–46, 49
  time required for, 11
  tomographic method, 8–12
  in vascular headaches, 29–33
  ^{133}Xe brain solubility, 6
  ^{133}Xe tracer in, 6–7, 15–20

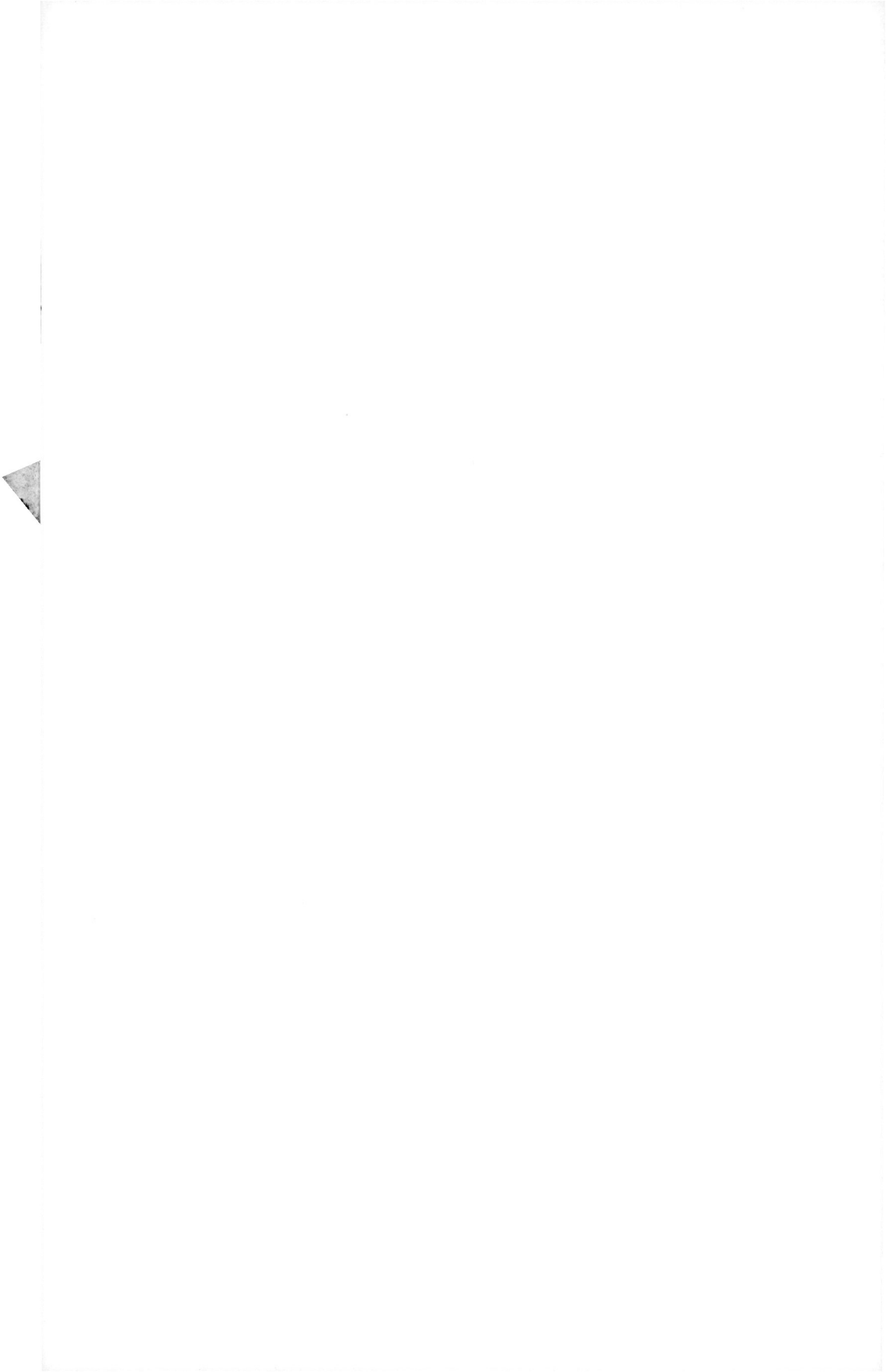

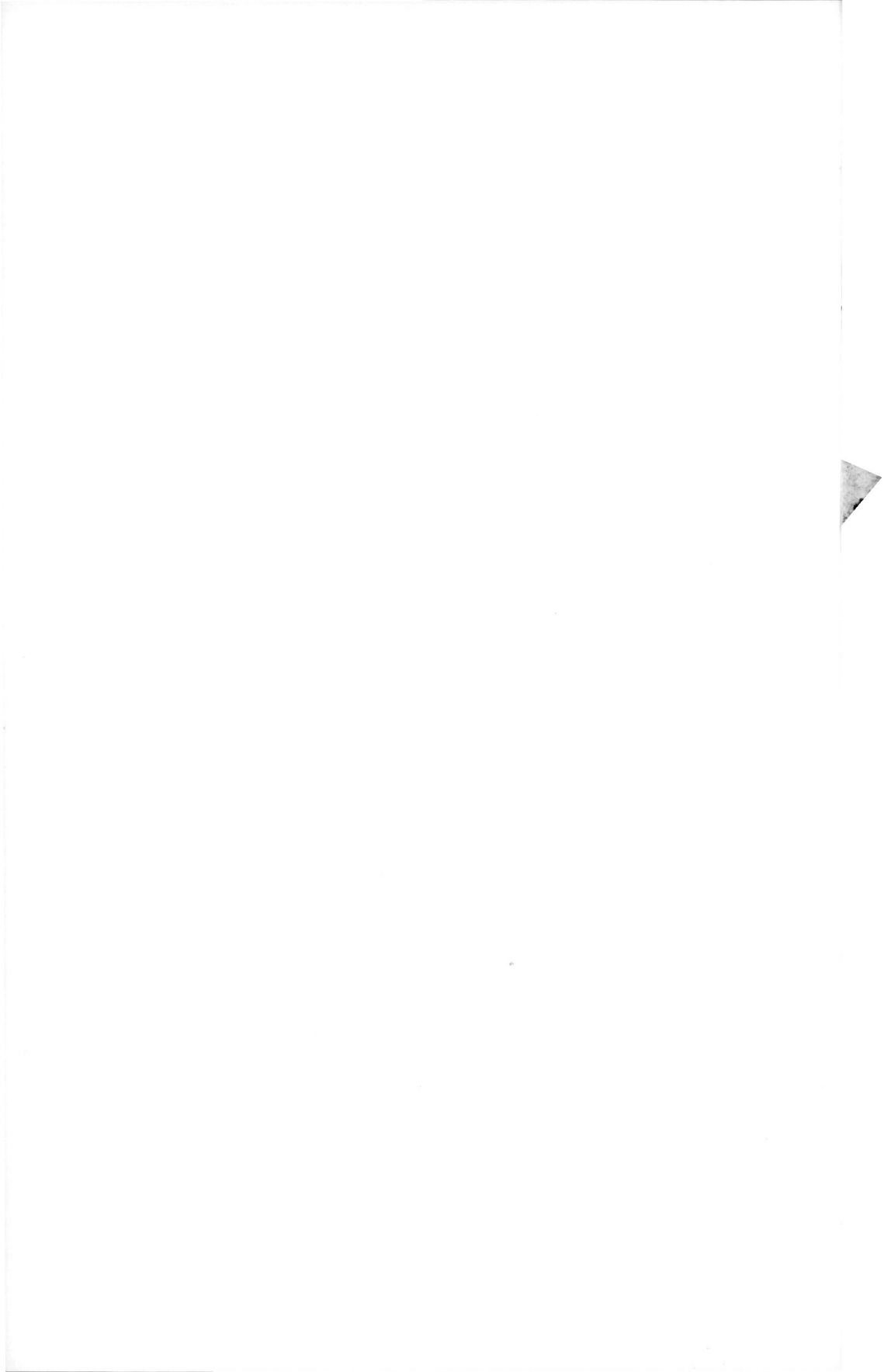

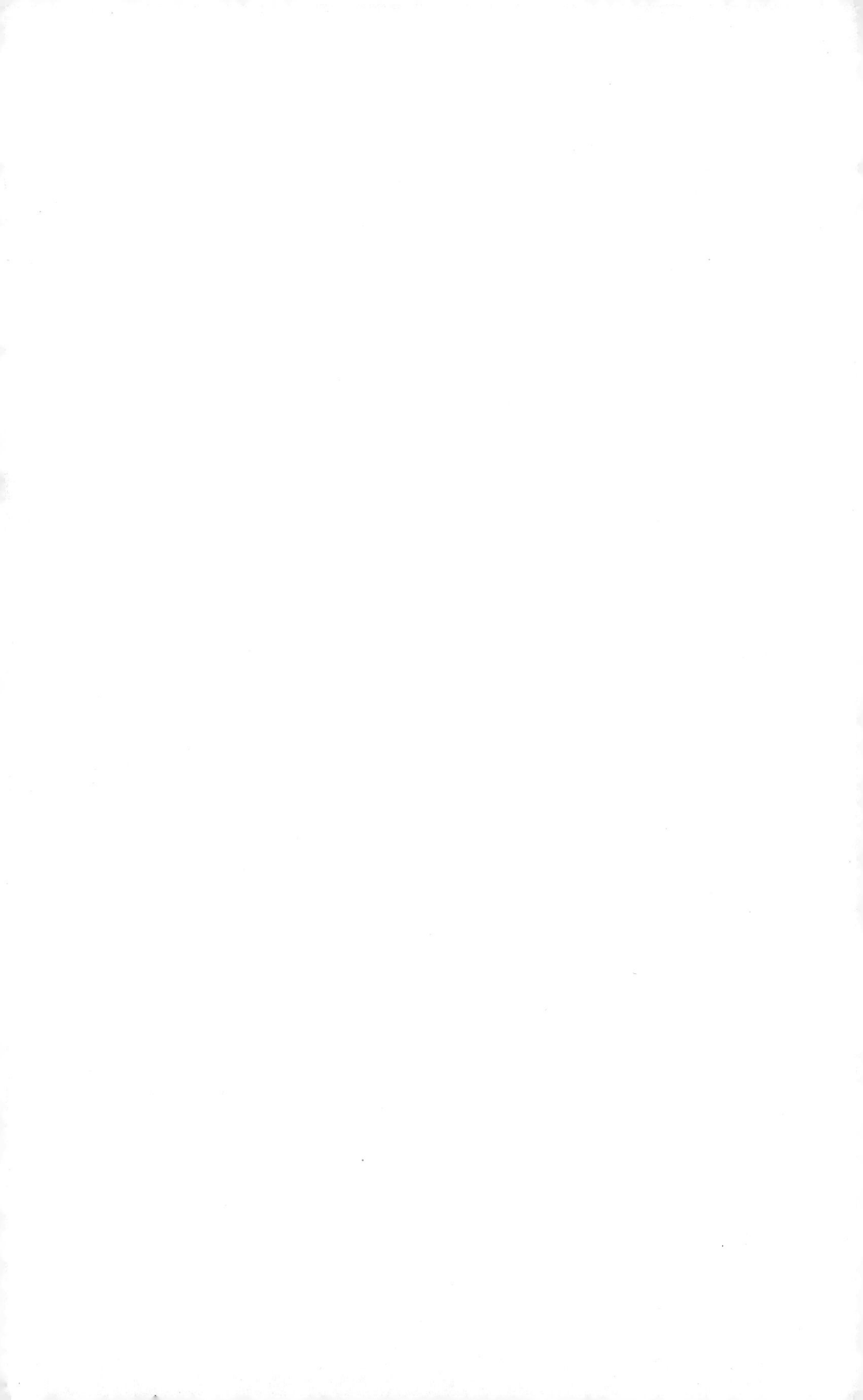